D0444183

Health and the Rise of Civilization

Mark Nathan Cohen

Health and the

Rise of Civilization

Yale University Press   *New Haven and London*

Published with assistance from the Louis Stern Memorial Fund.

Copyright © 1989 by Yale University.
All rights reserved.
This book may not be reproduced, in whole
or in part, including illustrations, in
any form (beyond that copying permitted by
Sections 107 and 108 of the U.S. Copyright
Law and except by reviewers for the public
press), without written permission from the
publishers.

Designed by Jill Breitbarth and set in Ehrhardt type
by Tseng Information Systems, Inc. Printed in the United
States of America by Vail-Ballou Press, Binghamton, N.Y.

Library of Congress Cataloging-in-Publication Data
Cohen, Mark Nathan.
Health and the rise of civilization / Mark Nathan Cohen.
p.   cm.
Bibliography: p.
Includes index.
ISBN 0-300-04006-7 (cloth)
      0-300-05023-2 (pbk.)
1. Medical sociology.   2. Health.   3. Civilization.   I. Title.
RA418.C664   1989
614.4—dc 19   89-5405
                                              CIP

The paper in this book meets the guidelines for
permanence and durability of the Committee on
Production Guidelines for Book Longevity of the
Council on Library Resources.

10 9 8 7 6 5 4 3 2

Contents

Preface

In recent months, a number of friends have asked whether the manuscript I was preparing had a name. When I responded that I was writing a book called "Health and the Rise of Civilization" I was met with a combination of amusement and disbelief at the scale of the undertaking.

I have, in fact, attempted to provide a broad overview of the impact of cultural evolution on human health. I am interested in exploring both the logical links between behavior and health and the links between civilization and patterns of behavior. The book proceeds in several steps. After a brief introduction (chapter 1), I consider how changes in human behavior affect health (chapter 2); I then review the major changes in human behavior that occurred during the evolution of human civilization (chapter 3). I "predict" the probable consequences of those changes for human health, using models from contemporary epidemiology and nutrition science and examples from recent history (chapters 4 and 5), and review ethnographic evidence about health and nutrition in the smallest, economically simplest (that is, the most "primitive") human groups, contrasting them with patterns of health and nutrition in recent history and the modern Third World (chapter 6). Finally, turning to the archaeological record, I adduce evidence for changes in health and nutrition in prehistory (chapter 7).

Such a broad overview required me to use and compare data from many sources and to combine the work of a number of scholarly fields. The project carries at least two risks: that these data, generated by different means in different fields, are not readily comparable and that within the limits of my own scholarship I cannot do justice to the full range of information available in any one field; nor can I fully appreciate, much less explain, all of the subtleties, debated by experts in each field, that cloud straightforward interpretation of the data.

I would nonetheless justify the attempt by pointing to several advantages of such a broad approach. First, it is my sense that any one line of scientific inquiry and any one study must be fraught with assumptions and potential errors, no matter how carefully it is done. Good reconstructions of history or prehistory, like good science, must develop out of the replication of observations; ideally those reconstructions must crosscheck conclusions derived by one technique with those derived by another. Most of the conclusions of science are validated not because someone designs a perfect experiment but because several different, imperfect techniques produce similar results.

Second, it is my perception that individuals working in particular fields often do not appreciate the value or importance of their results, either because they are unaware of questions that are of interest to other scholars or because they do not realize the extent to which their results can be compared to those available in other disciplines. An archaeologist by training, I was myself unaware of the degree to which the data of skeletal pathology might be used to test controversies in our interpretation of prehistory; when I began to talk to the skeletal pathologists, I realized that many were unaware of the questions archaeologists were asking.

Third, it seems to me that the members of individual disciplines often lack a sense of the limits of their own data and methods. A colleague once defined an academic discipline as a group of scholars who had agreed not to ask certain embarrassing questions about key assumptions. In my reading I have become aware that each of the disciplines involved here includes assumptions that need to be examined in the light of other disciplines. The analysis of prehistoric skeletons involves assumptions about the quality of samples that make historical demographers uncomfortable; but historians often use the documentation of a society about itself uncritically, giving insufficient attention to the differences between those records or statements and the actual behavior of the society. This failure to distinguish between words and deeds would unnerve any anthropologist. Moreover, much comparative analysis of recent history appears unaware of the much larger arena of potential comparison in anthropology and prehistory. Perhaps most important, the field of medicine often appears naive about the full range of human biological experience, basing conclusions about human health—even about what is "normal"—on the comparatively narrow experience of contemporary Western society.

Fourth, and most important, as a major tenet of my style of scholarship, I believe that patterns in data that are often not visible or noticed in more focused and specialized studies may be visible in broad overview. It is certainly my sense that the combination of methods summarized here provides a picture of the trajectory of human health and of human civilization that has not been visible to specialists working in any one of the specific fields incorporated in this work.

Finally, the particular broad synthesis that I have attempted has a justification of its own. We all operate, uncritically, within a framework of beliefs and stereotypes that might, like this book, be called "Health and the rise of civilization." This preexisting set of beliefs molds our writing of history and shapes our political decisions. Yet it receives critical review only rarely or only on the basis of incomplete information. I have aimed to make the subject more generally understood.

I have written a book that strives for careful balance between the scholarly and the popular, addressing a multidisciplinary audience and, I hope, an audience of educated lay public. Assuming, in any case, that not all readers will be versed in the basic principles in every field represented in the book, I have provided, in the first three chapters, an overview and review of some basic concepts in health and in social organization and cultural evolution. In subsequent chapters, which begin to deal in a more thorough and substantive way with data essential to the argument, I attempt to provide nontechnical explanations of the derivation of data, pointing where necessary to potential major pitfalls in data-gathering techniques. Particular attention is paid to problems in skeletal analysis (chapter 7), which will be least familiar to most readers.

The very breadth of the overview and the need to explain principles of analysis to a multidisciplinary readership have necessitated a certain amount of simplification of the data and interpretations in chapters 1 to 5. At the same time, because I am offering controversial conclusions that must be bolstered with substantial supporting evidence, I have attempted to provide in chapters 6 and 7 both broad and fairly detailed coverage of available data on the health of band societies and on the archaeological record.

In the interest of readability, the text follows the style of an extended essay that can be perused without reference to the endnotes. Readers who wish to pursue my arguments further or challenge the implications of the text will find extensive explanations, caveats or alternative hypotheses, data, sample sizes, and sources in the notes at the end of the book. The bibliography that follows the notes lists not only sources cited but others inspected during my research.

This project was initiated while I was a fellow of the Center for Advanced Study in the Behavioral Sciences (Stanford). The bulk of the research was completed at my home campus of the State University of New York in

Plattsburgh. Much of the research and the bulk of the writing were done while I was a fellow of the John Simon Guggenheim Memorial Foundation and a visiting scholar of the departments of physical anthropology and of archaeology of the University of Cambridge. I would like to express my appreciation to the heavily overworked department of Interlibrary Loan at Plattsburgh (Craig Koste and Mary Turner) and to the librarians of the Haddon Library of Cambridge University.

I would like to acknowledge the assistance and advice of Patricia Higgins in particular, and of George Armelagos, Jane Buikstra, Della Cook, Robert Foley, J. P. Garlick, Carrie Harris, Kristen Hawkes, Nancy Howell, Jim Oeppen, John Speth, James Woodburn, E. A. Wrigley, and Ezra Zubrow. Among these, Oeppen, Hawkes, and Woodburn were, together with Jim O'Connell, Kim Hill, R. P. Mensforth, Robert Bailey, and Nadine Peacock, kind enough to allow me to cite data in (then) unpublished manuscripts. The initial inspiration I owe to Alexander Alland, who first directed my attention to the interaction of human health and cultural evolution.

Chapter 1

Images of the "Primitive" and the "Civilized"

The escape from the impasse of savagery [hunting and gathering] was an economic and scientific revolution that made the participants active partners with nature.

V. Gordon Childe, *What Happened in History*

All cultures activated exclusively . . . by human energy have been . . . crude, meager, and of a low degree of development. For culture to evolve, to develop higher and better forms, judged from the standpoint of serving human needs, the amount of energy harnessed and put to work . . . must be increased.

Leslie White, "The Energy Theory of Cultural Development"

Rather than anxiety, it would seem that hunters have a confidence born of affluence, of a condition in which all the people's wants are generally easily satisfied.

Marshall Sahlins, "Notes on the Original Affluent Society"

Our perception of human progress relies heavily on stereotypes we have created about the "primitive" and the "civilized." We build our ideas of history out of images that we have projected on our past.

In fact, Western civilization teaches two conflicting images of the primitive and the civilized, and each has become something of a cliché. On the one hand, we teach admiration for smaller societies or simpler cultures, as exemplified by romantic portrayals of the American Indian. On the other hand, we teach disdain for the primitive and appreciation for science and civilization. These two themes intertwine in our poetry and our fiction. They complicate our sense of history and our political decisions, but neither is subjected to careful examination.

In the absence of such scrutiny, it is all the more dangerous that the two images have such unequal power. We associate the idea of progress with science and base our decisions on the assumption that human progress is real and well documented. We relegate our appreciation of the primitive to "romance," implying that it is nothing more than the stuff of poetry and legend. In the popular mind, at least, to be primitive is to be poor, ill, and malnourished; and group poverty is a demonstration of primitive lack of technological sophistication—lack of "development."

From this perspective we are convinced that we have, through our own inventiveness, gradually whittled down the list of problems and dangers once faced by all humankind. We reason that we ought to share unreservedly the benefits of our progress with those we view as less fortunate because they are less civilized. It is precisely because of this naive popular optimism about our progress that the actual record of cultural evolution and its effects on human well-being deserve a closer look. We may well discover that there is more romance to the "scientific" assumption of progress than we usually recognize and more empirical validity to the "romantic" perspective of the primitive than we usually concede.

The careful resolution of these conflicting images—sorting out the fact and romance on each side to obtain some reasonably clear picture of the actual path of human cultural evolution and its consequences—is of more than purely intellectual interest. At stake are decisions now being made concerning the modernization of many populations around the world. For these decisions, the economic and social histories of past populations can serve as a concrete and valuable guide. To those populations facing transitions, some of which have been faced before in one form or another, we owe a careful look at the historical record. Also at stake in some small part are our choices about our own future courses, although for these decisions the experiences of the past can only be a very general guide.

Anthropology and Images of Progress

Reconstructing the pattern of cultural evolution in detail is the province of anthropology. Branches of the field deal with both the analysis of small-scale contemporary societies and the reconstruction of societies of the past. But anthropologists themselves are ambivalent about progress, because their data are mixed and because their science, like all science, is influenced by the popular crosscurrents of our own culture as much as it guides those currents.

Anthropologists commonly profess attraction to the people they study. Their ethnographic descriptions, at least for most of the twentieth century, have reflected and reinforced the romantic perspective, expressing appreciation of the qualities of simpler lifestyles. Yet, anthropology grew as a discipline in an era of European colonial expansion and enormous optimism about the advantages of Western ways of life. As a result, although much of the theory developed in the discipline seems to value the structures of simple societies, it nonetheless celebrates the progress of civilization.

The latter tendency is particularly apparent if one considers the theories of social evolution offered by anthropologists or the descriptions they provided of the great technological revolutions of prehistory (the "broad spectrum" revolution, or the invention of such sophisticated tools as grindstones, sickles, small projectiles, and fishing equipment to obtain and process an increasing variety of wild foods; the Neolithic revolution, or the development of agriculture; and the urban revolution, or the rise of cities and the state).[1] Such models, at least until the last two decades, have generally celebrated our progress; the major transformations of human societies have been portrayed as solutions to age-old problems which liberated human populations from the restraints of nature—an image traceable to Thomas Hobbes some three hundred years ago. Thus, for example, in the last century, Lewis Henry Morgan described the three major stages of human cultural evolution as a progression from "savagery" to "barbarism" and then to "civilization"—terms hardly less prejudicial when he wrote than they are now. Far more recently, Leslie White portrayed human history in terms of progressive increase in efficiency, and Julian Steward characterized the technological changes of prehistory as "freeing" human beings from the "exigencies" of simpler lifestyles and "permitting" new organizational styles to unfold. In perhaps the most explicit statement of this progressive sense of cultural change, V. Gordon Childe described the major technological and social revolutions of prehistory essentially as great improvements in the adaptive capacity of the species.[2]

Explicit, or at least implicit, in all of these theories was the idea that progress could be measured through the increase in the numbers and power of the human population—an observation that few scholars would deny.[3] Also implicit in most of these theories, at least as they came to be understood by the public, was the idea that progress favored individuals and improved their lives. We assumed that the human workload became lighter, our nutrition better, our diseases fewer as civilization emerged. This image still persists most strikingly in descriptions of the history of human life expectancy, which commonly suggest a steady, if irregular, upward trend.[4]

This image has long been subject to challenge by Marxist scholars, who suggested that civilization meant progress only for the privileged because its machinery was usurped for their benefit. During the 1960s, however, different (and in some ways more basic) challenges emerged. Observations of hunting and gathering bands, technologically the simplest of observed human groups, seemed to suggest that they fared relatively well and worked relatively little. It became fashionable for anthropologists to refer to them as the original "affluent" society.[5] At about the same time, economist Ester Boserup[6] argued that many of the technological changes observed in history were not "progress" at all, but necessary adjustments—often with diminishing returns—to increasing population. Her vision was very much at odds with prevailing anthropological and economic theory and with popular understanding. Through her perspective, however, the primitive became interpretable not merely as a struggle to survive in the face of limited knowledge but as a successful, efficient adaptation to small population and small social scale. Critical to Boserup's idea was the realization that adaptive advances measured as numerical success might not offer benefits for individual people and might not be perceived as progress by the individuals involved.

The key issue, then, is whether forms of society that we call civilized and that are undoubtedly related to improved short-term adaptive capacity of the species as a whole necessarily imply an improvement in the health and well-being of members of society—whether they imply progress in the sense that we commonly use the word.

In the past few decades, another thread has been added to the debate about conflicting images of progress. Medical evidence has begun to accumulate concerning the relative health of individuals and populations, both modern and prehistoric, who have participated in different economic and technological systems. These data are important precisely because they give us a sense of how different technologies and episodes of technological change impinged on the individuals who participated in them. In short, the medical data provide measurable evidence of the quality of different lifestyles. For the first time, we have at our command empirical evidence to assess and perhaps resolve the debate about the meaning of progress that has divided anthropologists, historians, and philosophers and has confounded popular thought. Perhaps more important, we have evidence with which to begin to assess accurately and specifically how major technological changes in our history have affected human well-being.

The medical evidence takes three forms. First, detailed observation and laboratory analysis of illness in our own society have enhanced our understanding of patterns of illness and health. We have begun to understand the "rules" that govern the occurrence of various types of illness. We have then been able to extrapolate those rules to predict future occurrences of a disease (the essence of contemporary epidemiology) or to reconstruct health patterns of the past. In making such reconstructions, we assume that basic rules of biology, chemistry, and physics do not change; we suppose that, although biological organisms evolve, their requirements are unlikely to have changed inexplicably or "magically" within the short span of human prehistory and history. We assume, in other words, that the analysis of changing patterns of health can be carried out using the same principles of uniformitarianism or natural law that govern predictive statements in all sciences. These are the same principles that enable us to interpret the climate and geology of the past by observing geological processes in the modern world; they are the same principles that in the 1960s permitted us to design a rocket capable of taking off from the moon using calculations based on earthbound experience, before anyone had been to the moon itself.[7]

Second, these theoretical models of changing health through human history have recently been supplemented by actual field studies of the health of individuals living in technologically simple societies—the societies that are the source of our stereotypes of primitive life. Within the past twenty-five years, for example, medical teams have recorded health and nutritional data for such groups as the !Kung San of the Kalahari, the Hadza of Tanzania, the Pygmies of central Africa, and other groups of Africans retaining (or perhaps merely approximating) some aspects of an ancient hunter-gatherer lifestyle. Similarly, medical teams have conducted health studies on a variety of populations in South America and New Guinea living in small groups, some living by hunting and gathering, some fairly mobile in their habits, and some still largely isolated from world commerce. These data are supplemented by more scattered medical studies of such hunter-gatherer populations as the Aleut and Eskimo, the native Australians, and the hunter-gatherers of South Asia and Southeast Asia. Such evidence can be compared to studies of health in contemporary civilization and to the records of health of recent historical populations.[8]

Third, we can now make direct evaluation of some aspects of ancient health using techniques of human osteology and paleopathology. Human remains (skeletons and occasionally mummies) from archaeological sites provide clues to the health of prehistoric individuals. Comparisons of archaeological remains from different times and places, which reflect various ways of life, have enabled prehistorians to assess the impact of prehistoric economic, social, and political change on those individuals.[9]

None of these three modes of inquiry is an infallible guide in the evaluation of human progress. Each involves imperfect and incomplete information, and each requires us to make assumptions about the relationship between past and present that may be tenuous and that can never be fully evaluated.[10] The emerging conclusions are credible not because one technique is perfectly reliable but because several potentially fallible but independent techniques appear to suggest similar conclusions.

Taken together, the three lines of inquiry—the extrapolation of epidemiological rules, the study of contemporary groups, and the analysis of prehistoric skeletons and mummies—paint a surprising picture of the past.

They suggest a pattern of changing health associated with the evolution of civilization that is more complex than we commonly realize. If the evidence confirms some of our own proud image of ourselves and our civilization, it also suggests that our progress has been bought at higher cost than we like to believe.

Chapter 2

Behavior and Health

> Health is a state of complete physical, mental, and social well-being, and not merely the absence of disease or infirmity.
>
> > Preamble to the charter of the World Health Organization

> Health [is rather] a modus vivendi enabling imperfect men to achieve a rewarding and not too painful existence while they cope with an imperfect world.
>
> > René Dubos, *Man, Medicine and Environment*

I should begin by making two points about the nature of health and disease. The two points are relatively simple but are not widely understood or appreciated—and they are not always consciously applied, even by people who would surely profess to understand them. The first point is that human activities can create disease or increase the risk of illness just as surely as medical science reduces the risk. Most threats to human health are not universal, and many are not ancient. Most threats to health do not occur randomly, nor are they dictated solely by natural forces: most are correlated with patterns of human activity.

The second point, as the quotation from René Dubos suggests, is that human activity is never as successful in minimizing health risks as we would like. Despite the stated ideal of the World Health Organization, minimizing health risks is rarely our only or primary goal. Our activities—and their effects on health and disease—involve compromises.

The Role of Human Activity in Promoting Disease

The role of human activity in promoting disease can easily be illustrated by reference to examples from three broad classes of illness: infection and infectious disease, malnutrition, and functional or degenerative diseases.

INFECTION

Infectious diseases are those caused by the presence of microscopic parasites, including viruses, bacteria, fungi, protozoa, spirochetes, rickettsias, and worms. These diseases depend on the survival and spread of the infecting organisms. Each organism must enter the human body by one of a few routes (through the mouth, nose, or anus, the openings of the genital tract, or cuts and breaks in the skin surface). To produce symptoms of disease, the organism must survive in human tissues; if the infection is to spread, the organism must reproduce, and its offspring must leave the body. Once outside the body, offspring must survive, grow, and find a way to reach a new victim or "host."[1] (They may, for example, be transmitted by direct contact between bodies, be blown through the air, or carried in food or water.) In short "germs," like people, must complete their life cycles, generation after generation, if the species are to survive.

Human exposure to a disease depends in part on simple geography. Each disease-causing organism, particularly one that spends part of its life cycle outside the human host, has a geographical distribution limited by its tolerance for extremes of temperature and humidity. As a rule, the humid tropics are particularly permissive of parasite survival; cooler and drier climates harbor fewer parasites. Human beings can remain free of some diseases simply by avoiding natural environments that permit their survival, but expanding populations may encounter new diseases as they penetrate new environments.

Human exposure to a disease also depends on whether human habits are consistent with the survival and reproductive requirements of the organism involved. One gets an infectious disease not because one is, in some vague way, "unclean," "unhygienic," or "primitive" but because one performs (or fails to perform) specific acts that allow a particular organism to complete its life cycle.

A large number of organisms that cause infections, for example, pass from one human being to another by leaving one body in feces and reentering the body of another individual through the mouth, usually in contaminated food or drinking water. This mode of transmission (so-called fecal-oral transmission) is common in most, if not all, human groups, including our own. (It accounts for most cases of diarrhea.) But human habits increase or decrease the likelihood of infection. The modern practice of flushing away excrement after defecation undoubtedly reduces the risk of infection, unless sewage contaminates drinking water supplies, as has occasionally been the case in recent history. The civilized custom of washing one's hands after defecating also affords some protection, but the primitive practice of abandoning a village site at short intervals (before feces can accumulate) also undoubtedly reduces the risk. So, too, does the modern Islamic custom, not practiced in the West, of eating with only one hand and cleaning oneself only with the other.[2] Eating at home reduces the risk of encountering new infections; eating in restaurants (where employees apparently must be reminded to wash their hands) increases the risk.

Organisms vary enormously in their survival requirements and in their modes of transmission. Some organisms, such as the spirochetes that cause venereal syphilis (and its lesser known relatives—endemic syphilis, yaws, and pinta), cannot exist without contact with warm, moist human skin or other tissue and can only spread from person to person by the touch of the appropriate tissues.[3] Others, such as the virus that causes measles, can live for relatively short spans in moist droplets in the air. They can spread among individuals near one another even if those individuals never touch, but they cannot survive for long between human hosts.[4] Such other infections as the virus of smallpox may persist for longer (but finite) periods of time on inanimate objects and thus can spread among human beings whose only contact is touching a common object within a reasonable period of time.[5] At the other extreme are various bacteria and fungi that can exist indefinitely in the soil. These may only occasionally (and perhaps only accidentally) infect human beings; they require no contact among people for their transmission. But human activities that involve digging or inhaling dust increase the risk of exposure.[6] Changing human habits will affect the transmission of these different organisms in different ways. (A major problem facing us at the moment is to determine the precise requirements of the organism causing AIDS (acquired immunodeficiency syndrome) and to determine exactly what changes in our behavior might stop its spread.)[7]

In some cases, microorganisms live primarily off other animals, known as disease "reservoirs." Bovine tuberculosis, for example, is primarily a disease of cattle and their wild relatives, although it can infect people who drink contaminated milk.[8] In other cases, such parasites as the protozoan that causes malaria or the rickettsia that causes typhus rely on mosquitos, ticks, fleas, or lice (so-called vectors) to carry them from person to person. When a reservoir or vector species is involved, the risk of human infection depends on how people interact with those species and how our behavior affects their survival: whether or not we keep domestic animals, whether our management of soil and water encourages or discourages mosquitos and other insects. Throughout our history, human beings have made a number of economic and behavioral choices that have affected the survival and dissemination of reservoir or vector species. Some of these have been conscious decisions; too often they have not.[9]

Human habits, by affecting the time and the place at which an organism enters the human body, may influence the subsequent development of the disease. Many diseases, including such common "diseases of child-hood" as mumps, are known to produce more severe symptoms when they attack mature individuals.[10] Epstein-Barr virus is more likely to generate the symptoms of mononucleosis when it attacks mature individuals,[11] and poliomyelitis viruses are more likely to produce paralysis when they attack adults than when they attack infants or children.[12] Human activities often help to determine the age at which individuals are exposed to these diseases. "Good hygiene," for example, may delay (rather than prevent) infection with unfortunate results.

The difference between yaws or endemic syphilis (comparatively mild diseases of skin and bone) and venereal syphilis appears to result largely from the time and place of the infection. In warm, moist climates, the organism can survive on the surface of human skin, and because human beings in such climates commonly and sensibly wear little clothing, the organism is usually passed by casual skin contact, most often in childhood, resulting in yaws. In colder, drier climates, the same organism (or a relative so similar that distinguishing the two is difficult, if not impossible) can only exist on those parts of the human body that provide the requisite warmth and moisture. Under these conditions casual childhood contact produces endemic syphilis (the lesions of which are localized to such moist areas as the mouth and genital region).

If people in such climates change their rules about clothing, "hygiene," and body contact in a way that discourages casual childhood transmission of the parasite, then the disease can only spread in those more limited contacts —primarily sexual or "venereal"—in which appropriately unclothed warm and moist body parts are brought in contact with one another. The result is a disease (venereal syphilis) of internal systems of the body contracted primar-ily by adults and potentially passed to unborn children with consequences far more severe than those of yaws or endemic syphilis.[13]

In addition to altering the life cycle of the parasites or exposure to those parasites, human populations can alter the pattern of infections that they suffer by changing the condition of the human host. We now know that in-fection by some organisms does not always mean illness. Certain organisms may be ubiquitous, or at least more common than the diseases associated with them. Some illnesses seem to depend on whether or not the human host can fight off the infection. Illness may actually result from the reaction or overreaction of the human body as much as from the activities of the parasite—or more. The response of the body depends, in turn, on a number of factors, including nutritional state,[14] the presence of other infections,[15] and even the emotional state of the individual.[16]

Tuberculosis, in particular, may be a disease largely controlled in such a manner, at least in the modern world where the infectious agent, a bacillus (bacterium), has until recently been ubiquitous. In the generations now entering middle age or older, most individuals were "infected," as proved by the incidence of positive skin tests, but few got sick. In fact "illness" almost always resulted from the reactivation of bacilli stored in the body long after the initial spread of the germ. The reactivation appears to be correlated with malnutrition, chemical stresses on body tissues, and the social displacement and psychological disorientation of potential victims.[17]

NUTRITION

We can analyze patterns of nutritional stresses on human beings in similar terms. Each necessary nutrient—vitamin, mineral, amino acid, fatty acid, and fiber—has a defined natural distribution. Each must be eaten in certain quantities and must be absorbed by the body from the digestive tract. Many must be ingested in particular form or combination if they are to be absorbed from the intestine and used successfully. Some are stolen by our parasites either before or after they enter our bodies. Many can only be stored for a short period in the human body, and most have mechanisms by which they are excreted from the body. Similar rules govern the effects of natural toxins or poisons in our food.

Our behavior largely dictates whether we will obtain adequate nutrition. We can change our food habits or alter the natural supply and distribution of nutrients (either purposely or inadvertently), but our activities can also have more subtle effects, changing our bodily needs or affecting the rate at which nutrients are absorbed from the intestine or excreted.[18]

Iron, for example, although fairly common in nature, can only be readily absorbed by the body in certain forms and food combinations (particularly those containing meat or rich in vitamin C). Human food choices, the combinations of foods that make up meals, and even styles of food preparation, as well as the presence of parasites, play a major role in determining iron levels in the body (possibly resulting either in iron-deficiency anemia or iron poisoning).[19]

In contrast, iodine is comparatively scarce and is unevenly distributed in nature. It is present in the sea and in many seafoods; it is also present in the rock, soil, and water (and therefore in the plants and animals) of some regions but not of others. People who live in areas of iodine-poor soil and water are prone to iodine deficiency, which can cause goiter and the retardation of growth and mental development. Eating foods that interfere with iodine utilization in the body, such as cabbages, can make the problem worse, particularly if the foods are eaten raw. But the major factor controlling iodine intake is human movement or trade. People living in iodine-poor regions must obtain their supply from somewhere else.[20]

DEGENERATIVE DISEASES

We can apply the same kind of reasoning to a whole host of other diseases that have become prominent in the twentieth century as infectious diseases have declined in importance. These are diseases that, for lack of a clear understanding of their epidemiology, we have tended to consider either unfortunate but unexplained weaknesses in individual bodies or the inevitable results of getting older. I will refer to them collectively as "degenerative" diseases for lack of a better term.

We are discovering that such diseases as adult-onset diabetes (diabetes mellitus), multiple sclerosis (MS), and even appendicitis are not universal among human groups, nor are they randomly distributed. We are also discovering that such problems as arthritis, cancers, heart disease, hypertension, strokes, osteoporosis, varicose veins, and hemorrhoids are not universal functions of "growing old." Each of these diseases displays a pattern that enables us to begin to determine the factors controlling its occurrence. We can demonstrate that individual behavior has a significant effect on the chance of getting each.[21] Breast cancer, for example, may be associated with high fat, protein, and calorie diets, and with high levels of estrogen (whether produced in the body or added in diet or medication). The risk seems to be lower, however, for women who bear and nurse a number of children and higher for women who do not nurse or who bear their first child at a relatively late age. For whatever reason, a high incidence of breast cancer is clearly associated with women leading modern, Western lifestyles.[22]

Adaptive Compromise

The most important point that emerges when one compares the health of human groups from around the world is that the frequency of disease of all three of these types (infectious, nutritional, degenerative) varies markedly from group to group. This variation is partly a function of genetic differences between individuals and between populations, of course. A number of genetic variations among human beings have evolved as adaptations to the stresses of living in different styles or parts of the earth; many of these traits continue to affect the susceptibility of specific human populations to particular illnesses. (Such variations often act to the benefit of populations living in their historic homelands in traditional lifestyles, but to the relative detriment of populations geographically or culturally displaced in relatively recent history.)[23]

It is now a common observation, however, that populations of African, Asian, Australian, Amerindian, or European ancestry become more alike in the incidence of various diseases as their ways of life become similar. Most of the differences in our experience with disease appear to result from cultural factors: the incidence of a particular disease in any group seems largely a function of the group's behavior, not its genes. The task facing human societies is to design behavioral strategies that balance or minimize the risks.

But minimizing the risk is not easy. The human environment poses myriad adaptive challenges. Some forty-five substances (or more, depending on how one counts and classifies) are known to be necessary for human survival.[24] The number of potential sources of infection, toxicity, and other risks is too large to be enumerated. Some risks combine or compound each other in ways that create additional hazards. The sheer number of such dangers makes it unlikely that any human population could ever adapt successfully to them all, even if it could eventually accumulate sufficiently accurate knowledge and techniques to cope with some or even most dangers.

If adapting to a large but fixed number of risks to our health were the only problem we faced, however, we might hope, as the World Health Organization charter implies, that medical science would eventually perfect our health care. Unfortunately, the task is more complicated.

One additional problem is that human groups, particularly in the recent past, have often been faced with continuously changing circumstances. Human beings (with or without the scientific method) do recognize patterns of illness and often do, by trial and error, devise good solutions to health problems that become embodied in their cultural lore. Anthropological descriptions of human societies abound with examples of rituals, customs, and religious rules that appear, almost inadvertently, to help balance the diet or protect people from dangers.[25] But such patterns develop slowly; cultural adjustments often lag behind the appearance of new stresses.[26]

An even bigger problem is that the defense against any one health risk often makes another risk worse. The various substances that we require do not occur in the same foods. A food rich in one vitamin may be poor in another or may contain chemical "antagonists" to other vitamins (that is, substances that interfere with the work of other vitamins). An increased level of one nutrient may negatively affect absorption or utilization of another. Providing more calories often means accepting lower levels of other nutrients or incurring new risks of infection or poison. High quality protein from meat may be dangerous food to obtain, and it may increase one's risk of parasitic infestation. Eliminating one disease vector may aid the spread of another vector. Even eliminating one of our parasites often opens the door for another to attack.[27]

A further complication is that health decisions never take place in a social vacuum. Societies have limited resources, and they have other priorities that compete with health, so health is always played off against other goals. Social values can even interfere directly with finding solutions to health problems. For example, people may actually generate unnecessary malnutrition by maldistribution of available food, even within households, because of culturally held beliefs about "proper" food assignment.[28] And people around the world often choose to accept obvious risks to health for the sake of maintaining valued customs, much as American teenagers continue to take up smoking for social reasons despite widespread warnings about the risks they incur.[29]

The final point—and the one that seems hardest for us to recognize or accept—is that individual well-being is always being traded against group success. Health must always be balanced against politics. Until this point in human history, at least, each group has had to compete with other human populations for space and resources. Success has meant the competitive displacement of rival groups or, at least, the ability to hold one's own. In fact, such competitive success has been the bottom line of cultural survival. The "arms race" is a distraction from investment in health, and it has always been with us in one form or another.

But it is not clear that "success" has implied much more than this. It need not imply that a group maintain the welfare of all individuals. On the contrary, there is reason to argue that competitive success by populations has often (perhaps always) been bought at the expense of the well-being of some individuals. Every human group known has some basis for excluding certain members from full participation in health benefits and has had mechanisms to decide who will enjoy scarce resources and who will be bypassed in times of scarcity. In fact, all known human groups have mechanisms by which they eliminate some individuals outright: exile, exclusion, or execution of adults; neglect, abortion, or infanticide of the young.

In addition, throughout human history, successful populations have been, manifestly, those that subordinated the interests of whole classes of members to the power of the group. As civilization emerged, decisions made for and on behalf of the group have increasingly been entrusted to special elites concerned as much about collective power as about collective welfare.

The final point that needs to be made is that the compromise keeps changing. The central theme of this work is not primarily to point out that adaptation is compromise, but to call attention to the ways in which that compromise has changed through human history—to show how changes in the size, distribution, economy, and organization of human populations have altered the structure of adaptive strategies and of health. Most changes in health reflect these changes in our societies (and our numbers), not the progress of our medicine.

Chapter 3

The Evolution of Human Society

Before I pursue the theme of changing patterns of health, it seems advisable to sketch a brief (somewhat simplified and idealized) history of how human societies have evolved. This will provide a background for arguments pursued in subsequent chapters.

In attempts to understand human cultural evolution, anthropologists commonly divide human societies into categories that add a degree of scientific precision to our discussion of the primitive and the civilized and help explain why compromises in health change as society changes. Although a number of systems of classification have been proposed and there is some disagreement about the precise divisions to be made, such categories are usually defined with explicit or at least implicit reference to the size of the population involved. The smallest of human societies typically include no more than thirty to fifty people in any one local community or *band* and involve no more than a few hundred individuals in a larger, loosely coordinated network of bands that make up the whole society. At the next level are villages and small towns of several hundred or even a few thousand people, sharing a common language and culture, which may be linked in loose confederacies (*tribes*) or united in more formally organized *rank* societies or *chiefdoms* numbering many thousands of individuals. In contrast, what anthropologists refer to as *civilization* contains communities of various sizes, but at least some of those communities—the cities—contain many thousands (or hundreds of thousands) of individuals. These communities are typically integrated into larger units or *states,* in which large populations are unified by a common, centralized political organization but may no longer share a common language or culture.[1]

This classification of societies by size is also, at least in a very rough sense, a statement about the historical sequence or evolution of human cultures—the progress of human civilization. Perhaps the two clearest trends in the archaeological record of human society are the gradual increase in the overall size and density of the human population and the progressive displacement of small communities and small political units by larger ones.[2] Small-scale, autonomous social and political units—bands or autonomous villages—grow into larger societies over the scale of archaeological time, or they are engulfed by larger societies. They may be assimilated or become enclaves of specialists within the larger group. They may simply be displaced by larger societies and become extinct or survive only in marginal locations removed from the arena of direct and serious competition.[3] Independent bands and autonomous villages and towns, which once contained nearly all of the human population, now persist only as scattered remnants in such out-of-the-way and undesired locations as deserts, tropical rain forests, or the Arctic—and even those remnants are rapidly disappearing.

The size of communities serves as a good basis for classifying societies, because it appears to dictate—or at least to be correlated with—many other features of society. Despite their superficial variety, contemporary societies in each category share pronounced similarities in overall design. Differences in community size apparently explain many of the changes in economic and social organization that occurred during our history and account for many differences between behaviors that we call primitive and civilized.

Band Societies

Comparative analysis of the few remaining band societies suggests that they share many common features. Most band societies focus their economic activities on wild plants and animals. They hunt, fish, and trap small animals and gather or harvest wild fruits, tubers, leaves, and seeds in varying proportions; they do not farm, nor do they raise domestic animals.[4] In the modern world and in recent history, some such groups have traded hunted or gathered foods for farmed staples. In early prehistory they must have subsisted entirely on the basis of wild resources. Such groups appear, moreover, to consume most foods immediately—within hours, or at most a few days, of obtaining them.[5]

This dependence on wild foods, which are generally more sparsely distributed than farmed foods and thus provide fewer calories per acre of land exploited, appears to limit the density of band populations. Recent historic hunter-gatherer societies have only rarely exceeded an average of one person for each square mile of territory they exploited; in fact, most such societies were observed to have population densities of substantially fewer than one person per square mile. The exceptions were often in such locations as the northwest coast of the United States or Canada—or at such times as the late Pleistocene Ice Age in Europe—where wild resources were plentiful.[6]

The sparse distribution of most wild foods—and the fact that most bands have no means of transport other than their own labor—also helps to account for the small size of individual band communities. If the community were larger, foragers would have to seek food over an area too large to be searched with reasonable ease and would have to transport food impossibly great distances by foot.[7]

At least partly because they rely on wild foods that can easily be depleted in any one region, contemporary hunter-gatherer bands are usually much more mobile than other types of human society. Most bands observed in recent centuries have moved their camps every few days, weeks, or even months. The frequency of movement seems to be determined in part by the desire for new foods and in part by diminishing returns in foraging activities in the vicinity of the old camp. In contrast to our own preference for sedentary lifestyles, however, members of hunter-gatherer bands commonly appear to enjoy their mobility, and they use movement as a means of solving a variety of problems unrelated to their food supply. Mobility provides knowledge about the surrounding environment and hence a measure of economic and political security; it relieves boredom and provides a handy means of disposing of refuse and avoiding filth. And individual freedom of movement serves as a means of resolving social conflict: after a serious dispute, someone leaves.[8]

Probably because of their small community size and their mobility, contemporary hunter-gatherer bands are typically relatively simple in their social and political design. The most important aspect of this simplicity is the lack of economic specialization within the group. Men and women often perform different tasks, but households tend to participate equally in the basic tasks of subsistence and undertake the full range of activities performed by other households. Additional crafts are generally limited to those that each family performs for itself. An individual may specialize in something that he or she does well, but it is rare for anyone to specialize to the exclusion of performing the common basic tasks—and an individual is rarely so heavily dependent on a speciality that he must trade with others within the group to obtain food.[9]

Hunter-gatherer bands usually lack or minimize social distinctions that other societies employ—social clubs, classes, and formal kinship groups, such as clans. Apparently their small numbers permit individual, face-to-face interactions among members and eliminate the need to subdivide and classify the members of the group.[10]

Such groups tend to minimize their formal politics.[11] Group decisions are commonly made by consensus. To the extent that leadership is recognized at all, it is commonly informal, ephemeral, and limited to spheres in which individuals have demonstrated particular prowess. One man may lead a hunt; someone else will lead the dance. Such leadership is reinforced by the prestige and authority conferred by demonstrated skill and wisdom; it is rarely if ever reinforced by coercive power. Leaders retain their special position only so long as their leadership decisions satisfy their fellows.

In short, bands are typically small, informal networks of friends and kin who know one another personally, who deal with each other as individuals and as friends and relatives, and who remain together largely as a function of mutual dependence and positive feelings toward one another. They tend to operate much in the same manner (albeit with some of the same tensions) that similar small voluntary associations of friends and kin operate within our own society. The difference is that for them such associations comprise the whole community. Economic exchange (a type that anthropologists call *reciprocity*) usually takes place informally, on the basis of need, social obligations, and personal ties—rather than on the basis of market value and profit —just as it does among groups of friends and kin in our own society. An exchange carries with it the expectation that a friend or kinsman will return the favor in whatever manner he is best able (which may only be affection or respect) rather than returning an object of equal or greater value.[12]

The structure of hunter-gather bands means that patterns of care and responsibility are very different from those to which we are accustomed (or rather they resemble patterns that we associate with friends and family rather than patterns that we associate with society at large). Individual members of such bands exercise a high degree of control over their own group membership and their own economic welfare. Each adult has equal and direct access to resources, direct personal leverage on other significant individuals, and relative freedom to leave the group. Furthermore, the motivations for mutually supportive interactions are commonly strong, as befits groups of friends and kin.

Because of this relative autonomy of adult individuals and the kin- and friendship-based ethic of sharing that commonly prevails, such groups have often been characterized by anthropologists as egalitarian. And it is clear that these same features—group size, the friendship ethic, and the power of individuals to move—tend to guarantee that the group will be responsive to individual needs and comparatively evenhanded in its fulfillment of those needs. Exploitation of members either by other members of the group or by outsiders is difficult. Members of hunter-gatherer bands can easily withstand an attempt by another member of the group to wield undue power or influence: they simply leave. For the same reason, within recent history hunter-gatherers have been comparatively difficult to conquer or incorporate into civilization, despite their relative lack of political muscle, although they are easily displaced.

But just as there is a lack of other specialized activities, there are no special agencies besides family and friends to assist individuals in trouble. No agency protects against dangers too great to be faced by the family, and no agency replaces family and friends should they withhold their aid. Therefore, whereas fit adult individuals may exert more autonomy than their counterparts in other societies, dependent children (or such other dependents as the elderly, the crippled, or the sick and injured) may be comparatively vulnerable to the potential loss of parental services.[13] Moreover, it is clear that such societies are not "egalitarian" to all of their members. As in all other societies, those with power (in this case, healthy adult providers) are capable of making decisions at the expense of powerless individuals, who by virtue of extreme youth, age, or incapacity are unable to exercise independence.

There is one other problem with such informal organization: it apparently only works for very small groups in which individuals can recognize and deal with one another on a personal basis. The same style of organization does not work when each individual must deal with too many others (a pattern readily verifiable by psychological experiments within our own population).[14] This fact, as much as the relative scarcity of wild resources, explains the small size of hunting and gathering bands. Observation of contemporary hunter-gatherer bands with rudimentary economic and political organization indicates that groups of more than fifty to one hundred people (which occasionally form for seasonal rituals or the exploitation of certain resources) are unstable because social tensions inevitably fracture the group, whether or not food is in short supply.[15]

Economic Adjustments to Growing Population

If the population increases, human groups will have to make economic adjustments to accommodate their greater numbers. The primary economic need is to find or generate larger supplies of food and other materials necessary to survival. This can be accomplished in several ways.

First, groups can exploit more territory to obtain the needed resources.

Home or camp can be moved more often or moved farther, and individuals can walk farther from home to obtain food each day. Of course, these solutions only work if there are no competing populations in the vicinity. Members of the group can also be less selective about what portions of the neighboring environment to use, making fuller use of areas hitherto deemed dangerous, unpleasant, or unprofitable. The group can split in two, a portion moving entirely into an area once unexploited and perhaps considered unsafe or unfit for habitation and exploitation. The archaeological record of early human groups clearly documents such expansion from preferred to secondary parts of the environment and suggests that this type of expansion was among the earliest strategies employed by our ancestors to expand their food supplies.[16] Ultimately, access to new territory through the movement of individuals and even whole communities is bounded by the limits of human speed on foot and human transport.

The second type of adjustment that can be made is to exploit existing territory more intensively, using types of food or other resources hitherto considered unacceptable, uneconomical to obtain, or difficult to prepare or process. The early human archaeological record in various parts of the world clearly documents a shift in the range of foods exploited (beginning about fifteen thousand years ago in the Old World, about eight thousand years ago in the New World) as population density, and often community size, increased—the so-called broad spectrum revolution. Vegetable foods apparently increased in importance in the human diet, in proportion to animal foods; small animal trapping increasingly supplemented big game hunting; fishing and marine gathering increasingly accompanied land-based foraging; such small seeds as cereals were added to the diet.[17] Special tools, such as grindstones to process these foods, seem to have become increasingly common.

The third strategy a large community can employ is to adjust or even out natural fluctuations in the daily, seasonal, or annual availability of food. Like any animal population, a human community is limited in size by the amount of food available in the leanest season. If a community can store food for sparse seasons it can support a larger population. Many human communities, including very small groups of the type just described, rely on stored foods during some lean seasons, and large human communities must rely heavily on such storage. In fact, it is becoming increasingly clear in the archaeological record that prehistoric hunting and gathering communities in many locations achieved substantial size by storing wild resources.[18]

The fourth, and perhaps historically most important, strategy that a group can adopt is to increase the productivity of the territory it exploits (that is, to increase the amount of food produced per acre) by farming—a series of techniques that human groups are thought to have first adopted ten thousand years ago or fewer, during what has come popularly to be referred to as the Neolithic revolution.[19]

Farming is the investment of human labor to assist the growth of selected plant and animal species. Such selected species might be ornamental plants or such utilitarian plants as gourds, medicinal (or hallucinogenic) plants, or special spices. Through human history, however, an increasing proportion of farmers' effort appears to have been devoted to promoting crops—particularly cereals and tubers—that would produce calories prolifically and could then be stored. The agricultural staples wheat, rice, corn (maize), rye, barley, millets, sorghum, sweet potatoes, yams, and manioc all share these two qualities.[20]

The investment produces changes in the landscape. We assist our chosen crops by displacing their competitors and detractors: destroying the parasites and predators that eat them, removing the weeds that compete with them for space or food, clearing the forests that block their access to the sun. We also modify the physical world to create conditions more suitable for their growth: we level the ground, break up the soil, and adjust the supplies of water and other nutrients through fertilization and irrigation. Because part of the purpose of manipulation is to have selected plants and animals to grow outside their original, native habitats, the investment in the landscape may ultimately become sizable, and the crops may become heavily dependent on our intervention.[21]

The investment often also implies changes in the crops themselves. Given so much attention, many plants and animals become domesticated. Their life cycles are brought fully under human control, and their physical and genetic structures changed through intentional or inadvertent selective breeding to suit human needs and to meet the requirements of cohabitation with human populations and manipulation at human hands. Many of our domestic species are so altered by the new relationship that they could no longer grow independent of human care.[22]

But the relationship is a mutual or symbiotic one.[23] Human populations also become dependent on their domesticates, and human habits come to be dictated by the reproductive needs of their domestic species.

Any community, even one of only moderate size, that relies on farming (or even significant storage of wild resources) to provide its food needs to adjust its pattern of movement. A significant dependence on storage requires sedentism or permanent occupation, rather than mobile camps. Domestication of crops increases the need for sedentism. Because crops require protection before harvesting as well as after storage, human groups may be forced to remain in the vicinity of their fields or gardens throughout the year. And because storage from one season overlaps the investment in the next season, permanent occupation of longer duration is encouraged. Permanent villages become the rule, and the relatively flimsy dwellings of temporary or seasonal camps may be traded for more substantial and permanent houses.

One result is likely to be an increase in trade. Sedentism means reduced access to varied sources of food and other natural resources (such as stone or metal for tools) that are available to mobile hunter-gatherers through their patterns of movement. Farmers or sedentary hunter-gatherers[24] must do without such variety or develop alternate means of attaining these additional resources, and trade is the solution. In addition, individuals who remain in one place can accumulate possessions in a manner not possible for mobile populations. They may, therefore, be more inclined to trade for exotic materials.

Domestication also implies a change in the perception of labor and ownership. Individuals must invest or commit their labor well in advance of receiving any reward. This need for prior investment in resources to produce future food supplies promotes a sense of individual ownership. In societies that eat farmed foods, individuals often own their produce even if they do not own the land. Produced food becomes personal or family property. Moreover, in a small farming community it is common for rights of use to specific resources, such as land, to be assigned with some care. Land may be temporarily owned while in use, even though ownership is not permanent. In addition, the right to membership in the local community that owns the land is likely to be assigned with greater selectivity and care than in hunting and gathering bands. Groups investing in agriculture often show a greater concern with defining group affiliation and with rules of inheritance and descent (membership in a particular clan or lineage) than do hunting and gathering bands.[25] Groups become more rigid, and the increasing rigidity tends to produce both greater identification with individual communities and more pronounced tensions between communities.

Social and Political Adjustments to Increasing Community Size

Sedentism and rigid group definition, in combination with larger group size (whether associated with intensive foraging or farming),[26] have further effects on the social structure of the group. If human beings are to live permanently in groups of more than fifty to one hundred people, they apparently have to change their own rules.

People who live in large permanent groups must find ways of dealing with neighbors too numerous to be known individually. One of the major steps facilitating progress to larger group sizes appears to have been the development of systems to categorize, identify, and stereotype group members.[27] Large communities of farmers are commonly divided into subgroups. Individuals are treated according to the category to which they are assigned. Membership in the groups or categories often supersedes individual friendship and personal familiarity as a basis for social and economic transactions. The categories may include such economic specializations as blacksmith, but in simple sedentary communities, such specialists are still relatively rare. Almost all people are farmers (or foragers), distinguishable only by the same categories of age and sex that are universal to human groups. In order to get around this difficulty, these communities invent distinctions among otherwise relatively similar individuals, including elaborate and formal divisions based on kinship and descent, age, sex, or initiation into special clubs. Clans and lineages are not only resource-owning groups; they provide a major means of classifying unknown individuals.

In addition, individuals cannot move away from social tensions and disputes, as all individuals are locked to their investments. This may explain why farming groups (and large, permanent groups of hunter-gatherers) commonly became involved in complex formal networks of social and political institutions usually based on principles of kinship.

For example, larger group size creates problems of informational flow and decision making. Consensus may become difficult to attain because the group is too large for discussion, and it may be difficult to identify common leaders on the same ad hoc personal basis that is used in smaller bands, because individuals are unfamiliar with other members. Disputes will be difficult to settle because the participants do not know one another and may have no common friend or relative that they can turn to for fair judgment.

If the society is small enough, disputes can still be handled informally within each lineage (or *segment*) of the society, whereas disputes between segments can be negotiated by the leaders (elders) of the two groups. Larger groups need to designate permanent leaders—headmen or chiefs—to whom people regularly turn when decisions must be made or disputes settled. To simplify the demand on those individuals, which might otherwise become overwhelming, formal channels of appeal are established within the group. Individuals may communicate with leaders only through defined intermediaries (usually the senior members of their own group).[28]

Large group size also means that informal reciprocal exchanges between friends and kin may not suffice to move food (or other goods) from where they are available to where they are needed. As a result, "big men" or chiefs commonly operate as the foci of relatively formal exchange systems that collect the wealth of the society in a central location and redistribute it to group members. Central collection and redistribution provide a powerful mechanism for the movement of goods. (But in a society with few specialists such redistribution may do little to provide a safety net for individuals whose crops fail and may play only a minor part in the lives of individuals who for the most part remain economically self-sufficient.) Central collection is, however, also a powerful mechanism for stimulating the production of extra food or surplus to be used for such common purposes as large-scale building projects, ceremonies, or collective feasts.

A final significant change in social structure associated with increasing social scale reflects the relationship of the individual to the community as a whole. Community membership replaces self-sufficiency and friendship between individuals as the basis for determining access to services and resources. Access to land is determined by membership in the community and its various segments, and economic well-being becomes geared to community systems of storage and redistribution. One result is the elaboration of community projects, such as storage systems that serve the group and small joint efforts at improving the land. A second result is what might be called increased patriotism. Large communities must invest an increasing proportion of their resources in reinforcing feelings of membership and commitment to the group. Much of the effort of the group becomes directed toward both occasions that celebrate group membership, such as feasts and festivals, and symbolic monuments and tombs that seem intended to reinforce group ties and celebrate the status of central individuals. The community diverts increasing amounts of energy from individual welfare to celebration of group identity.

To function effectively, for example, leaders must be readily identifiable; so they are allowed to wear special ornament or dress. Individuals may wear costumes or ornaments that signal their affiliation and tell other individuals how to behave. The association between large social scale and fancy clothing or luxury ornaments is more than coincidental. Sedentism does not merely permit individuals to accumulate luxury goods; it stimulates their acquisition because they play a new, necessary social role.

In short, tribes and chiefdoms trade some of the flexibility of band society for more formal rules; they trade some of their sense of individual reciprocity for an emphasis on group membership. They lose some of the sensitivity to individual needs that characterized simpler bands. The reorganization also entails some increase in principles of segregation and exclusion, limiting the right and ability of individuals to pursue their own welfare and the responsibility of individuals to care for their neighbors. In addition, the resources of societies become diverted more and more from immediate application to individual needs and toward celebration of community membership and defense of the community, celebration of privilege and authority, and, perhaps, privileged consumption by leaders.

Most such groups are still relatively egalitarian. Although economic distinctions based on skill may occur and distinctions of birth or other fixed status may confer privileged access to luxury goods, leaders rarely enjoy much economic privilege or much power. Their privilege is likely to be measured more by their ornaments than by the quality of their diets.[29] The various groups in the society may also be fairly equal in their access to important resources, even if distinguished by their clothing or their paraphernalia. Basic differences in access to such essential resources as food usually do not occur, and no individuals (other than those condemned or driven out for crimes) are denied access to means of livelihood.

These systems contain, however, the seeds of more complex and less egalitarian society. Redistribution systems can grow to claim larger and larger shares of societal production; headmen or chiefs, initially nothing more than the first or most central of equals, can assume increasing power. Centrally collected, stored produce is liable to expropriation by outsiders or by the chiefs themselves.

The Structure of Civilization

Truly large-scale societies—the civilizations that begin to appear in the archaeological record of various parts of the world about five thousand years ago—need to make a number of additional economic and social adjustments.[30]

First, further increases in the size of the population generate further demand for food production. (Demand for extra production may also have been stimulated by the incentive to trade or by the political demands of redistributor-chiefs.)

Increased demand can be met in only three ways: further increases in the density of growth of desired plants, increases in the frequency of cropping (that is, in the number of times per decade, and ultimately per year, that a given piece of land is harvested), and extensions of the total area under cultivation. All of these initiatives imply an increase in the investment that must be made in farming before sufficient food can be obtained. An increase in the density of growing crops or in the frequency of cropping implies a significant increase in the application of fertilizer and an increase in the effort needed to clear and prepare the land.[31] And extending the area under cultivation commonly implies the need for improvements that overcome such barriers to cultivation as poor soil, poor drainage, excessively steep slope, or lack of water. Civilizations commonly move water from place to place, raise swampland so that it will drain, level the land to facilitate irrigation, or terrace hillsides.

The need for such investments has, in turn, a number of effects on the structure of society. Many of the investments needed to extract further increases in production using irrigation or leveling schemes exceed the power or organizational capacity of individuals, families, or small-scale networks of friends and neighbors. They may even exceed the capacity of whole communities of moderate size. These tasks involve massed and coordinated labor. But they also require the application of specialized skills and the attention of skilled, full-time managers.[32]

Perhaps the most fundamental difference between civilization and simpler forms of society, long recognized by anthropologists and sociologists, lies in the way civilization arranges and distributes the various economic functions necessary to support it. Civilization by its very nature is a mechanism for assigning specific economic tasks to specialists and then managing their economic interactions. No longer does everyone produce some food. An increasing proportion of the population provides other goods and services and relies on the mechanisms of the society rather than its own efforts to provide basic nutritional needs. Food producers are comparatively few and are themselves economic specialists, who are often dependent on the work of other specialists even to carry out their basic farming tasks.

This new organization is reflected in basic spatial arrangements of the society. Communities are no longer self-sufficient. They, like individuals, come to be specialists that carry out various functions.

The new mode of organization also gives rise to a new type of community —the city—which is larger in size than other communities and serves a different purpose. Cities are basically aggregates of specialists and managerial personnel. These individuals may be supported by an indigenous group of farmers, but they may be wholly dependent on outside sources to provide their food, as in the case of modern Western cities. They grow larger than other communities for two reasons. First, they are freed from the constraints that limit the size of food-producing communities, in which each worker must be able to walk or ride to where he works the land. Second, there are new incentives for aggregation: specialists can often work most efficiently in the immediate vicinity of other specialists whose efforts complement their own or provide their raw materials.

Trade and transport, which are peripheral in the economies of simpler groups, play a central role in civilization and are major determinants of its design. Redistributive systems account for an increasing proportion of the production and wealth of the group—and become more central to each individual's survival as the numbers of specialists and special projects increases. Dependence on storage facilities and the machinery of transport increases; trade networks are expanded. Access to trade networks may become more important for the survival of communities than access to natural resources. Trade patterns and specialized resources become more important in determining community locations than local food resources. A permanent community might for the first time exist where there was no resource to harvest except salt or iron ore, which could be traded for food grown elsewhere. A community might exist at an otherwise barren crossroad.

Perhaps because communities are dependent on one another, the political boundaries of the society may be defined with relative care. The boundaries of civilizations are often legally defined and rigidly fixed in geographical terms (becoming lines on a map) rather than flowing with the movement of people, the expansion or contraction of family units, or changes in the environment, as do the boundaries of simpler groups. The unification of communities into permanent and rigid political units is one of the hallmarks of civilized organization.

The new mode of organization may also change the basis and rationale for interactions at the individual level. Small-scale societies maintain at least the fiction of interaction on a personal basis. Individuals are, and perceive themselves to be, similar in purpose and style; they are friends or kin, at least in a loose sense. In civilizations, individuals are, and perceive themselves to be, different from one another, although kinship often remains important for some relationships. Their ties are those of trading partners, individuals whose relations with one another are based primarily on the exchange of goods. In addition, as a result of the sheer size of many civilizations, the movement of specialists, and the militant origins of many civilized groups, civilizations may come to include individuals of varying ethnic background who lack common cultural roots. They may lack a basis for understanding one another or any motivation for cooperation. It is no coincidence, nor is it simply progress, that such civilizations commonly develop written systems of record keeping to document and regulate transactions.

Leaders take on an increasing range of functions: responsibility for warfare and defense, control of trade, management of dispute, coordination of the efforts of specialists, management of cooperative and communal efforts, and coordination of the more elaborate system of storage and redistribution. Management itself becomes a full-time job, widening the gap between leaders and followers.

A further major organizational principle that distinguishes civilization from the societies that preceded it is social stratification or division into social classes representing distinctions in wealth and power far more profound than those characterizing the earlier groups.[33] It is a regular feature (in fact, for most anthropologists, a defining feature) of civilizations that they are organized into social classes in which elites own essential resources (land, water, and more recently, factories) and one or more lower classes must earn the right to the fruit of those resources through their labor. The lower classes of all civilizations pay rent or taxes, surrender a share of their crop, or surrender a fraction of their labor in exchange for the privilege of eating—a privilege that the ruling class has the right and power to deny.

Class stratification completes what ethnic distinctions and economic specialties began: to create a society of groups and individuals whose interests are not only divergent but competing. Civilization becomes an uneasy balance of conflicting interests. It cannot be attributed to coincidence or progress that civilizations produced sets of rules that were literally and figuratively written in stone. Codified and written laws add predictability to interactions between strangers, at the expense of personal flexibility. Nor is it surprising that civilizations substitute formal adjudication before professional judges (perhaps with values of blind and abstract justice) at the expense of more personal and informed judgments by friends and kin or local chiefs, as practiced by smaller groups.

This new structure—the amalgam of divergent and competing interests —in turn underlies another major transformation that characterizes civilization: the transformation from a society based on consensus, peer pressure, prestige, and authority to one based on power or physical force. Civilizations rely on controlled use of force to regulate the interactions of strangers and to assure the resolution of conflicts of interest that are not bounded by friendship or kinship, and it is characteristic that civilization employs specialists in the use of force as a means of maintaining social control—professional armies and police. It is this specialized apparatus for control by force that anthropologists refer to when they speak of the emergence of the "state."

Paradoxically, this inequality and the power to back it up underwrite most of the monuments and accomplishments of civilization. The power to coerce labor and extract surplus produce are inseparably linked to the investments that are the hallmark of civilized production. Coerced labor is converted to irrigation ditches, aqueducts, or leveled, drained fields, and it provides for the support of individuals who assume full-time responsibility for weather prediction and medical care (to name just a couple of applications appropriate to the theme of this book). Of course, it is also converted to monumental constructions—like pyramids—which have no function other than to aggrandize the managerial class or celebrate the power of the state, just as the less impressive monuments of simpler societies do. Thus, the very process that creates the potential of civilization simultaneously guarantees that the potential is unlikely to be aimed equally at the welfare of all of its citizens.

Most anthropologists and historians would agree, I think, that the new style of government combines necessary managerial functions and the exploitative potential of the class system. We disagree about whether the power of states first grew out of needed management functions or out of more purely exploitative conquest of vulnerable sedentary populations.[34] We also disagree about whether the adaptive benefits of large-scale management outweigh the costs of exploitation. That is an empirical question that I will address with medical evidence.

Modern civilization, the industrial nation state, has not really changed the basic design of civilization but has, if anything, exaggerated a number of the principles just elaborated. The political boundaries of states and the enclosed populations have grown progressively larger.[35] Systems of storage and transport account for an ever-higher percentage of food and other goods consumed and move those goods progressively greater distances. The ratio of nonfood producers to food producers, and hence the ratio of urban to rural people, has increased, as has the size of cities. Specializations have become narrower, their interdependence more complex; even the proportion of the population devoted to food production has become so specialized as to be self-sufficient for no more than a tiny portion of its own array of dietary needs. The scale of investment and the fruits of prior investment have increased enormously. Human labor is supplemented increasingly by forms of power and energy resulting from such previous investment; simultaneously, there has been a large increase in our dependence on this investment, such that individuals without access to the means or fruits of investment may be increasingly unable to command resources. A contemporary farmer with good land and water but no capital can not compete.

Modern states embrace an increasingly broad spectrum of ethnic groups, intensifying problems of communication and cooperation—despite the ideology of nationalism, which attempts to reassert a sense of unity and a cooperative basis for interaction. In states built on the Western model, at least, the market mentality and the profit motive increasingly replace patterns of interpersonal cooperation as a basis for social interaction; market value increasingly supersedes traditional obligations of trade and sharing as a basis for the movement of goods. Modern civilization commonly proceeds much farther than its ancient counterparts in using economic specialization as a basis for interpersonal relations, to the almost complete exclusion of kinship. Despite any ideology to the contrary we may hold, we have not eliminated the class structure by which some individuals may be prevented altogether from producing their own food or from commanding it in the arena of exchange. We have, however, begun to restructure social classes along international lines, replacing indigenous lower classes with populations from the Third World.

Chapter 4

The History of Infectious Disease

Changes in the size and density of human populations and in the design of human societies are likely to have had fairly profound effects on the distribution of infectious diseases. Studies of the habits of various parasites, analyses of historical patterns of disease, and mathematical simulations of disease processes all suggest that early primitive human groups were probably exposed to a different—and much more limited—set of diseases than modern civilized populations. Almost all studies that attempt to reconstruct the history of infectious diseases indicate that the burden of infection has tended to increase rather than decrease as human beings adopted civilized lifestyles.[1]

Probable Patterns of Infectious Disease in Prehistoric Band Societies

Parasites must complete their life cycles *repeatedly* and must spread from person to person (or they must spread repeatedly from the soil or animals to people) if they are to pose a threat to human populations: if the chain of reproduction and dissemination is ever completely broken, the disease disappears.[2] When a human population is small, a parasite is afforded only a limited number of opportunities to spread; if a group moves frequently it may threaten and ultimately break the chain of infection. Given these constraints, only certain types of parasites can persist and infect small and mobile bands. These diseases appear to be of two types: either the organism must rely primarily on other plants or animals (or the soil) rather than people, for its survival; or it must be a slow-acting or chronic disease designed to make maximum use of the limited available human fuel while affording itself a long period of time to effect successful transmission from host to host.[3]

Diseases in the first of these categories, the so-called zoonoses, more than any other type of disease, are likely to have varied fairly profoundly in importance from one environment to the next, posing new threats to human populations as they moved into new environments and shaping the patterns of human expansion (favoring expansion away from the tropics to cooler, drier environments where parasites are less common and discouraging penetration of tropical rainforests in which parasites abound). Diseases of the second category, chronic diseases contained within the human population itself, are likely to have been fairly cosmopolitan, traveling with people as they moved.

ZOONOSES

Zoonoses or zoonotic infections are diseases caused by organisms that normally complete their life cycles in one or more animal host without human involvement. They do not require human bodies for survival and often thrive in environments where human beings are only occasional intruders. Human beings are accidental victims, and from the point of view of the parasite they are likely to be dead-end hosts; although the parasite can infect a person and produce symptoms of disease or even death, it cannot survive, reproduce, and disseminate its offspring from inside the human body, so the disease spreads no further.

Human beings expose themselves to many of these diseases through contact with wild animals or their carcasses. For example, rabies cycles among wild animals in some parts of the world. Infected animals tend to behave aggressively, and their bite spreads the infection to a new host. Human hunter-gatherers confronting wild animals in areas with endemic rabies must have been exposed at least occasionally.[4] Tularemia, a disease related to bubonic plague and dangerous but quite rare among modern populations, may have been a significant cause of sickness and death among American Indian populations who regularly handled game and fur-bearing animals.[5] Handling wild animals or their remains can also result in infection with such other diseases as toxoplasmosis,[6] hemorrhagic fevers,[7] leptospirosis,[8] brucellosis,[9] anthrax,[10] salmonellosis,[11] and a long list of lesser-known infections.[12] In addition, people can encounter a variety of highly lethal anaerobic bacteria, including the agents of gangrene, botulism, and tetanus, if they expose themselves to the intestinal contents of animals while butchering a kill.[13]

Eating wild game also involves risks. Trichina worms (trichinosis) occur in wild animals and may be encountered by hunters. Animals get trichinosis by eating one another, and people can be infected by eating the meat of any of a variety of mammals that are at least partly carnivorous—often pigs, but also a number of other species (bears, dogs, wolves, foxes, cats, and even rodents). The disease still infects a few bear hunters in the Northern United States, and it is a common problem for hunters in other parts of the world. It is particularly a problem for Eskimos and other arctic hunters forced to rely heavily on carnivorous or partly carnivorous prey because of the scarcity of strictly herbivorous animals.[14]

In addition, wild animals can harbor a variety of tapeworms and other worm parasites whose life cycles do not normally include human beings. These can, however, still inflict damage ranging from mild skin irritations to convulsions and death if ingested.[15] Moreover, the meat of wild animals, particularly if scavenged rather than killed, can carry staphylococcal infection and salmonellosis, as well as botulism.[16]

In addition to those diseases transmitted directly from animals to man, others can be carried from animals to people by vectors that do not discriminate in their choice of hosts, alternately biting human beings and other animals. Bubonic plague, which is normally transmitted by fleas among wild rodents, could have infected the occasional prehistoric hunter or trapper (in a few isolated parts of the world), much as it infects the occasional park ranger or incautious camper in the United States today who handles the flea-infested carcass of a dead rodent.[17] Fleas also transmit murine (or zoonotic) typhus from rodents to people.[18]

Mosquitoes transmit a number of infections from wild animal or bird populations to human beings. Yellow fever and malaria can be transmitted between monkey and human populations in this manner and undoubtedly afflicted early human populations, at least occasionally. Mosquitoes and other arthropods also transmit various forms of encephalitis that are often localized in their distribution and such lesser-known local infections as sindbis or West Nile fever.[19] (Many of the latter localized mosquito-borne infections generate few clinical problems in populations accustomed to them. Early childhood exposure to many such infections seems to provide immunity at the cost of only relatively mild symptoms.)

Mosquitoes and other arthropods also transmit a variety of filarial worms between humans and wild animal hosts, although the majority of filarial infections appear to be primarily human diseases that would therefore require large human populations to maintain them.[20]

African trypanosomiasis, the protozoan parasite of sleeping sickness, appears originally to have been an infection transmitted among wild ungulates (such as gazelles) by a few species of tsetse flies whose natural habitat was an unmodified bush/savanna terrain. The type of sleeping sickness that these flies transmit is far more lethal to occasional human hosts than the milder domestic form of sleeping sickness that has recently begun to affect larger numbers of people through fly transmission within human settlements.[21]

Ticks, another type of vector, are particularly common in wild landscapes. Even today, they are most likely to transmit infection to hikers and campers, and it is reasonable to assume that they would have transmitted disease to early hunter-gatherers. The large number of distinct local tick-borne diseases from which human beings occasionally suffer in different parts of the world is a kind of testimony that our own activities have had relatively little positive effect on the spread of these vectors or the diseases they carry. We know of at least fifty localized forms of tick-borne viral diseases for which the normal hosts are birds or small mammals but that can infect a human host who accidentally encounters a tick in the wild.[22] Far better known are the tick- and mite-borne rickettsias—Rocky Mountain spotted fever, Lyme disease, and a host of similar infections around the world, including Q fever, scrub typhus, and tick typhus.[23]

In addition to infections cycling in wild animals, some infections are capable of attacking isolated human beings because they can be preserved for various lengths of time in the soil. Anaerobic bacteria, such as the clostridia causing gangrene, botulism, and tetanus, are among the most serious of these infections, but a variety of fungal infections (mycoses) can also spread from the soil. Many of the latter are only minor irritants,[24] but such mycoses as the coccidioidomycosis of the American Southwest can be a serious threat to health.[25]

As a group, the zoonotic and soil-borne diseases have some important characteristics in common. Because they strike only rarely and cannot spread directly from person to person they do not claim many victims. But zoonotic diseases often have a relatively severe impact on the body. Because they are rare, an individual is not likely to have built up any individual immunity to the disease through prior exposure, and the population to which the victim belongs is unlikely to have evolved resistance to the organism. In addition, because the disease organism does not depend on the human host to house or transmit it (and has not depended on human transmission in the past), there has usually been no selection for a strain of the parasite that is less virulent or more compatible with human life. Parasites often evolve to be relatively benign toward their main hosts, as the survival of the host is to their advantage; an accidental host does not benefit from such evolution.[26]

Moreover, many zoonotic diseases attack adults more than they attack children, particularly in societies where it is the adults who venture out of camp. The age of the victim may contribute to the severity of the disease. In addition, the loss of an adult provider may be far more threatening to a small band than is the loss of a young child who, from a biological point of view, can be replaced with relative ease. By attacking the productive (and reproductive) adult members of the population, infrequent zoonotic diseases might still have relatively severe economic and demographic consequences for the group.[27]

Perhaps most important, in a world without rapid transportation or transportation over water, most zoonotic diseases would have had a very limited distribution—limited by the dispersal rates of wild host and vector species. Rabies may have been fairly cosmopolitan in prehistory given the number of different host species and the ability of bats, a major reservoir, to fly. But even rabies has been successfully prevented from reaching such islands as England during the past fifty years despite large-scale trade because of strict quarantine laws.[28] In contrast, bubonic plague is thought to have had a relatively narrow geographic distribution in Asia until it was spread by human transportation within the span of recent, recorded history.[29]

CHRONIC INFECTIONS

The other major category of infection likely to have attacked early human populations consists of infections that would have been able to persist and maintain themselves using only the small and mobile populations of hunter-gatherers themselves as hosts. Such organisms would need to be able to survive for long periods of time, perhaps indefinitely, in a single person. They would also need to be able to pass easily and reliably from person to person, whether by touch, by droplet (sneezing and breathing), or in food, without needing to complete any portion of their life cycles in the soil or in other animals.

These diseases are chronic, often relatively mild, infections, which neither kill the human host nor stimulate the host to generate complete immunity and which are therefore not self-limiting in their host. Yaws, a persistent infection of simple human societies in the tropics (and the cousin and probable ancestor of the syphilis of civilizations), is one such infection.[30]

A list of infections likely to have afflicted early human groups can be compiled in part by noting which chronic infections human beings share with other primates. When recent reinfection of apes and monkeys by human hosts or vice versa can be ruled out, such shared infections are likely to be those that human beings have carried throughout their evolutionary history and geographical range. Various classes of bacteria (staphylococcus, strepto-coccus, gonococcus, pneumococcus, diplococcus, meningococcus, and some types of salmonella) are considered likely to have been ancient human infec-tions on this basis, as are a number of intestinal protozoa, including various forms of amoeba.[31] The herpes virus, as well as several other groups of viruses that produce chronic infections in human hosts, are also considered possible fellow travelers of early man.[32]

Some of these infections are commensal microbes that commonly live in various parts of the human body without producing symptoms of disease or provoking a reaction on the part of the body—until they are accidentally introduced into a different body system or until there is a breakdown of the normal immune response. Some bacteria of the genus *Staphylococcus* are normal, fairly common, permanent inhabitants of human skin and mucous membranes and are commonly transmitted from mother to child at birth, but they are capable of producing serious infections of bone if introduced into wounds.[33]

Apes also suffer from a variety of worms and other intestinal parasites (in-cluding types of hookworm and pinworm) that affect people; the list of their afflictions is often considered a model of the parasite burden of early human groups.[34] Apes generally move less rapidly and less widely than do people, however, and they generally inhabit moister habitats—hence more parasite-tolerant soil regimes—than did early man. Comparison to the apes may thus overestimate the probable burden of worms and other fecal parasites in early mobile human groups.

THE POSSIBILITY OF HITHERTO UNKNOWN PREHISTORIC DISEASES

In addition to evaluating these two categories of known disease likely to have afflicted simple human societies,[35] we must also consider the possibility that early primitive human groups may have suffered from some diseases that no longer occur in human populations or at least are not recognized by modern science. The early explorers occasionally referred to unusual disease symptoms among the indigenous populations they observed, although few of these reports are well documented.

The existing evidence suggests, however, that such unknown diseases are unlikely to have been of great importance or, at least, unlikely to have been more important than those we know about. Uniformitarian logic and obser-vations on the diseases of other animals suggest that any unknown disease would have to belong to one (or some blend) of the two classes of disease just discussed. In addition, although there have been a number of chances for civilized human beings to catch such diseases from their small-scale contemporaries, there is little evidence of such transmission. Africa has shared a large number of diseases with the rest of the world in the last several hundred years, including many of those just discussed, but they are its zoonoses. They do not appear to originate with or have been confined to its most primitive human populations or to be a product of technologically simple lifestyles. Most of these diseases have long been part of the disease burden of the whole civilized world, in any case, and have long been recognized by science. There is little evidence to suggest that expanding civilizations encountered much in the way of new diseases through contact with small-scale societies in other parts of the world.[36] With the possible and highly controversial exception of syphilis, few diseases are known or thought to have spread to Europe or Africa from American Indians;[37] few new diseases have been encountered in recent contacts with the Australian native population,[38] the Indians of the Amazon basin,[39] or the relatively isolated small bands of African hunter-gatherers.[40]

One prominent exception—an example of previously unknown disease (and a previously little-known mechanism of survival and transmission) associated with the lifestyle of a primitive group—was Kuru, discovered in 1957, a slow virus transmitted by ritual cannibalism among natives of New Guinea.[41] AIDS may be another example of a disease passed from small-scale society to large, but its origin is in dispute, and in its dangerous form it appears to be a very recent phenomenon.[42]

Because diseases often evolve toward less virulent forms in coevolution with their hosts, however, we must also consider the possibility that some diseases that we now recognize as mild afflictions (and even some commensal or symptomless infections) may have evolved from diseases that once produced more severe or acute symptoms in human populations. This possibility is hard either to evaluate or to rule out.[43]

The Transition from Nomadism to Sedentism

When early human societies adopted sedentary habits they undoubtedly altered the balance of their parasites. Sedentism has some advantages in warding off infectious disease. Nomadic bands are likely to encounter a wider range of zoonotic diseases than do more settled populations. In addition, a single species of parasite may display minor local variations in chemistry that can fool the human immune system. A different local strain of a parasitic species from only a few miles away can act like a new disease.[44]

Sedentism would not only reduce the variety of infections but would also enable a group to get a head start adjusting to its local parasites. Human groups do tend to adjust to local parasites that may produce morbid symptoms in strangers; hence the well-known sense of travelers that some diarrhea is likely to affect them in new places even when the natives show no obvious symptoms of disease. The immunity of local peoples may reflect genetically evolved immunity; more often it represents immunity acquired in childhood. Such acquired immunity could follow an earlier bout of illness, but it might follow an almost symptomless bout of infection if the individual is first affected while supported by maternal antibodies provided in mother's milk.[45]

In addition, people may be protected by the natural populations of commensal microorganisms already inhabiting their intestines that can hold their own against incursions of other local, potentially pathogenic organisms.[46] Such microorganisms protect their human host from other infections in the process of fighting off their own competition.[47] But these local flora, like their human hosts, do not have a proven ability to fight off new competitors introduced through the movement of populations, and they may be less successful in the attempt; so people may be relatively susceptible to new strains of infection. In addition, movement of people and the introduction of new diseases also tends to undermine such cultural protective mechanisms as appropriate habits of hygiene that groups of people have developed to protect themselves against familiar infections.

Of course, sedentism has one other major advantage: it makes it easier to care for the sick and helps reduce the risk that a sick individual will die.

But sedentism has several disadvantages that may well outweigh any advantages it confers. The first of these is that sedentary populations typically increase their investment in trade. Even local trade reintroduces the problem of travelers' diarrhea because local microvariants of common diseases are transported to new hosts, disrupting both established patterns of immunity and established cultural standards of hygiene. As soon as a population begins to trade, it may lose any advantages in averting infectious disease that it gained by settling in one place.

In addition, sedentism encourages the spread of many diseases. If the climate is mild, nomads typically build relatively insubstantial shelters and make minimal use of them, conducting most of their activities in the open air. Sedentary populations often build more substantial houses and undertake more activities indoors because a large investment in housing makes more sense to people who will be staying longer in one place (and also perhaps because sedentary people who can not move away from their neighbors need more privacy).

More substantial shelters provide better protection against the elements

—precipitation and extremes of temperature—but they probably encourage disease transmission. Permanent houses tend to attract vermin, including insects and rats, so that the diseases carried by these vectors may become constant rather than occasional threats to health. Several species of mosquitoes (culicine mosquitoes carrying a variety of infections including encephalitis and aedine mosquitoes carrying both yellow fever and dengue fever) like to live near human houses and are encouraged by the construction of permanent dwellings. The diseases that they transmit then tend to become more common with the establishment of sedentary villages or towns. Urban yellow fever is transmitted by a mosquito that lives almost entirely around water stored in human dwellings.[48]

Moreover, sunlight is one of the best disinfectants known, and conducting one's activities out of doors reduces the transmission of many diseases. Conversely, substantial, permanent houses also provide enclosed air circulation that facilitates transmission of airborne disease. The influenza virus, which does not survive readily out of doors, is easily transmitted within the safe, substantial houses that sedentary people build for themselves.[49]

Refuse associated with sedentary communities can also increase the disease load by attracting wild animals to human settlements. This attraction is the major means by which rat-borne bubonic plague is brought into human communities. The attraction of rats (and therefore of rat fleas) to human settlements, and ultimately their attraction in large numbers to human cities, creates the danger of infection in plague proportions. Rats may also bring hemorrhagic fevers and a series of lesser-known infections into human settlements. Wild canids (dogs and wolves) attracted to garbage might bring rabies; wild felids (cats) bring toxoplasmosis. Common flies attracted by garbage act as mechanical vectors transmitting various diseases, particularly fecal-oral infections, from place to place and hence from person to person within their flying radius. Such flies, however, seem to be common even in the camps of mobile populations with minimal refuse buildup.

Sedentism also results in the accumulation of human wastes. Nomadic human beings periodically leave behind their own germ- or worm-bearing residues and reduce their chances of reinfecting one another. Fecal-oral transmission, as well as the transmission of any germ that can survive on the ground, in soil, or on inanimate objects, is reduced by group movement but encouraged when a group settles down. For example, ascarid worms, whose eggs leave the body in feces and can then reinfect food or water or be transmitted to food via the hands of infected individuals, are more likely to spread among sedentary groups than among nomadic bands, and they are likely to spread more intensively, giving each individual a larger dose or heavier worm burden. Similar principles apply to essentially all other fecal-oral diseases, including the various protozoan and bacterial species that produce diarrhea.[50]

Sedentism is particularly likely to increase disease transmission of any parasite that must complete essential phases of its life cycle in the soil (or elsewhere outside a human host) before its offspring can reinfect a new individual. If human beings abandon a campsite at intervals shorter than that necessary for the development of the parasite, they should effectively prevent successful completion of the cycle. Hookworm (infection by worm parasites of the genera *Ancylostema* and *Necator*) is discouraged, although not always prevented entirely, by group movement because the worms, deposited in the soil by human feces, must mature in the soil before they can reinfect a new individual. If the group moves on before the worms mature, the cycle of infection may be broken. Sedentary habits increase the proportion of larvae that successfully reinfect a new host.[51]

Sedentism also increases the transmission of any disease carried by a vector whose life cycle is interrupted by human movement. Fleas, for example, often do not parasitize nomadic people—or animals—because their larvae, which are not parasites, live in the animal's nest or house rather than on its body. If the house or nest is abandoned frequently, fleas and the diseases that they carry are discouraged or eliminated.[52]

A similar principle operates in the case of two other families of infections that are two of the most important infectious diseases remaining in the world today: schistosomiasis (bilharziasis) and malaria. The fluke or flatworm that causes schistosomiasis is excreted in human feces or urine (depending on the particular species of the parasite) and must then pass through a developmental stage in a fresh water snail before it can reinfect another human host. From the point at which it is first deposited by a human host in water, the organism can only move as far as it can swim, be transported by the host snail, or be moved by water currents before it reinfects a new human host. Its survival depends on the probability that it will encounter a new host within that radius. People who settle in one place encourage its transmission because they permit the cycle of infection—from people to snails and back —to continue.[53]

Malaria, which may have caused more deaths in human populations than any other human disease, is also likely to have become increasingly important as a consequence of sedentism.[54] Mobile human groups commonly move outside the flying range of individual mosquitoes and thus tend to break the cycle of transmission, as an individual mosquito must bite two or more people at defined intervals for the disease to spread.[55] For the same reason, most significant filarial infections—including elephantiasis and river blindness, which are primarily transmitted from person to person by insect vectors—will also become more common when groups become sedentary.[56]

Human Alteration of the Landscape

Human alteration of the landscape associated with farming is at best likely to have had mixed effects on disease. Land clearance may have helped to alleviate some types of infection. By simplifying the natural landscape, farmers may well have eliminated some of the zoonoses to which their ancestors were exposed. As already noted, some types of insect vectors, particularly ticks and some kinds of tsetse flies, prefer habitats undisturbed by human activity. These vectors and the diseases they carry may have been more common, posing a greater threat to human beings, when they intruded into a wild landscape.[57]

But human alterations to the landscape apparently aided parasites and vectors of some of the most important diseases. Although both malaria and schistosomiasis are capable of persisting in the wild and infecting wild animal populations, they are significantly increased by human modification of the landscape. In both cases, the vector species are encouraged by human activities.

The snails that carry schistosomiasis tend to like shallow fresh water that is not turbid (that is, that has very little current and hence little suspended silt or mud). They also thrive in water rich in dissolved solids, dissolved oxygen, and weeds. The required combination of conditions is comparatively rare in natural waterways but more common in man-made ponds and irrigation ditches. Hence, schistosomiasis is primarily a disease of irrigation farmers and paddy rice cultivators who work in intimate contact with such bodies of water.[58]

Species of anopholine mosquitoes that are the most important vectors of malaria enjoy the delicate mix of light and shade and the frequent small bodies of stagnant water that human farming communities tend to create.[59] Land clearance associated with agriculture aids the mosquitoes. Historically, land clearance also decimated populations of nonhuman primates that had previously been the primary hosts of both mosquito and malarial parasites, forcing these organisms to rely on human hosts. There is a significant correlation between the evolution of farming economies and the incidence of malaria;[60] data suggest that genetic adaptation to malaria (the sickle cell trait and other forms of abnormal hemoglobin)[61] is far more common in tropical farmers than in hunter-gatherers. Most authorities agree that falciparum malaria, the most severe of human malarias, is a relatively new disease—one that almost certainly postdates the development of agriculture in the tropics. Other, milder forms of malaria, such as vivax malaria, are generally considered more ancient diseases of primates and possible occasional afflictions of early man, but Livingstone has recently argued that even these milder forms have exerted their important influence on human populations only since the Neolithic revolution.[62] In the last two centuries, extensive swamp drainage and clearance has reversed the trend—but primarily only in temperate parts of the world where the life cycles of the appropriate mosquitoes are relatively fragile and the countries in question have the wealth to make large-scale investments.[63]

Several other mosquito-borne diseases are also affected by human alteration of the landscape. Farming not only increased populations of aedine mosquitoes, which carry yellow fever; it also helped bring the disease within reach of human populations. The disease, which naturally circulated at tree-top level among monkeys and high-flying mosquitoes, was brought down to ground level by human clearance of forests and the creation of farms that attracted foraging monkeys to the ground. From there, the disease was transmitted to human beings by low-flying mosquito species.[64] Onchocerciasis ("river blindness"), an infection of filarial worms carried by simulium flies, has similarly increased in importance in recent history because dense, sedentary human settlements on river banks generate wastes that fertilize the rivers and make them better breeding grounds for the flies. Similarly, modern damming of the rivers has increased fly breeding.[65]

Agricultural intensification relying on increasing doses of fertilizer has also tended to increase the transmission of fecally borne diseases, particularly in those parts of the world in which human feces are a major form of fertilizer.

Changes in Food-Related Technology and Food Storage

Variations in the handling of food associated with sedentism and civilization have also had important effects on disease transmission. Undoubtedly, the most important technological improvement in food processing was the use of fire to cook and, incidentally, to disinfect foods. In its most rudimentary form, the use of fire in food preparation appears to be several hundred thousand years old, predating the appearance of the modern human species.[66] Some cooking has therefore been part of the human repertoire throughout the portion of the archaeological record on which this book focuses; cooking is known and practiced by all of the groups whose health is under consideration.

Changes in the style of cooking linked with the emergence of civilization have, however, affected disease transmission. The biggest of these changes was probably the development of pottery with the adoption of sedentary life-styles. Ceramic pots are both bulky and heavy, and their use is incompatible with frequent group movement, so their appearance in the archaeological record is correlated (at least roughly) with sedentism. The importance of such pots is that they permitted foods to be stewed instead of roasted or not cooked at all. More thorough cooking would have helped reduce the risk of infection from foods, particularly game. Anyone who roasts meat on an open fire knows how difficult it is to cook things thoroughly. In fact, roasting, as it is practiced by many known band societies, is often extremely rudimentary, barely heating internal portions of the game.[67] There may also be a disadvantage to cooking in pottery, however. The pots themselves, particularly porous vessels before the invention of glazing, may have encouraged the growth of such bacteria as salmonella and transferred them from food to food.[68]

Further improvements in cooking technology are likely to have had mixed results. On one hand, our ability to cook thoroughly and to sterilize by cooking has clearly improved, particularly in the century since Pasteur elucidated the principles of sterilization. On the other hand, by adding additional steps to food preparation we often increase the risk of infection by salmonella and other organisms. In fact, salmonella poisoning may gradually have increased in human history as trade in food, as well as commercial or institutional preparation of food, has become more common.[69] Moreover, by centralizing and commercializing much food preparation—that is, by making food preparation a task for specialists—we increase the risk that individuals will be exposed to unfamiliar, hence dangerous, organisms. Home food preparation and home cooking at least have the advantage that one is likely already to be exposed to whatever infections the cook may introduce.

Food storage also has a number of consequences for disease transmission. Storage may discourage transmission of some parasites that live in fresh edible foods or adhere to them as a result of contact with soil or other contaminants. Storage will be particularly helpful in reducing infections if such preservative techniques as toasting, drying, and pickling (or more modern methods of sterilization and preservation) are applied to increase the shelf life of the stored products. Reliance on stored foods may also tend to reduce the likelihood of infection because it forces people to rely more on storable, dry vegetable products that are relatively infection-free rather than on fresh meat, which is probably the most dangerous source of food-borne infection. Yet, stored foods may also accumulate bacteria and fungi that can both infect human hosts and poison them with their by-products. Ergotism, poisoning with toxins generated by a fungus growing on stored rye grain (which became a significant problem in historic Europe), is probably the best-known example.[70]

Such fungal or bacterial contamination of stored foods may also provide unexpected health benefits. Mold growing on stored foods can produce such antibiotics as tetracycline and penicillin as well as toxins; archaeologists are just beginning to realize that intentional fermentation, which may also produce antibiotics, is an ancient and widespread means of preservation.[71] Inadvertent fermentation of stored grain may have produced tetracycline in Nubian (southern Egyptian) storage bins.[72]

Stored foods have another disadvantage. Like garbage, they tend to attract wild animal reservoirs of disease, increasing the risk that various zoonoses will enter the community. Stored foods tend also to accumulate the feces of rodents and the bodies of insects, either living off the grain or on the rodents. Both may be the source of new infections. For example, hymenole-pid tapeworms cycle between beetles and rodents in stored grain and can produce accidental infections in people.[73]

Modern canning techniques, of course, eliminate some of these problems of secondary infection of stored foods and the attraction of pests, but they also introduce some increase in the risk of such highly lethal anaerobic infections as botulism.

The Role of Domestication of Animals

The domestication of animals has probably increased the range of infections to which the average human being is exposed. Domestic animals do provide some advantages for human hygiene. Both pigs and dogs act as scavengers that remove human waste and recycle garbage, helping to offset some of the other dangers of sedentism.[74] In addition, a controlled meat supply eliminates some of the risk of encountering the parasites of wild animals. But the risks balance—and may outweigh—the advantages because domestic animals themselves are a major source of human disease. Domestication forces human beings to deal at close range with animals throughout their life cycles and to encounter their body fluids and wastes, as well as their carcasses. Domestic dogs, as well as wild ones, can transmit rabies. In fact, they are the major source of human infection.[75] Domestic cats may harbor toxoplasmosis, and their feces in contemporary human homes pose a risk of infection with potentially serious consequences for unborne babies.[76] Tetanus, one of the most dreaded diseases of recent history, is spread by domestic horses and to a lesser extent by cattle, dogs, and pigs. It can also spread to the soil, but soil that has never been grazed or cultivated is generally free from the bacteria.[77] Moreover, domestication often implies the creation of artificially high population densities among domestic animals and their confinement to enclosures—factors that facilitate the spread of disease among the animals, just as they do among human beings. Such diseases as anthrax, hoof and mouth disease, and brucellosis, which human beings can contract from animals, may pose a particular risk to both animal and human health when animals are confined.

Domestication also creates the danger that certain species become so intimately involved with human beings that they enter into cycles of mutual infection with human hosts. The most important tapeworms affecting human health cycle between human beings and domestic animals. Human beings become infected by eating imperfectly cooked meat; the animals are infected, in turn, by exposure to human feces, and the worm successfully completes its life cycle. Although one might occasionally kill and eat a wild animal that had previously been infected by eating grass or other food contaminated with human feces, the chance of such an infection occurring is slight. The risk is so slight, in fact, that the chances of the parasite's life cycle being reliably maintained in this manner are very slender. The chances increase substantially when the animals spend the bulk of their lives in intimate association with relatively large human populations. The result has been the appearance of worms, particularly the tapeworms of pigs and cows, that make their living entirely between human beings and domestic animals.[78]

For the same reason, today ocean fish are comparatively safe to eat (raw or cooked); freshwater fish living in water exposed to human feces are much more likely to bear tapeworms; and cultivated fish, essentially domesticated fish reared in man-made enclosures, can pose an even greater risk unless ponds are protected from fecal contamination.[79]

Trichinosis is today primarily a health risk associated with domestic animals, although for a slightly different reason. Pigs are infected, just as people are, by eating infected meat. The most common source of infection is scraps of pork from infected pigs that show up in the garbage fed to other pigs, just as they may show up in the human diet. Pigs that are truly "corn fed" are safe.[80]

A variety of parasites, such as the hydatids of echinococcus, cycle in the wild between herbivores and their canid predators (for example, wild sheep and wolves). The transmission of these parasites, or at least the risk to people, is increased by our joint domestication of such herbivores and of dogs. Even the presence of domestic dogs alone can apparently increase the likelihood of such parasites cycling in wild herbivorous animals living in the vicinity of human settlement. Human beings can serve as occasional hosts for some of these parasites; in fact, under certain conditions echinococcus can create a significant disease burden for human populations with domestic animals.[81]

Many of these parasitic worms, although they can spread as far as infected meat is transported, are at least limited in their effects. One infected human being cannot infect another directly but contributes to the spread of the infection only by reinfecting farm animals. Although they can affect large numbers of city dwellers through the dissemination of infected meat, these infections are not self-perpetuating in human cities. But other diseases associated with the crowding of domestic animals and with continuous human contact have potentially more serious effects. Various species of salmonella are maintained by domestic animals living under crowded conditions but can spread from person to person once a cycle of human infection has begun.

We believe that many diseases that now travel primarily from person to person originally came from domestic animals. Measles apparently originated as rinderpest among cattle or distemper among dogs; smallpox came from cattle (but possibly from monkeys); influenza from pigs or chickens; the common cold from horses; diphtheria from cattle. Most human respiratory viruses probably had their origins only after animals were domesticated.[82] Tuberculosis may be another case in point, but its derivation is in dispute. It was assumed for some time that human tuberculosis was derived from bovine tuberculosis in domestic cattle; but the recent realization of its wide distribution in wild animals plus the fact that it was apparently present in the New World before Columbus, when no domestic cattle or other domestic bovids were present (see chapter 7), suggests that it may have been derived from some other source—buffalo, wild bird populations, or perhaps from several sources in different places.[83]

Increasing Population Size and Density

Perhaps the most basic point of all is that the survival and dissemination of any parasite is likely to be assisted by an increase in the number of available hosts. Like all organisms (including people), parasites generate more offspring than are likely to survive. Most parasitic organisms produce many offspring and "hope" that a small percentage of those offspring will be successfully transmitted to new hosts. The odds against the survival of any one offspring are extremely large, and only a few do survive, but the odds improve significantly when the number of potential hosts and their proximity to one another increase.

The increasing density of the human population should therefore improve the transmission of essentially all parasites that pass from person to person, whether they are carried between hosts in the air, in water, in food, or in soil. It should also affect diseases that are transmitted by vectors, providing that the vectors also depend on biting a succession of human hosts. A variety of fecal-oral diseases (worms and intestinal protozoa or bacteria) commonly appear to thrive in crowded human settings and to increase with increasing population density, as do diseases spread through the air, such diseases as tuberculosis, which may spread by a number of routes, and mosquito-borne malaria.[84]

If human societies get larger, parasites spread more readily. This means that a higher percentage of individuals will be infected. But it also means that each infected individual is likely to receive a higher dose of the parasite (that is, to be infected by more organisms) as a result of repeated acts of infection. An individual may get a more severe illness, since the outcome of the infection often depends on the size of the dose received (as well as on the success of the organism multiplying in the body). In short, both the number of infected individuals and the proportion of severe cases should increase.

In addition to this general intensification of existing infectious diseases, high population densities and large population aggregates (particularly large populations united by rapid transportation networks) can have another effect. Large populations make possible the survival and transmission of certain diseases that could not have survived at all (at least in their modern form) in a prehistoric world populated only by relatively small and isolated human groups. There is apparently a threshold effect by which gradually increasing human population density reached a critical level, permitting new infections to thrive, spread, and attack human hosts.

Many of the so-called epidemic diseases of recent history—the infectious diseases that move easily from person to person and spread as great waves —depend on rapid and continuous transmission to new human hosts. They rarely, if ever, attack other animals or, at least, are not transmitted by vectors or stored to any significant degree in animal reservoirs. They must be handed directly from person to person because they have little or no capacity to survive outside the living human host. They are relatively acute (incapacitating) and of short duration in each human host. They are rarely if ever carried for long in any single human host. And they result either in death or in lifelong immunity in each individual. In short, they depend on human beings but rapidly run out of human fuel. They can survive only in very large populations in which production of new babies (or arrival of immigrants) keeps pace with their spread.[85]

The measles virus provides a good (and well-documented) example. Measles is known to attack almost all available human hosts, to incapacitate them, and to leave them dead or with lifelong immunity (and freedom from further infection) within a matter of weeks. The virus must be passed on within that brief span; it must go directly from individual to individual because it does not survive long on inanimate objects and apparently cannot live in other organisms; unlike many other viruses, it is apparently never stored for long periods of time in human "carriers" (that is, individuals who display no symptoms, produce no immunity in their own bodies, and remain infective longer than the normal human host), and it never, or almost never, attacks the same individual twice.[86]

Scholars have speculated about the size of population necessary to permit measles to survive and spread. If the infection could conserve its fuel, proceeding from host to host one at a time in an unending chain, it would require about one new host every two weeks or approximately twenty-five to fifty individuals per year. But the disease tends to radiate in all directions from a given host, infecting an ever-increasing circle of individuals. It has been estimated that anywhere from five thousand to forty thousand new hosts per year would be required to maintain an epidemic of the disease radiating in this manner. If one were to assume that the population were on an island or were otherwise cut off from immigration and emigration—and were thus dependent on new births to supply the fuel—this would imply a total population of at least three hundred thousand to five hundred thousand individuals, the number necessary to provide enough new babies each year to keep the disease from burning itself out.

Epidemiologists have attempted to test and refine their predictions by studying the epidemiological records of island populations or of other populations enjoying varying degrees of isolation as a result of geographical barriers or as a result of low population densities and poor transport. The studies suggest that measles does indeed tend to be self-limiting (that is, to burn itself out and disappear) in isolated populations smaller than the suggested threshold size.[87]

The implication of these studies is that measles is a modern disease whose origins must be related to the growth of the human population and its coalescence into dense aggregates or widespread and efficient trade networks. It is, in effect, a disease of civilization. Measles may have come from a virus of dogs or cows, but the critical mutation apparently occurred after the emergence of civilization. If the new virus had appeared among early hunter-gatherer groups (even those that were relatively large and sedentary) or small farming villages it would almost immediately have disappeared again. It might have proved devastating for one or a few neighboring bands (as it now does when introduced), but it would almost certainly have been incapable of spreading very far.[88]

Many other diseases share enough of the attributes of measles to suggest that they, too, must be recent diseases. Diseases commonly assumed to be of recent origin are mumps, rubella (German Measles), and smallpox.[89] More surprising inclusions on the list are rhinoviruses (including the common cold) and the influenza and parainfluenza viruses ("flu"), which we consider common, repetitious, and often relatively mild.[90] Each new cold or flu strain still requires a large pool of potential victims to spread. Each strain is self-limiting and immunity-producing in its victims, so each tends to burn itself out in much the same manner as measles. Influenza, of course, can be lethal, just as measles can, particularly in populations without prior exposure. Observations on modern island communities suggest that these diseases do not persist, and in fact, they do not occur except after contact by boat or airplane with larger populations.[91]

Identifying other diseases dependent on large group size and high population density has proved more problematic. It was once thought that chickenpox had a history similar to that of measles because it seemed to have similar epidemiological properties.[92] This proposition is now disputed on the grounds that, after its acute phase, the disease can persist in the human body almost indefinitely and then reemerge as shingles. Shingles sufferers can reinfect children or other previously unexposed individuals with chickenpox. One adult with a case of shingles could therefore introduce chickenpox to a new generation of children forty years or more after the last chickenpox epidemic. Chickenpox could be transmitted perpetually across generations even in very small and isolated groups.[93]

Polio was, in contrast, once considered an ancient disease. The most common consequence of infection with polio virus is a mild or symptomless infection of the intestine, not the acute nervous-system affliction that made it famous. Individuals can apparently spread the virus for months following an infection. But each strain of polio does give lifelong immunity to surviving victims (hence the efficacy of polio vaccines), and studies among Eskimo[94] and Amazonian populations[95] have documented its failure to persist in small isolated communities. It may well be a modern disease.

Francis Black has recently proposed several additions to the list of density-dependent infections—diseases of civilization—including two strains of streptococcal bacteria, as well as the agents of diphtheria and whooping cough. Some of the more acute fecal-oral diseases that tend to kill their hosts or to be eliminated from the body, such as cholera and shigella, may also belong on the list.[96]

The historians of the early empires, including Herodotus in Greece and others in ancient China and India, make it clear that major epidemics were already a feature of civilized life as long as four to five thousand years ago, at which time populations of sufficient size and density to maintain the diseases in question were in existence. Subsequent records show that epidemics have continued to be a common feature of human history in regions of civilization.[97] Unfortunately, early descriptions are often too vague to provide clues to the specific nature of the disease in question. Moreover, what seems in historical reports to be a sudden emergence of epidemics at the dawn of civilization may reflect the invention of writing and the keeping of historical records more than the actual appearance of new diseases. We will have to rely on mathematical models and studies of contemporary populations to reconstruct the early prehistory of these diseases, aided by the indirect testimony of archaeological skeletons.[98]

Expanding Networks of Trade and Transportation

Finally, we must consider the effects of the evolution of transportation networks that move people (and their food resources, pests, and parasites) increasing distances with increasing speed. Under conditions of limited travel and low population density, such infectious diseases as existed would have remained within a relatively restricted radius, either chronically or occasionally reinfecting the same populations but rarely spreading to new groups.

As the scale and speed of trade increases, so does the number of infections. Within individual countries in the modern world, civilized patterns of transport associated with craft specialization and labor migration plays an important role in the dissemination of disease. For example, the seasonal migration of labor associated with such specialized tasks as mining in South Africa has been implicated in the dissemination of a range of diseases, including tuberculosis, influenza, syphilis, and even malaria.[99] But transportation associated with civilizations also spreads disease to new locations on an international and intercontinental level, increasing both the range of disease endemic to each location and the risk of sudden exposure to new epidemics.

William McNeill has suggested that the recent history of human disease can largely be written as the history of such population movements; he suggests that three major waves of disease in recent history can be linked to three major events of transmission: the linking of China, India, and the Mediterranean by sea and by land early in the Christian Era; the spread of the Mongol empire in the thirteenth century; and the beginning of the era of

European seaborne exploration in the fifteenth century. The Mongol expansion is thought to have transported bubonic plague from its initial focus as an endemic disease of rodents somewhere in central Asia to other parts of the Old World, paving the way for its eventual transmission by shipping to other continents. McNeill and others have described the importance of shipping in transmitting new diseases back and forth from Old to New World during the age of exploration.[100] Many of the great epidemic diseases of civilization —measles, mumps, smallpox, German measles—are thought to have been introduced for the first time to the American Indians after the voyages of Columbus. Bubonic plague is likely to have spread to the New World at the same time (or later) as did at least some strains of malaria and possibly also yellow fever. Some populations of Africa, Asia, and Mediterranean Europe display specific genetic adaptations to malaria, and many Africans display a less well-defined relative immunity to yellow fever, suggesting a long history of experience with the disease, but no native New World populations display such traits. Moreover, the ecology of the vector mosquitos and of other reservoir species in the New World, compared to that of the Old, suggests that these infections are relatively recent arrivals in the New World.[101]

More controversial is the history of syphilis, which first becomes prominent in historical medical writings in Europe shortly after the time of Columbus, leading to speculation that he may have brought it back with him from the New World. But much debate has centered around whether syphilis was indeed new in Europe at that time or simply newly recognized as a distinct disease. Some authors argue that Old World syphilis is already visible in biblical accounts.[102]

Cholera is even more recent as a widespread disease, its history largely confined to the past two hundred years. Originally confined to India early in the nineteenth century, it spread rapidly in association with two patterns of populations movement: the movement of Islamic pilgrims to and from Mecca and to various parts of the world, and the deployment of British military forces to various parts of their empire. Cholera, in fact, continues to spread, arriving in new parts of the world, often accompanying industrialization, even since 1960.[103] Prior to 1980 the most important recent movement of infectious disease associated with civilized transport and aggregation of combat troops in Europe and the United States was probably the cycle of pandemics of influenza. AIDS is the newest threat clearly associated with intercontinental transport.

Less well known, partly because the effects are more subtle and partly because they affect parts of the world to which less attention has been paid, are the spread of schistosomiasis through Asia, Africa, and Latin America through the movement of workers between major irrigation systems (albeit possibly assisted by the spread of migratory birds); the spread of dengue fever to the islands of the Pacific and a number of locations in Asia; and the role of colonial-government-mandated movements of people in spreading malaria, sleeping sickness, cattle rinderpest, and possibly other infections through Africa in the nineteenth and twentieth centuries. Tapeworms of cattle and pigs apparently spread around the world when domestic animals were exported from Europe in the seventeenth and eighteenth centuries.[104]

The importance of transport in spreading disease both within and among political units and, conversely, the power of small group size and isolation to protect human groups from infection may perhaps best be illustrated by a relatively recent event. Even within a densely populated country with a well-developed system of commerce (France in the eighteenth century), small size and relative isolation from major trade links apparently had striking protective effects against bubonic plague, despite the fact that plague transmission is facilitated by insect vectors and a highly mobile reservoir species. In France during the plague epidemic of 1720–22, only 12 percent of villages of under one hundred people, which were commonly relatively isolated, were affected.[105] But cities of more than ten thousand people, which formed the major nodes in the trade network, were all severely affected; and for communities of intermediate size and levels of outside contact, the chances of being hit were directly proportional to community size. In other words, despite the relatively cosmopolitan nature of the French nation in the eighteenth century, nearly 90 percent of small villages were spared an epidemic that killed 30 to 40 percent or more of the populations of large towns and cities. A similar distribution of plague-related deaths has been reported elsewhere in Europe.[106]

Conclusion

If we now look back over the range of changes in social organization and economy implicated in the evolution of civilization and consider the consequences of each for infection, it appears that the general trend is likely to have been one of an increasing load of infection through time. Larger groups of people, sedentism, food storage, domestic animals, and trade and transport all exact a price in addition to conferring benefits. The evolution of civilization has probably broadened the range of infections to which human beings are exposed and has probably increased both the percentage of individuals infected and the size of the common dose of infection by tending to increase the reproductive success of the various parasites.

Since the presence of any one parasite in the body often lowers the body's resistance to new infections, this increase in disease is likely to be self-compounding. The influenza virus often opens the way for bacterial infection of the lungs; the presence of either malaria or hookworm increases the probability that an individual will die from measles.[107]

Large-scale populations do have one important advantage in dealing with epidemic diseases. A so-called virgin soil epidemic is one occurring in a population in which no one has had the disease before. Typically, many people of all ages are sick at once, and there is no one to provide food and basic hygiene. The death rate can be extremely high. A detailed description of such an epidemic of measles among Yanomamo Indians of Venezuela has been provided by Neel et al. (1970). Once epidemic diseases become a common fact of life, as they do in civilized populations, however, the group can adjust. Genetically susceptible families have already been weeded out, and people may have learned important lessons about how to help the sick. The most important advantage of civilization is that only children are in danger because their parents have already survived a previous epidemic wave and are now immune. Children may have some basic biological advantages in fighting off these diseases, many of which appear to be more severe in adulthood. But their biggest advantage is that they have healthy parents to care for them. Whether one dies of measles largely depends on the quality of hygiene and nutrition that are maintained through the illness. Many epidemic diseases apparently declined in importance in recent European history for reasons such as these, before scientific medical intervention can be claimed to have played an important part.[108]

Aside from medical technology, which has been a significant factor in health care for fewer than one hundred years, this adjustment to epidemic disease is probably the biggest advantage that civilizations enjoy in terms of infectious disease, and it is a powerful advantage, not only in terms of health but of politics. As McNeill has noted, once civilization has begun, the disease load that it harbors becomes one of the major weapons of its expansion.[109] The worst position in which one can find oneself from this point of view is to be a member of a small group within reach of emergent civilization. Disease harbored by civilization eliminates competitors in large numbers, demoralizes them, and convinces them of the superiority of the conquering or colonizing system. As McNeill has pointed out, epidemic disease—which visibly kills the conquered while leaving the conquering carriers untouched —becomes a powerful demonstration of the superiority of civilization and its gods. The disease load of civilizations paradoxically becomes a major feature of their competitive success.

Chapter 5

Changes in the Human Diet

When human subsistence strategies change (from foraging focused on large game animals and selected vegetable foods to broad spectrum foraging of small game, small seeds, and aquatic resource, then to subsistence farming, and finally to intensified farming and trade by specialists), there are likely to be a number of changes in human diet and nutrition. These changes affect the efficiency of food production in terms of the number of calories produced and eaten per hour of work. They also affect the nutrient quality of the diet, the reliability of food supplies, and the texture of foods consumed.

The Economic Efficiency of Food Production Strategies

There is a long standing debate among economists and anthropologists about whether improvements in human technology actually increase the efficiency with which people get food.[1] The available data suggest there may have been less progress in food-producing efficiency than most people assume.

Several estimates of the efficiency of hunting and gathering techniques[2] suggest that—when they are encountered or available—large mammals are the wild resource likely to provide the highest caloric return for an hour's work. The high efficiency of taking available large game compared to other foraging activities is evident in tropical savannas, semi-deserts, tropical rain forests, temperate forests, and northern latitudes—that is, in almost all environments in which tests have been conducted.[3] Hunting available large mammals also appears to be a relatively efficient strategy regardless of whether foragers use stone or iron weapons, whether they have nets, blowguns, or only spears, and whether they have fishhooks, sickles, or grindstones to help them catch and process food.[4]

In game-rich environments or when large animals are available, hunters may average 10,000 to 15,000 kilocalories or more per hour of work even with only relatively simple weapons. In poorer environments, large animals, once encountered, can still provide 2,500 to 6,000 kilocalories per hour. The only other wild resource that can be harvested at a rate competitive with large game animals are some varieties of nuts (which still require much more time-consuming preparation) and anadromous (migratory) fish that can be caught en masse in nets or traps. The choicest of vegetable resources (other than nuts) may be harvestable at rates of 5,000 to 6,000 kilocalories per hour, but the average return from all wild vegetable resources is commonly less than that provided by large game when it is available.

Economic activities associated with the broad spectrum revolution commonly produce far smaller returns for labor even when the appropriate technology, such as nets or grindstones, has been developed. Caloric returns from hunting small animals or birds are usually fairly low—perhaps only a few hundred to 1,000 or 1,500 kilocalories per hour of work. Small seeds of the type that ultimately became our agricultural staples also provide poor returns. Estimates of caloric returns from obtaining and processing such seeds range from 700 to 1,300 kilocalories per hour of work. Fishing with hooks and lines is usually less productive than hunting large animals; and shellfish, although easily obtained, cannot be gathered with an efficiency that approaches big game hunting. Estimates of the efficiency of shellfish harvesting suggest that it provides 1,000 to 2,000 kilocalories per hour of work.[5]

The implication of these figures is that the transition from hunting to broad spectrum foraging is a process of diminishing returns probably motivated by growing population, expansion into game-poor environments, and the disappearance of large game animals, rather than by improving technology.

In contrast to the figures just provided, subsistence cultivators in various parts of the world (most of whom now use metal tools) seem to average about 3,000 to 5,000 kilocalories per hour of work.[6] This figure represents a clear improvement in efficiency over previous exploitation of the poorest of wild resources but still suggests an unfavorable return in comparison to hunting in game-rich environments. Farming apparently restored some efficiency that foragers had lost but probably represents no net improvement over once-rich hunting economies. It seems likely that hunter-gatherers blessed with a reasonable supply of large animals to hunt would not have bothered to farm but that broad-spectrum foragers increasingly forced to rely on small animals and seeds might well have been motivated to adopt farming—which is, in fact, what the archaeological record suggests.[7]

Whether caloric returns for an individual farmer increased as agriculture was intensified is also questionable. Boserup pointed out more than twenty years ago that the productivity of labor in agriculture should be expected to decline as more marginal land was used and as good land was used more frequently, because heavier and heavier investments in land clearance, fertilizer, and tilling would be required just to maintain production.[8] Boserup argued that such improvements in food production technology as the hoe, fertilizer, and the plow were actually means of maintaining levels of productivity (or delaying its decline) in the face of increasing demands on the soil.

Improvements in the quality of tools (such as the substitution of metal for stone) would be expected to have helped offset this decline, Boserup herself noted. So, too, would increases in efficiency associated with specialization of labor and regional specialization in different crops.[9] In addition, large populations coordinated by centralized leadership might have been able to undertake such improvements in the land as irrigation, drainage, leveling or terracing, which were impossible or unprofitable for smaller groups.[10] Land that had already been improved by prior collective investments of labor might then have been expected to provide relatively high yields. Boserup argued, however, that in most cases these improvements were probably insufficient to offset diminishing returns.

Other scholars have been critical of her conclusions and more optimistic about economic progress. Bronson has suggested that, although shorter fallow periods might initially result in reduction in efficiency, intensive annual cropping and irrigation agriculture generate higher yields than primitive farming.[11] Simon and Harris have each argued that the improvements in agricultural technology and efficiency associated with specialization and large-scale production have generally been sufficient to generate a net increase not only in the total food supply but in the efficiency of the individual farmer.[12] The available data do tend to suggest that farmers blessed with a well-developed irrigation system (let alone tractors and chemical fertilizer) can obtain caloric returns several times those of subsistence farmers.[13]

Regardless of whether Boserup or her critics are theoretically correct, however, the real question is whether individual farmers and the populations they supply actually obtain and eat greater returns for their labor. Whether anybody gets more food may depend on whether the increasing efficiency of farming keeps pace with the growth of population and the increasing proportion of people who are employed in other occupations. Whether the farmers themselves get more food depends on their access to improvements in land and tools and on how much of their produce they are able to keep. Farmers who have no access to improved technology or improvements in land—or who pay too large a proportion of their crop for the privilege of using the improvements—may receive no benefit. Geertz has provided a graphic description of growing population and declining productivity among historic and recent farmers in Java deprived of the chance to reinvest their surplus production;[14] Boserup suggests that the substantial differences between the productivity of agricultural labor in Europe and India largely reflect different levels of prior investment in improving the land.[15] In sum, improving efficiency of food production (or, at least, improving per capita availability of food) is by no means an obvious or universal feature of human history.

Dietary Quality

Dietary quality may well have been adversely affected by the major changes in our subsistence strategies. First, the proportion of animal foods in the human diet is likely to have declined as human populations grew, large animals disappeared, and the declining efficiency of hunting forced people to devote more of their attention to other resources. Sedentary habits associated with farming would have further reduced access to animal foods by restricting group movement and accelerating the disappearance of game in the vicinity of human settlements.[16] Domestication of animals may have offset these losses to some extent, but it is not clear that the initial domestication of animals fully restored what had been lost. Nor is it clear that subsequent improvements in the breeding or use of animals (including the development of milking as an alternate food source) were sufficient to keep pace with the demand of growing human populations.[17]

A decline in per-capita consumption of animal foods would have had a number of negative effects on the diet. Animal foods are the best sources of complete protein (protein with the best balance of amino acids for human needs). Animal foods are also the main source of vitamin B_{12}, and they are among the best sources of vitamins A and D. Various minerals, including iron and zinc, are most readily available in meals containing meat. In addition, animal fat has probably been a scarce and valuable nutrient for most populations throughout most of human history.[18]

In addition, the quality of vegetable food resources may have declined in the course of our history. Small groups of hunter-gatherers can be relatively selective, picking foods that are nutritious as well as easy to process;

larger groups cannot be so choosy. The broad spectrum revolution may initially have increased dietary variety, but the foods added are likely to have been those previously avoided. Moreover, growing population and the disappearance of preferred resources would ultimately have forced human groups to focus on "third choice" foods—those that are relatively plentiful but neither flavorful nor nutritious. Some, such as acorns and buckeyes, the third choice foods of several American Indian groups, are toxic unless carefully processed.[19]

The third choice foods that ultimately became our staples (cereals and tubers chosen for their prolific growth, their shelf life, and their ability to respond to human manipulation) are not particularly rich sources of nutrients other than energy. Most are poor sources of protein, vitamins, and minerals when compared to meat and to the variety of wild vegetable foods eaten by modern hunter-gatherers.[20]

The major cereal grains, for example, all contain a class of chemicals called phytates that tend to form insoluble bonds with metals in the human intestine causing them to pass out with the feces rather than being absorbed. As a result, significant dietary elements, including iron, zinc, and calcium, can be relatively hard to obtain from diets that depend heavily on some cereals, including wheat and maize, even if other dietary sources of the minerals are available. Similarly, the oxalates and phosphates common in staple tubers and in cereals inhibit iron absorption. The result may be an increase in anemia and other mineral deficiencies associated with diets focused heavily on these foods.[21]

In addition to their common drawbacks, the various cereals each have specific nutritional shortcomings that become important when they become a staple of the diet. Maize is poor in the amino acids lysine and tryptophan and in the vitamin niacin, as well as in iron content. It contains an antiniacin substance that may actually increase the need for this vitamin; and it contains a poor balance of two amino acids, leucine and isoleucine. Eaten exclusively or as a very high proportion of the diet, maize may promote such deficiency diseases as anemia and pellagra.[22]

Wheat is poor in the amino acids lysine, threonine, and tryptophan. In addition, in parts of the Middle East, wheat-rich diets are associated with zinc deficiency.[23] Rice is poor in protein, and populations that depend heavily on its consumption are often deficient in protein. The low protein content of rice also inhibits the activity of vitamin A in rice-eating populations, even when the vitamin itself is available in the diet.[24] Excessive dependence on rice can produce beriberi or thiamine deficiency, although in this case it is the processing of the rice rather than the cereal itself that is the key.

Other cereals less well known to Western populations are also associated with nutritional problems. Sorghum, an important staple grain in north Africa, can produce pellagra. Although it is richer in niacin and tryptophan than maize, its high leucine content may interfere with niacin utilization. Pennisetum millet, another staple grain in northeast Africa and India, is associated with thyroid gland disfunction (and goiterous enlargement of the thyroid gland similar to that caused by iodine deficiency) because it contains a chemical that interferes with thyroid hormone production.[25]

The various tubers and vegetable starches that are the staple crops of populations of the moist tropics—yams, sweet potatoes, potatoes, manioc, sago palm, bananas, and plantains—are relatively poor sources of protein and some vitamins and minerals for the number of calories they provide (even when compared to cereals), and many contain mild toxins that can have serious cumulative effects.[26]

Domestication—prehistoric and modern genetic manipulation of the crops—is not necessarily associated with improvements in the nutrient value of plants; indeed, quite the reverse may be true. Wild wheat, for example, contains more protein than most domestic wheat, although some modern hybrid wheats bred specifically for improved protein content may equal or surpass wild wheat.[27] Selecting domestic crops for good taste does, however, tend to breed out some of their toxic qualities.[28]

Reliance on stored food is likely to mean a further reduction in nutrient quality, partly because crops are chosen with storage rather than nutrition in mind and partly because the storage process itself tends to reduce vitamin content. Vitamin C and other water-soluble (B) vitamins may disappear in storage, as stored goods dry out. Intentional drying and cooking of foods in preparation for storage can result in further loss of these vitamins.[29] But some techniques of preservation may actually have increased the vitamin content of various foods. Pickling can increase the amount of vitamin C in foods. Fermentation, which helps make foods immune to spoilage, may also add to the nutrient value. For example, brewing beer from grain (which we now believe may date back several thousand years) also adds to its vitamin content.[30, 31]

If populations must become sedentary to live off stored staple foods, further nutritional problems may arise. Mobile foragers tend to sample a wider range of water and soils than sedentary farmers; thus, they have a far greater chance of avoiding dietary deficiencies (not only iodine but also fluorine and selenium) associated with particular soils.[32] Mobile populations also enjoy a wider variety of food species than sedentary populations because they cover a wider geographical range. So, sedentism is likely to reduce dietary variety and increase the risk of vitamin and mineral deficiencies associated both with a limited range of foods and with a limited range of soils.

In sum, the transition from small mobile hunting and gathering groups to larger sedentary populations relying on storage and agriculture is likely to have been accompanied by a reduction in the proportion of animal products in the diet, a reduction in the proportion of foods eaten fresh, a reduction in dietary variety, and, consequently, a decline in the overall quality of the diet.

Small-scale farming populations in many parts of the world have developed techniques to overcome some of the economic and nutritional problems associated with the adoption of storage and sedentary agriculture. They have employed innovative methods of food processing, as well as "clever" cooking and eating patterns. American Indians seem to have known for several thousand years that eating maize with beans compensated for the dietary shortcomings of the maize alone. Baking maize and other cereals in ash helps to increase their calcium and iron content, as well as the availability of niacin, as does grinding cereals on stone grinding implements.[33] Making tortillas may help to improve the nutritional value of maize meal by increasing the availability of lysine, tryptophan, and niacin while improving the isoleucine/leucine ratio.[34]

Old World populations have grown and consumed various legumes or pulses with cereals since very early in the history of agriculture, providing a dietary balance like that of maize and beans. The process of leavening bread, discovered early by Old World farmers, reduced the phytate content of wheat, facilitating mineral absorption in high-wheat diets.[35] Populations in both the Old and the New World had techniques for introducing vitamin C into diets otherwise poor in ascorbic acid. Chili peppers, an ubiquitous flavoring among American Indian populations utilizing maize, are a rich source of the vitamin. Garlic and onions played a similar role both as flavoring and as a source of vitamin C in the Old World.[36]

Subsistence farmers also employ other means of maintaining variety in their diets. Many cultivate gardens that retain as much variety as possible, despite an increasing focus on specific staple crops. "Primitive" gardens, in contrast to modern fields, are often eclectic mixes of plants of different types (the boundaries between crops and weeds may, in fact, be relatively blurred). Many plants that are not actively cultivated are tolerated in the garden and end up on the menu or in medicine.[37]

A third solution employed by subsistence cultivators is to continue to rely as much as possible on gathering additional wild resources. The archaeological record of early farming communities in both the New and Old Worlds suggests that early farming was accompanied by substantial reliance on wild foods that added protein and other essential nutrients to the diet. In much the same manner, contemporary subsistence cultivators commonly obtain a small but significant portion of their foods from wild resources—a fraction of the diet that contributes a disproportionate share of vitamins and minerals even if it does not make up a significant proportion of the calories consumed.

The intensification of agriculture, however, can create a number of new problems. Intensification means that land once left to support wild foods is gradually converted to grow more of the dietary staples. By taking up space once left for wild plants and animals, the new economy may undermine access to wild foods, resulting in a substantial decline in dietary quality.[38] The intensification of agriculture may also sharpen the boundary between crops and weeds. While improving the growing conditions of crops, this process may eliminate the weeds entirely, often with extreme nutritional consequences.[39] In addition, intensification may result in elimination of variety foods (such as chilis or onions) that cannot be grown efficiently, that compete for space, or that have growth requirements inconsistent with the investment in intensified agriculture.

When farmers become specialists within a larger political and economic system, they may regain needed dietary variety through trade; but they may also be particularly vulnerable to loss of dietary variety and quality because they may be forced (or given economic incentives) to focus their production on specific crops. They may grow a far smaller range of crops—and have less access to dietary variety—than do independent subsistence farmers.[40] Intensive agricultural systems also tend to promote agricultural specialization and reduce crop variety because crops must be chosen to meet the needs of the technology applied. A good example is a modern, pure field of grain designed neither for the nutritional balance of its product nor for the protection of the soils but for the convenience of harvesting machines.

Specialists at other tasks, who grow no food at all, depend on patterns of trade and transport (and the economics and politics of the society) rather than on their own nutritional needs to determine what foods they will receive. Even with relatively primitive technology, trade systems can usually move some goods farther and faster than people themselves can migrate, so they can provide dietary variety that rivals or exceeds that of hunter-gatherers.[41] When transportation is fast enough (as in the very recent past in affluent parts of the world), trade networks may also reintroduce continuous access to fresh foods, helping to offset nutrient losses associated with food storage.[42]

But trade networks may not solve the problem entirely. Traded food is likely to be comparatively scarce and expensive. In addition, trade puts a premium on transport efficiency, which means that foods should weigh as little and take up as little space as possible. Nutritious but perishable or bulky items cannot be moved (or can be moved only at great cost), and foods may have to be processed to reduce their bulk or increase their shelf life, often eliminating part of their nutritional value. Vitamins best obtained from fresh foods are likely to be particularly hard to get, unless sophisticated processing preserves them. Scurvy is most commonly a disease of specialized populations that cannot afford to obtain high quality fresh foods in trade or that are cut off from trade altogether (historically, most often on slow-moving ships or in cities under seige). Pellagra, the disease associated with excessive reliance on maize, is not primarily a disease of subsistence farmers; it is a disease of poor specialists who are not given (or who are not able to buy) appropriate foods.[43]

Elite social classes commonly manipulate trade systems for their own purposes. They use trade to increase their own political leverage, or they simply obtain a disproportionate share of scarce resources.[44] The decline in human consumption of animal fat and protein, resulting initially from human population growth and the decline of animals, can be reversed for privileged individuals by means of trade. But their privilege tends to exacerbate the deprivation of the poor.

In fact, trade systems often result in the movement of necessary resources *from* rather than *to* populations in need. It is a fairly commonplace observation that modern Third World farmers may be deficient in nutrients that they themselves produce because of the insidious effects of such exchange systems. In much of Central America today, for example, animal protein consumption has declined at the same time that production is increasing, because of the demand for the export of beef.[45] Deficiency of vitamin A is common in Indonesia, even though papaya, a rich source of carotene (from which vitamin A can be made by the body), is grown. The papayas are essentially all grown for export. In parts of Africa, people who eat lots of green vegetables rich in carotene (or other precursors of vitamin A) fail to obtain sufficient vitamin A because they export the fats and oils needed to facilitate the absorption of the vitamin from their own intestines.[46]

In sum, a net loss of dietary variety and nutritional quality could accompany the growth of human civilization, particularly if the organizational capacity of the society is not fully brought to bear to meet the nutritional needs of all its people.

One final point needs to be made about the quality of the diet. The quality of nutrients actually available to the body depends in part on the individual's parasite load. Some parasites actually produce vitamins for us, enhancing our nutrition.[47] But the most important impact of increasing infection rates on human nutrition is negative: our parasites increase our nutritional requirements and interfere with our ability to absorb food.[48] They do this in several ways. Some, such as hookworm, destroy human tissues, which require repair and replacement. Some, such as tapeworms, consume the products of our digestion within the intestine before we can absorb them for use in the body. Many force the body to devote its limited resources to the production of special substances (such as immunoglobulins) and even special cells (such as phagocytes) for defense. Some discourage food consumption by creating nausea or lassitude. Some inhibit absorption by increasing the rate of flow of material through the intestine or by imposing physical and chemical changes on the digestive tract. Diarrhea, measles, chickenpox, hookworm, and tuberculosis are all known to have a negative effect on levels of vitamin A. Malaria restricts food intake, causes vomiting and anorexia, promotes anemia, and, like all fevers, promotes protein loss. Hookworm infestation results in iron deficiency anemia and protein loss. Since the evolution of civilization is likely to have been accompanied by increasing rates of parasitization until the very recent past, we are likely to have experienced increasing nutrient requirements at the same time that the quality of foods was declining.

The Reliability of Food Supplies

Perhaps the most controversial question is whether the evolution of civilization has made hunger and starvation less common. Populations dependent on foraging for wild foods are vulnerable to hunger or starvation because of seasonal fluctuations in wild resources or major episodes of drought or other natural disasters. If a group is small enough to be selective about what it eats, it will have back-up foods available in case choice foods fail. In addition, such groups keep track of alternate food sources in other locations through group movement and through contact with other bands, and they use their mobility to escape local food shortages.[49] But their information may be imperfect, and they can only move as far and as fast as they can walk. If the disaster is widespread, they may not be able to escape. And because they rely on mobility to get food, they are unlikely—indeed unable—to have food stored for such contingencies.

Whether or not more civilized inventions are likely to have improved matters is debatable, however. Sedentary populations may well be at greater risk of food shortage or famine than are mobile groups because they are limited to a smaller territorial range and variety of foods and because they lack the fail-safe mechanism of mobility itself: they cannot easily move away from failed resources.

The development of storage technology may compensate for the loss of mobility. In theory, storage can guarantee food supplies through lean seasons or even the failure of natural or domestic harvests. In the modern world, storage systems involving refrigeration and other sophisticated food preservation techniques clearly have that capability. For those populations to whom the benefit of modern storage and transportation systems are extended without reservation, the risk of starvation is undoubtedly less than it has ever been in the past. But it is not altogether certain that in history, or even in the modern Third World, storage systems have actually worked so efficiently. The shelf life of most food stuffs is inherently limited in the absence of refrigeration (which is still relatively expensive to apply on a large scale and is not commonly available on such a scale). Stored crops are prone to rot and to losses from insect and rodent pests. In many parts of the Third World they may barely be able to last until the next harvest, let alone provide for years with no harvest at all.[50]

Storage also brings with it another important problem. Living wild plants and animals are relatively difficult either to destroy or expropriate; so the food reserves of hunter-gatherers are largely beyond the reach of raiders and conquerors, who can appropriate territory but cannot seize accumulated resources. Once human populations begin to centralize and store produce in which their labor has already been invested, the stored produce becomes an obvious target, even an attraction for raids by other human groups.

Our naive expectations notwithstanding, it is therefore an open question —or one for empirical investigation—whether sedentary populations with storage systems have typically been better buffered against hunger than mobile populations.

Quite apart from problems of storage, switching to domesticated food species does not necessarily make the food supply more reliable. Chosen for their productivity and their preference for human protection, our staple plant foods are not the hardiest of naturally occurring species. Moreover, when we manipulate the breeding of plants and animals to make them more manageable, more productive, or better tasting, we often distort their original design selected by nature for survival. Our domestic species often produce edible parts that are out of natural proportion to other structures, making them vulnerable. When we select animals that are docile we eliminate their natural protection; when we select crops for good taste, we are often breeding out chemicals that the plants use as defense against their own pests and predators.[51]

Human beings also tend to concentrate their selected plant species, creating unnaturally high densities of individual species. Such densities increase levels of competition for soil nutrients, reducing the size and viability of specific plants and threatening soil depletion. The high density also increases the potential that parasites and diseases will spread among the crop, increasing the risk of blight.

Domestic animals may suffer from crowding and confinement, as noted in the last chapter. This not only increases the risk of infection but also presumably increases the risk that the animal population itself (and hence the human food supply) will be destroyed.

The viability of domestic plants (and the reliability of a human diet based on them) is also threatened by human alteration of the natural distribution of the species through the domestication process. We commonly remove plants from their original habitat or extend their ranges so that most of the domesticated crop is living outside the ecological conditions in which it evolved. Often such transport of crops to new climates is successful in the short run or in a run of average years. The new crops compete successfully in their new locations and expand the food base of human populations. For example, wheat spread through much of the Old World in prehistoric times, just as maize spread through the New World, presumably because of their perceptible contribution to human food supplies. The introduction of maize and potatoes to the Old World and cattle to the New World after Columbus had dramatic effects on food supplies on both sides of the Atlantic.[52]

But even where the new crops are successful, there is a potential drawback. The wild plants of any region have generally been tested by natural extremes of climate and local parasites. They survive not only the run of normal or average years but extreme or bad years as well. Domesticated plants, newly introduced (and perhaps newly altered as well), may not survive bad years or new challenges—as the historic European potato famine attests.

People protect their domestic plants and animals against these risks, of course. We weed, fertilize, and eliminate parasites and predators. Our intervention has been successful enough to have produced a continuously increasing food supply capable of feeding a growing population through most of our history. But our technology has not been able to eliminate the risk of occasional crop failure or even to offset other factors that have tended to increase the risk. Episodic and even frequent failure of crops in the face of such natural stresses as irregular rainfall is a common feature of farming systems; because people are increasingly committed to advance investment in the food supply, failures cannot easily be recouped.

As agriculture is intensified, the risk of crop failure may get worse. A broad-based food economy is protected against crop failure by sheer variety. Some resources may survive when others fail. A focused economy—one with a single staple crop—is riskier, even if the crop is reasonably hardy.

Increasing the percentage of land farmed, the density of growing plants, the productivity of individual plants, and the frequency of harvest all impose new risks. Because planting usually begins in choice locations, the expansion of the planted area commonly means bringing more and more marginal (and risky) areas under cultivation. Increasing the density of plants or the frequency of cropping the same soils is likely to accelerate the depletion of soil nutrients. And plants designed for high productivity are often fragile and demanding crops.

Adding irrigation, fertilizer, or pesticides and breeding hardy crops can help protect against crop failure; large-scale storage and transport can provide extra insurance. Developing roads and other means of transport to move stored produce from one location to another may buffer whole populations against famine to an unprecedented degree. McAlpin suggests, for example, that the development of railroads in India had this effect.[53]

But although many of these improvements forestall immediate crises, they also generate new risks. Irrigation systems tend to become clogged with silt. More important, they tend to destroy irrigated soil through salinization (the buildup of salt residues from evaporation). This problem, in fact, seems to have plagued large areas of early civilization in the Middle East.[54]

As food production becomes more and more dependent on these investments, the food supply becomes vulnerable to economic and political crises as well as natural ones.[55] Food scarcity may result from the inability (or unwillingness) to maintain the investment. Many of the modern hybrid seeds on which intensive agriculture is based need more fertilizer than primitive varieties. If a population cannot afford fertilizer, its plight may be worse than before. The deterioration of roads and railroads, as much as fluctuation in climate, affects the capacity of many Third World nations to feed themselves.[56]

Specialization of labor is also a mixed blessing. Specialists (including specialized food producers) are particularly vulnerable to famine. They depend on systems of transportation and storage to provide all of their food; they depend on social entitlements or rights to food—determined either by their trading power or by social and political obligations—to feed them.[57] Their problem is that entitlements are fragile, whether based on market mechanisms, political obligations, or government guarantees. Markets, which operate on the basis of supply and demand, may fail to provide for individuals who generate no demand—who have no political power and nothing to trade (that is, who are without land or resources, who are unemployed, or who produce something that is of no interest to anyone else). Government guarantees or planned economies may also fail to provide for such groups, because governments are more concerned with such political objectives as maintaining an elite, supporting an army, or placating urban mobs than with feeding the needy. Most modern famine and much of historic famine reflect the failure of entitlements at least as much as they reflect crop failure; much contemporary hunger occurs when food is available but individuals have no money to buy it and no "right" to receive it.[58]

Occupational specialization also undermines another protection against famine enjoyed by primitive people. If specialization replaces kinship as the basis for social organization, people lose their primary claim on the support and aid of others. It seems to be universal among human groups that kinship creates both positive feelings among individuals and a sense of mutual obligation and concern. In societies where kinship provides the major organizing principle, mutual obligation pervades the system; the right to call on one's kin in times of need offers a major principle of insurance against want. In a system of specialists, freedom from want is much more likely to depend either on one's ability to force assistance or to entice it by the exchange of other goods and services. Specialization may also replace mutual obligation with intergroup tension, particularly if specialists are ethnically distinct, heightening both lack of concern for others and distrust of one's fellows.[59] In short, at the same time that civilization replaces self-sufficiency in food production with entitlements to food delivery, it tends to remove what are, in simpler societies, the most powerful and secure bases for entitlement.

Specialization, entitlement, and large-scale trade also add to the risk of hunger or starvation by introducing new sets of market factors that are beyond local control. Changes in supply and demand in other parts of the world can affect a group's ability to sell its own products or to buy food (or fuel and fertilizer necessary to make food). Such fluctuations in world demand are a significant source of economic hardship and hunger in modern Third World countries.[60]

In addition, people dependent on large-scale investment to feed themselves are subject to political manipulation. Farmers turn over the control of production decisions—and ultimately decisions about the distribution of the produce—to a managerial elite who may lack knowledge of, or concern for, local nutritional problems (and who may be motivated by different concerns). As the state grows and comes to consist of many different ethnic groups, the gap between the managers and the farmers gets larger and the corresponding ignorance or indifference becomes more important.

Investment, no matter how well managed, implies taxation, which may undermine the individual farmer's ability to develop his own surplus as a buffer for his family in crisis and may exacerbate existing crises.[61] And such investment may be mismanaged or converted to luxury goods, pyramids, or other monuments for the elite, rather than to productive resources.

The power of the elite not only affects the quality of food for the poor but may undermine their access to food, their very right to eat. Because they exert disproportionate demand, the privileged can distort production in the direction of luxury goods for themselves at the expense of subsistence goods for others. In Ethiopia, famine among pastoral populations has been heightened because these populations must compete with the increasing demands of commercial agriculture for export.[62] In Honduras, subsistence agriculture is threatened because farmland is being converted to grazing land to grow beef for export to the United States.[63] (The same is true of the Maya in Belize, with whom I work.) In much of Africa, subsistence farming has been displaced by production of such luxury products as coffee and tea. Similar patterns can be observed historically. In eighteenth-century France, amidst general shortage, the growing of cereal was forced to compete with the growing of grapes for wine.[64]

Finally, the organization of states with fixed (and often arbitrary) geographical boundaries may contribute in a significant way to the risk of famine —largely offsetting the capacity to transport food. State boundaries create artificial limits to the movement of food supplies and people. The problem may be particularly acute in the modern world because state boundaries are now commonly drawn with little regard either for the distribution of kinship or social groups (which might otherwise support one another in times of need) or for the distribution of ecological zones that historically complemented one another to support human populations.[65] Nationalism also promotes wasteful rivalry, and large-scale investments in the production and storage of food invites expropriation and destruction by one's enemies. In the historic and modern world (and presumably in the prehistoric world), wartime destruction of transportation, dams, and other improvements (or of food supplies themselves) has emerged as one major cause of famine.

Like the quality of the diet, the reliability of human food supplies is likely to have had a more checkered history than our images of human progress usually suggest.

The Texture and Composition of Diet

Although trends in dietary quality and reliability are uncertain, the pattern of changes in the texture of food is relatively clear. Hunting and gathering populations eat foods that are coarse and tough in two senses: they are tough to chew, and they contain a high proportion of inert, indigestible matter or fiber that must be processed by the intestine. In the evolution of civilized diets, foods have gradually been altered—first eliminating much of the need for chewing and, much more recently, eliminating bulk. These changes produce mixed consequences, at best, for health.

The first major steps in the process are associated with sedentism and farming. Compared to many wild vegetable foods, domestic grains and tubers are relatively soft concentrated packages of calories. In addition, sedentary populations with grindstones and with pottery can soften foods by boiling, producing mush or gruel—foods easier to chew, although they retain their fiber.[66] Much more recently—particularly with the past century —incentives for efficient transport and storage have resulted in further refinement of food, producing ever-more concentrated packages of calories with the indigestible fiber removed.

Coarse foods have important effects on jaws and teeth. The development of the jaws during childhood depends on the chewing force exerted. Strenuous chewing is necessary for the development of facial muscles and bones.[67] It may also determine alignment of the teeth. Apparently, human jaws initially evolved to meet in such a manner that the cutting edges of incisors met directly. It is only since the adoption of relatively soft diets following the rise of farming—and the adoption of modern eating utensils—that human beings developed the slight overbite that we now consider normal.[68]

In addition, coarse-textured foods result in heavy wear on teeth. Toothwear is likely to be a far more serious problem for hunter-gatherer populations than for more civilized groups; hunter-gatherers may face the problem that their teeth literally wear out (without ever decaying) before they otherwise succumb to old age. But the same coarseness means that there is little tendency for food to stick to the teeth and thus little tendency for cariogenic bacteria, dependent on adherent food, to attack tooth surfaces. Moreover, the constant abrasion of coarse-textured foods tends to clean tooth surfaces and scour away incipient caries, so hunting and gathering populations are rarely caries-prone. With the adoption of softer foods, tooth abrasion becomes less of a problem, but rates of caries increase.[69]

Coarse diets also pose a problem for toothless individuals—the very old and the very young. Elderly individuals may have to put great effort into food preparation; infants must be weaned onto animal or vegetable foods prechewed by their parents, or they must be given very special and relatively scarce products, such as the soft marrow fat contained in animal bones. If scarce or hard to prepare, however, these foods are relatively nutritious.

Cereals and starchy gruels increase the range of foods available to the elderly and facilitate weaning, but they are not particularly nutritious.[70]

One result of a coarse diet may be a far greater reliance on human breast milk to supply the nutritional needs of infants and toddlers than is the case among more civilized societies which enjoy the benefits of cereal gruels, other refined foods, and, more recently, animal milk as alternate foods for young children.[71] Reliance on breast feeding is almost certainly relatively healthy for the child.[72] Prolonged nursing, however, may be a serious caloric drain, as well as a mineral drain, on the mother, potentially threatening maternal health if nutritional intake is already marginal.[73]

A diet of coarse foods also helps to limit the accumulation of body fat. Most wild foods contain relatively few calories in proportion to their volume.[74] With the advent of starchy staple crops and refined foods, individuals can obtain more calories per mouthful and more calories per volume of stomach or intestinal content. Up to a point, this change may be an important and positive one, making it easier for the body to maintain energy reserves.[75] But the change also marks the first step in the progressive separation of calories and other nutrients. Hunter-gatherers may be lean despite otherwise good nutrition.[76] More civilized groups, paradoxically, by choosing calorie-rich foods and refining them, may be able to store more fat while being less well nourished in other ways.

Coarse diets may also affect human fertility in one of two ways. Hunter-gatherers may naturally be relatively infertile, either because of the comparative leanness of their diets and their bodies or because of the requirement for prolonged nursing. The proposed mechanism linking body fat to fertility is controversial.[77] The effects of nursing are better documented.[78] One clear implication of this, of course, is that human fertility may have increased as our diets became more refined.

In recent years, refinement of foods, carried to an extreme, has produced some new health problems—those associated with obesity, excess intake of fat and sodium, and lack of dietary bulk and fiber.[79]

Obesity is unlikely to occur (although it is not unknown) without the refinement of foods, because without such refinement it is hard for the body to process enough food to obtain a large excess of calories. Modern refinement frees calories and provides them in concentrated packages, making overconsumption possible. Given the costs of transportation and handling, low bulk, high-calorie foods are comparatively cheap, so there is an incentive for people to eat them.[80]

Obesity, which is quite rare among primitive societies that do not process food extensively, is associated with a number of diseases, most of which are recognized as diseases of civilization. Adult-onset diabetes, for example, although in part genetically determined, seems to be triggered by high caloric intake. (It may also be triggered by the intake of refined foods that the body processes much more rapidly than bulky foods, resulting in periodic massive doses of sugar instead of a steady flow.) Even the genetics of diabetes may be related to this dietary shift. It is postulated that diabetes may be an inherited condition that is insignificant or even advantageous to individuals living in a low-calorie regime but dangerous during exposure to high-calorie civilized diets.[81] Obesity is also associated with the production of excess cholesterol in the body and hence with atherosclerosis, coronary heart disease, high blood pressure, and a range of cancers.

The lack of dietary fiber seems to have other negative consequences.[82] The human intestine appears to be designed to process a larger volume or bulk than modern civilized diets provide. Healthy bowel function may, in fact, call for much more frequent defecation than we consider normal. Many people around the world who suffer from fewer bowel complaints than we do consider themselves constipated if they do not defecate more than once a day. Lack of fiber is associated with constipation and a series of constipation-related conditions, including diverticular disease, hiatal hernia, hemorrhoids, and varicose veins.

In addition, the lack of fiber appears to change the nature of the intestinal environment in ways that promote diseases, including cancer. The elimination of fiber from the diet increases the time that stools take to pass through the intestine and therefore increases the exposure of the intestinal wall to microbes associated with decay. These microbes and their byproducts are associated with both appendicitis and cancers of the large intestine, colon, and rectum.[83]

Loss of fiber also contributes to elevated blood sugar levels and rapid release of dietary sugars contributing to the appearance of diabetic symptoms; it tends to raise serum cholesterol levels by increasing the efficiency with which cholesterol is absorbed from the intestine. Low dietary fiber is thus also associated with the production of gallstones.[84]

Other aspects of modern food processing are also associated with diseases, particularly high blood pressure (and hence cardiovascular disease and stroke). Processing alters the balance of sodium and potassium in the diet. Excess sodium intake has long been implicated in the onset of these conditions, but recent studies have suggested that the balance between the two elements may also be important.[85]

Wild plants and animals contain sufficient sodium to meet human needs, and there is no reason to assume that a diet without extra salt as a seasoning would be deficient in sodium.[86] Fresh fruits and vegetables contain relatively large amounts of potassium. In addition, wood ash used in primitive cooking techniques may be a rich source of dietary potassium. As a result, hunter-gatherer groups are likely to ingest a healthy balance of the two elements.[87]

Since the adoption of agriculture, salt seems to have become increasingly important as a condiment (perhaps because cereals make pretty dull fare).[88] In any case, probably because sodium intake is addictive and one's taste buds gradually demand more and more, salt intake has risen. But salt is also a commonly used preservative associated with food storage and transport; in the modern world, sodium also occurs as a common element in a number of preservative compounds. This pattern of consumption of sodium added to foods (perhaps combined with the decline of fresh foods as sources of potassium) and the tendency toward obesity apparently underlie the emergence of hypertension as a disease of civilized populations.[89]

Modern diets also suffer from excessive fat intake, a pattern popularly associated with immoderate consumption of meat. Such a diet has several negative consequences that must be added to the problems of high fat diets and obesity already discussed. A high fat-to-carbohydrate ratio in the diet contributes to glucose intolerance and diabetes; moreover, atherosclerosis and coronary heart disease are associated with diets high in meat, total fat, animal fat relative to fats of vegetable origin, and saturated fats. Diets high in fat, particularly animal fats, also exacerbate the problem of intestinal and colon cancer because dietary fat alters the nature and concentration of biliary steroids and provides a substrate for carcinogenic bacterial action in the intestine. Dietary meat alters the bacterial flora, increasing the proportion of anaerobic activity that produces carcinogens. Diets rich in fat also promote ovarian cancer, leukemia, and breast cancer. The latter may also be associated with tall stature, suggesting, according to contemporary Western folk wisdom, that it is a function of good nutrition.[90]

These health problems are associated not primarily with animal products per se but with modern domestic animals. The key to this paradox is that domestication and particularly some of our modern improvements in domestication drastically alter the fat content of animals.

Wild grazing and browsing animals (at least those living on land) are normally quite lean—like well-exercised human beings—because they must exercise continuously to obtain food and because wild foods available to them are not particularly rich sources of calories or fats. Typically, wild African mammals have a total body fat content of about 4 percent. In contrast, domestic animals, whose food supplies are increasingly provided by humans —particularly modern domestic animals, which are fed grain, a relatively rich source of energy—often have body fat levels approaching 25 to 30 percent. In addition, the fat of wild animals contains a relatively high proportion of polyunsaturated fat, commonly about five times as much polyunsaturated fat in proportion to saturated fat as domestic food animals. Polyunsaturates in the diet may actually decrease serum cholesterol. It is for these reasons that domestic animals contribute to the modern risk of high blood pressure, atherosclerosis, heart disease, and stroke, whereas the meat of wild animals, even eaten in comparable quantities, apparently does not.[91]

In this instance, social class stratification in diet tends to work against the wealthy. Diseases associated with excess consumption of animal protein and animal fats but also of calories are primarily diseases of the affluent.[92] Citizens of affluent nations typically ingest anywhere from 35 to 40 percent of their calories in the form of relatively expensive fats as opposed to inexpensive carbohydrates. In contrast, uncivilized diets may contain only about 15 percent fat. In addition, among the affluent a high proportion of the fats are from domestic animals, meaning that they will contain a relatively high percentage of saturated fats.[93]

Early in our history, changes in the texture of the diet significantly altered the nature of stresses on human teeth. They may also have made a wider range of foods available both to the old and the very young, facilitating weaning (albeit often to foods of lesser nutritional value), and they may have helped to alter patterns of human fertility by affecting levels of body fat and patterns of nursing. More recent changes in the texture of foods seem to have contributed to the emergence of a number of degenerative diseases of civilization.

Chapter 6

Health among Contemporary Hunter-Gatherers

Observations have now been made on a number of contemporary human groups whose lifestyles approximate those of the smallest prehistoric human societies—that is, small, mobile, fluid groups (usually numbering fifty or fewer) foraging for wild foods.[1] None of these groups is a pristine remnant of ancient life. All exist in the modern world, and all are affected by its contact. None of these groups—nor even all of them together—provides a complete or unbiased picture of early human lifestyles. We should, perhaps, consider them twentieth-century experiments in small-group foraging, rather than remnants of the past. But they, along with the evidence of archaeology discussed in chapter 7, are the best evidence we have—and the only evidence we have ever had—about hunter-gatherers in the past. They provide hints about the epidemiological consequences of mobile small-group living and the nutritional consequences of eating wild foods. Moreover, these groups are the source of popular images of primitive life, and it is important to evaluate their health and nutrition, even if we no longer accept them uncritically as representatives of our past.

Several peculiarities of contemporary hunting and gathering bands should be noted at the outset. First, most such groups now live in environments from which the bigger game animals have largely disappeared. Some combination of changing climate and human hunting itself seems to have eliminated a substantial proportion of the large game from every continent that human beings inhabit—a process of extinction that apparently began shortly after the first arrival of human hunters in many locations.[2] Second, almost all contemporary band societies now inhabit what anthropologists refer to as "marginal" environments—such areas of the world as deserts and the

Arctic, comparatively useless for farming or even herding, or portions of rain forests that they possess because other more powerful societies do not want them. Perhaps more important, judging by the archaeological evidence, these are environments that hunting and gathering bands themselves did not choose to exploit until forced into them by the pressure of competition.[3] In addition, most contemporary hunting groups suffer the continued progressive encroachment of larger societies, but, paradoxically, they may now actually benefit from drastic recent reductions in their own numbers as a result of disease, which reduces competition for some resources.[4]

Third, all of these groups interact to varying degrees with larger-scale societies. They often have access to materials, tools, and weapons (particularly metal tools and primitive guns) that their ancestors did not have. Many now participate in trade networks associated with larger societies or even operate as specialists within those societies.[5] (There is one report of a group in Sri Lanka that has been playing the part of primitives for tourists for more than a century.)[6]

Members of some groups appear to have the option to move from the smaller to the larger society, either foraging or finding other kinds of employment, as conditions warrant.[7] Many are, however, subject to legal restrictions on their movements or their activities (particularly regarding the hunting of large game), and they often participate in market economies at a disadvantage, trading their goods to more powerful groups that can set prices through monopolistic practices.[8]

All of these groups are in contact with civilized diseases, in some cases only because missionaries and anthropologists have visited them but most often because they share more extensive urban contacts. Some even have access to bits and pieces of civilized medicine.[9]

There is not sufficient room in a book of this length to provide a detailed analysis of observed health patterns in all such societies. Instead, I propose to make a detailed presentation of one example and then compare the health of members of that society to that of individuals in other small-scale societies and in a range of historic and modern populations.

I will focus initially on the !Kung San and other San hunter-gatherers of South Africa who became famous during the 1960s as examples of primitive "affluence." I choose them not because they are typical nor because they are affluent—in many ways they are neither (nor do I consider them more pristine than other groups)—but precisely because they are famous and controversial, and consequently the subject of intense scrutiny and extended discussion. They are the group to which most others have been compared or contrasted.

The San of the Kalahari

Bands of San or Bushmen hunter-gatherers of southern Africa are actually part of a larger network of related populations extending in and around the Kalahari desert in South Africa and Botswana. During the 1950s the network was estimated at approximately fifty-three thousand people. A large percentage of these were settled in various outposts of civilization, such as the cattle ranches that were gradually taking over the territory. Richard Lee has estimated that perhaps 60 percent of the population were full-time hunter-gatherers as late as the turn of the century but that by 1976 fewer than 5 percent still relied on hunting and gathering for a living.[10] However, it is now recognized that the group as a whole has a longer history of economic interaction with outsiders than has commonly been assumed.[11]

But in more inaccessible and inhospitable parts of the desert, a small percentage maintained a relatively independent foraging lifestyle until quite recently. In these regions small bands of individuals, commonly numbering between fifteen and fifty people, continued to depend largely on hunted and gathered resources, which they exploited with a pattern of frequent movement of camps. There is evidence that San-like peoples practicing a similar way of life have inhabited some portions of the desert for at least eleven thousand years. There may be more pressure on food and water resources in the desert now than would have been true in the past. Although the San have been able to hold onto parts of the desert because more powerful groups lack interest in this relatively inhospitable area, the remaining San population may be more concentrated in space—deprived of some critical water holes by competitors and forced to inhabit other waterholes more steadily than in the past—as a result of encroachment by more powerful populations on portions of their territory. It is also apparent that the density of game has declined in recent years as a result of the arrival of firearms and the construction of fences for cattle control, leading the San to develop techniques for taking smaller game. In fact, as far back as 1928, D. F. Bleek reported that, as a result of declining game and restrictive game laws, the San were being forced to focus on smaller animals, much against their will.[12]

The concentration of San populations around a few reliable sources of water presumably increases problems of finding food in an already inhospitable desert; it should increase the transmission of infectious disease in the population as well, even though the desert itself tends to discourage the survival of parasites and their vectors. The presence of larger Bantu-speaking populations and their cattle in the vicinity, as well as increasing contact with the world network of urban civilization, presumably also increase the range and severity of diseases to which the San are exposed. All observers agree, for example, that the relatively large and permanent cattle posts that the San visit have more severe problems of feces and garbage disposal and of flies than do the small temporary camps of the San themselves. Moreover, there is general agreement that the San who frequent these larger settlements appear less healthy than those living in the desert in nomadic camps.

But the presence of the cattle posts also offers an alternative lifestyle and may help to relieve pressure on wild resources by siphoning some population; the posts may permit individuals to survive periods when wild resources are scarce. During the 1960s most adult San, even those then living in hunting camps, were found to have spent at least part of their lives at cattle posts. The cattle posts also serve as a possible haven for the old, the sick, or the infirm; it is an unresolved question whether the higher frequencies of various illnesses and pathologies at the cattle posts noted by most observers reflect harsher conditions of life there or the convenience of the cattle posts as places for the afflicted to congregate.

A number of groups of San living by hunting and gathering have been the subject of fairly careful observation and analysis, which often includes quantitative as well as qualitative assessments of workload, nutrition and health, and patterns of fertility and mortality in the populations. Perhaps the most thoroughly studied and documented group are the !Kung San of Dobe, which Lee, Nancy Howell, and a large interdisciplinary team of scientists have studied for years.[13] The descriptions of the Dobe !Kung provide the bulk of what follows, but they can be compared with descriptions of the /Gwi and //Gana San of Kade provided by Tanaka,[14] the /Gwi San provided by Silberbauer,[15] the !Kung of Nyae Nyae provided by Marshall,[16] and the wider network of !Kung provided by Harpending and Wandsinder.[17] In addition, a number of short-term or specialized medical studies of San groups are available to help flesh out the picture of their health.[18]

NUTRITION

In his pioneering and startling quantitative analysis and description of the !Kung economy, Lee kept detailed records of food consumption in one band, weighing food to assess the quantities of various foods eaten and obtaining chemical analyses to assess their nutrient value.[19] He found that wild vegetable foods made up roughly 75 to 80 percent of the food consumed and hunted meat accounted for the remaining 20 to 25 percent. He also found that the !Kung relied primarily on twenty-three species of plant foods representing only a fraction of approximately eighty-five plant species growing in the vicinity that we (and the San) know to be edible. Similarly, they regularly hunted only seventeen species of animals from among the fifty-five species they considered edible. Their diet was thus both highly varied, even eclectic, and surprisingly selective from the larger menu of available species. Although some of their dietary choices appear unappetizing to us, the San contradicted our stereotype of primitive foragers who would eat anything.

Despite the likely underrepresentation of actual food consumed (because it probably left out snacks eaten in the course of foraging), Lee's analysis also suggested that, with the possible exception of the total calories it provided, the !Kung diet was reasonably nutritious. Their diet was notable for the range of wild vegetables and meat consumed and the fact that foods are eaten fresh with a minimum of processing. Several of their vegetable foods compare favorably to all but the most nutritious of modern domestic foods in nutrient quality. The mongongo nuts that are a staple of the !Kung diet rank with peanuts and soybeans in terms of the quality of protein, vitamins, and minerals they contain; several other of their vegetable resources have been found to be rich sources of vitamins.[20]

According to Lee's assessment, !Kung protein intake averaged 93 grams per person per day, of which 34 grams came from animal sources—figures comfortably within recommended daily allowances and well above Third World averages. Similarly, Lee's theoretical calculation of nutrient values of foods consumed suggested that the diet of the !Kung exceeded recommended dietary standards for all minerals and vitamins. Caloric intake, which Lee estimated at 2,140 kilocalories per person per day, was low by our standards but average by Third World standards and, in fact, adequate, according to prevailing scientific standards, for people of small stature and moderate workload.

Tanaka has painted a similar picture of the //Gana San he studied at Kade, describing their vegetable resources as abundant and varied and suggesting that they exercised a high degree of selectivity in the choice of foods —this in an environment where for three hundred days a year there was no standing water and water had to be obtained from melons and tubers. Tanaka estimated that the Kade population averaged 2,000 kilocalories per person per day. He also suggested that individuals in these groups ate 150 to 200 grams of meat a day, even though game was considered particularly scarce in that part of the Kalahari. In a third study, Metz and his coworkers found other groups of San to be adequately nourished on a diet consisting of about 20 percent hunted game and 80 percent gathered vegetables.[21]

Silberbauer suggests that the /Gwi San of the central Kalahari were efficient hunters who could hunt more than they do and who were highly selective in their choice of prey. Silberbauer's account is slightly less sanguine regarding dietary quality. He asserts that the /Gwi diet was "depressed" during some periods and, because of the apparent positive response of the people to vitamin pills, that some water-soluble vitamins may have been marginally deficient in the diet. He suggests that the most common deficiency may have been of fat.

Wilmsen's description is also less optimistic.[22] He reported that the San diet varied markedly with the seasons. He found that caloric intake averaged 2,260 kilocalories per person per day between April and August, but that intake declined substantially (to an unspecified level) between October and January. He also reported that meat intake fluctuated from a high of 220 grams per person per day in June (representing about 40 grams of meat protein) to a low of 15 grams of meat per person per day (representing only 2 to 3 grams of meat protein) in December. But he found that good vegetable sources of protein and minerals were reasonably distributed throughout the year.

With the exception of the reservations expressed by Silberbauer there is, thus, general agreement among all workers that the San diet is theoretically well balanced, providing at least adequate amounts of protein and various vitamins and minerals. The diet of San babies and children also appears to be relatively good. They are nursed for relatively long periods (often several years) and when weaned are placed on a diet of pulp made from a variety of wild vegetable foods that are often relatively good sources of protein, in contrast to the cereal gruels to which neighboring farmers wean their children.[23]

The major controversies about San diet concern not the quality of the diet but quantity and reliability. Lee, for example, argued that his studies, conducted during drought years when many surrounding African farms were failing, indicated that the !Kung diet was not only adequate but reliable. He suggested, in fact, that it was better buffered against crop failure than that of the nearby farmers. Others, however, have remarked that San resources may not be as reliable as Lee has suggested. Harpending and Wandsnider argue that Lee's conclusion may be misleading. They point out that the growth of the edible portions of plants favored by the !Kung and the ease with which they can be located may actually be assisted by drought conditions. The plants they eat put more of their growth into edible portions during a drought and may produce less edible material during the rainy season. The rains also foster growth of grasses that may obscure visible clues to the buried roots that the !Kung eat. Hence, the !Kung diet appeared sound during a drought but would be more seriously threatened in a wet year. Also in contrast to Lee, Silberbauer reports some history of famine among

/Gwi associated with periods of severe drought in the central Kalahari. Lorna Marshall suggests that food-related anxiety is widespread among the !Kung of Nyae Nyae, although she herself concludes that food of one sort or another is generally available.

A similar controversy surrounds interpretation of the relatively small caloric intake that is common to the groups studied. Several workers have argued that the low caloric intake is a matter of cultural choice, not a lack of food. Lee pointed to both the high selectivity of Dobe !Kung diet and the fact that lots of food went to waste as evidence that the low caloric intake was voluntary. He concluded, essentially, that the !Kung were not lacking calories, but rather that our standards for caloric intake were unrealistically high. Howell further asserts that the caloric intake is not restricted by limits on food potentially available in the !Kung environment or by any limits on !Kung ability to obtain food.[24] Rather, in her estimation the low intake is a cultural choice expressed in lack of attention to food preparation. Tanaka also emphasized specifically that the //Gana San were not scraping by on the brink of starvation. Like Lee, he argued that the observed caloric intake of the //Gana San exceeded calculated nutrient requirements for people of their small size and moderate work habits. Marshall has the impression that food of one sort or another was generally sufficient for the group—even if not sufficient for them to get fat.

Others working with the !Kung have been less sanguine in their interpretation of low caloric intake, suggesting that hunger is common among the San, as is seasonal loss of weight in periods of relative scarcity. Silberbauer noted that at the beginning of the summer the /Gwi San diet was only marginally adequate, producing complaints of hunger and thirst and some weight loss. Recent comparative observations suggest that the San appear far leaner than other foragers. Hausman and Wilmsen have suggested that seasonal variations in food supply were sufficiently severe to promote weight loss among the San, as have Harpending and Wandsnider. Blurton-Jones and Sibley suggest that heat may limit San foraging at some times of the year.[25]

Lee suggests that seasonal weight loss averaging 600 grams (about 1.3 pounds) is observed among Dobe !Kung; Wilmsen observed seasonal weight loss closer to 2 kilograms (4.4 pounds) representing about 6 percent of body weight. Howell has noted that the growth of !Kung children is seasonally slowed by reduced food intake, although she notes that children ordinarily do not actually lose weight seasonally. Howell has also observed that there is little evidence of mortality resulting from food shortages among the !Kung.

The low caloric intake of the San may be associated with their small size. !Kung males living as hunter-gatherers average 162 centimeters (about 5 feet, 4 inches) and females 148 centimeters (about 4 feet, 10 inches). Their children are relatively large at birth (suggesting good nutrition in utero) and maintain normal patterns of growth through the period of nursing but commonly fall behind Western patterns of growth after weaning. There is evidence that children grow more steadily in the period after weaning and achieve greater stature on the richer diets of the cattle stations.[26]

In contrast, Lee has pointed out that there are few negative health effects of the !Kung diet, which though poor in calories is rich in all other nutrients;[27] the various observers agree that, at the cattle posts where San children grow more rapidly to taller statures, they are also more likely to display clinical signs of qualitative malnutrition than are those at the hunting and gathering camps, apparently because they sacrifice dietary quality while obtaining more calories.

MEDICAL STUDIES OF NUTRITIONAL STATUS

The general picture of good nutritional quality can be confirmed—and some of the controversy about dietary quantity and reliability resolved—by reference to medical studies that have been undertaken on various groups of San.

As part of the overall research strategy at Dobe, Lee invited a medical team to visit the Dobe !Kung and to check clinically for signs that either confirmed or refuted the dietary calculations. Truswell and Hansen, the team who visited the !Kung in 1967 and 1968, conducted a variety of tests, including physical exams, urinanalyses, electrocardiograms, and analyses of blood samples.[28] They were ambivalent about the low caloric intake and overall leanness of the group, which displayed low weight-for-height ratios and very small skinfold thickness measures (the latter measuring subcutaneous fat deposits). But they observed no clinical signs or symptoms of serious malnutrition. They saw no manifestations of marasmus or kwashiorkor. Anemia was very rare, and they saw no signs of mineral or vitamin deficiency. They saw no signs of scurvy. (There was one partial exception. They observed craniotabes or incipient rickets secondary to vitamin D deficiency in infants, which they attributed not to dietary deficiency but to excessive protection from exposure to the sun. The condition was found to disappear spontaneously as soon as the infants were exposed to the sun as a normal part of their social maturation.)

In blood tests, measured levels of iron, vitamin B_{12}, and folic acid were all healthy. Total protein in the blood was a reasonably healthy 7.4 grams per 100 milliliters, although the fraction of infection-fighting immunoglobulins was slightly elevated. Serum albumin levels were generally within normal limits at 3.5 to 4 grams per 100 milliliters. Urinary nitrogen and potassium were better than those of healthy control (comparative) populations; calcium, zinc, and copper levels were found to be within normal limits.

Similar results have been reported by other health teams. Studying other !Kung San, Bronte-Stewart and his associates found that signs of protein malnutrition or vitamin deficiency were very rare and that there were no signs of protein deficiency, or kwashiorkor, associated with weaning (elsewhere a common problem in Africa).[29] Metz and coworkers reported the San to show few clinical signs of malnutrition.[30] Robert Hitchcock suggests that signs of malnutrition were rare among nomadic hunting and gathering Kua San but more common in Nata San living sedentary lifestyles around cattle posts, where wild foods were depleted and where they were second-class citizens with regard to access to domestic foods.[31] Even Silberbauer, who expressed reservations about the quality of !Kung diet, saw no clinical signs of vitamin or mineral deficiency.

Philip Tobias reported blood serum protein in three groups of San to be relatively high, averaging 7.9 to 8.2 grams per 100 milliliters, comparable to healthy Western values (and well above values common among black Africans).[32] As with the values reported by Truswell and Hansen, however, a higher proportion of the protein was concentrated in infection-fighting immunoglobulins than is considered ideal among Westerners. Tobias found albumin levels to be low. Metz and his coworkers reported that San in their study had normal serum iron levels.[33]

In sum, observations by several different teams of scientists and in several different San populations living as hunter-gatherers all seem to confirm that qualitative nutritional health is good—and that such hunger as is reported, although it may result in significant seasonal undernutrition and weight loss and substandard skinfold measurement, is not associated with other clinical symptoms of malnutrition.

Truswell and Hansen did report that the Dobe !Kung appeared to have relatively low serum sodium and that they had low urinary phosphorous levels, the latter a "deficiency" that they attributed to low cereal intake and to which they attributed no significance for health. Silberbauer also reported low sodium intake for the /Gwi San in combination with relatively high levels of potassium, resulting from the high percentage of potassium in certain fresh vegetables consumed, as well as from potassium in wood ash accidentally consumed with cooked foods. He noted also that the taste for salt was much lower than among Europeans and that this reduced desire might be an advantage in water-poor environments.[34]

One of the disadvantages of the eclectic San diet may be a relatively high rate of sporadic reactions to toxic qualities of the foods eaten. Nurse and Jenkins report studies of liver enzymes suggesting that the San and other hunger-gatherers may be more highly selected for efficient detoxification of items in the diet than are their neighbors, since they display uncommonly high levels of a rapidly acting form of an enzyme, liver acetyltransferase, which functions in detoxification.[35] The same enzyme also accelerates the production of glucose, however, and may be nothing more than an adaptation to a diet in which carbohydrates are not otherwise easily obtained.

Various authorities have also reported that the !Kung and other San appeared little affected by several common modern health problems.[36] Diabetes mellitus does not occur, although some San showed irregular reactions to glucose tests, suggesting that they might display diabetic symptoms if placed on a diet rich in fats and sugars. High blood pressure (or progressive increase in blood pressure throughout life, which until recently we took for granted as a natural phenomenon) does not occur among the !Kung or the San at Kade. The !Kung diet, focused on vegetables and lean meat of wild animals, also appears to supply relatively little saturated fat and lead to little buildup of excess cholesterol. Measured levels of serum lipids and cholesterol were low.

Coronary heart disease appeared scarce or absent. According to Truswell and Hansen, the !Kung reported no angina and no memory of sudden death of the type associated with heart attack; Singer also reports that angina, cardiac abnormalities, and heart attack are rare but not unknown among San. The !Kung do, however, display mitral valvular disease, a rheumatic condition presumably secondary to streptococcal infection. Varicose veins, hemorrhoids, and hiatal hernia were also relatively scarce or absent among the !Kung. The !Kung did not display the general decline with age in visual acuity that is common in more civilized society, although cataracts, injuries, and the sequelae of infection took their toll on eyesight. The !Kung were found to experience no hearing loss with age—a function, at least in part, of the absence of loud noises in their environment.

The !Kung do have their own culturally promoted medical stresses, which result from bad habits: individuals older than sixty commonly display bronchitis and emphysema, probably as a result of their habitual heavy smoking.

One side effect of the coarse diet is that the !Kung display few dental caries but are prone to extreme toothwear, particularly at advanced ages, and may literally outlive their teeth, not from decay but from abrasion. A further consequence of the extremely high-bulk diet is the challenge to the physical capacity of the gut, particularly in children. The diet produces characteristically distended bellies, which reflect high gut volume not malnutrition, as such distension often implies when combined with other symptoms. The high-bulk diet presumably protects the !Kung and other San against diseases associated with constipation and long transit time in the gut.

INFECTION

The !Kung record of infectious disease is more complicated and more difficult than nutritional status to interpret because of their level of contact with outsiders. When tested, their blood samples show antibodies to a series of local arbovirus infections, including Sindbis, West Nile, and Wesselbron fevers. These diseases, part of a world network of related infections that circulate commonly among wild animals and birds through the action of mosquito vectors, are presumably ubiquitous features of the natural environment to which hunter-gatherers would naturally be exposed. These diseases, however, appear to vary in importance with climate. San populations have been found to have higher antibody rates to such arboviruses in better watered regions but relatively low rates in the desert interior.[37]

Both rabies and toxoplasmosis are encountered from interaction with wild animals, although both appear to be more severe problems among sedentary groups because human refuse tends to attract the canids and felids that transmit the disease. Trachoma and streptococcal infection (with its secondary rheumatic manifestations) were observed among !Kung and other San and may reflect ancient indigenous health problems.[38]

Various studies have found the !Kung and other San to be relatively free from a range of intestinal worm parasites, either because their small numbers, hygienic habits, and frequent movements tended to discourage the parasite or because the dryness of the Kalahari sands was not conducive to the survival and transmission of soil-dependent parasites.[39] Ascarid worms and other fecally transmitted worms common to more sedentary populations of the region have generally not been found in nomadic San populations. Truswell and Hansen found, somewhat surprisingly, that the !Kung did suffer from the hookworm Necator (but not from Strongyloides); in no case was the infection sufficient to reduce iron or vitamin B_{12} to levels inducing anemia, the chief danger of hookworm infestation.

Presumably because they keep no animals, the !Kung and other San have generally been found free of tapeworms and hydatid disease, which most commonly cycle between human beings and their domestic herds and flocks. There is little evidence of schistosomiasis among the !Kung or other San, although in this instance freedom from disease presumably reflects the dry habitat as much or more than San habits. In addition, although approximately 40 percent of !Kung display eosinophilia (elevated levels of eosino-phils—white blood cells characteristic of parasite infestation), the levels encountered generally suggested mild infestation.[40]

Various groups of San do display a range of intestinal bacteria and proto-zoa similar to those of other rural Africans (such organisms as chilomastix, iodamoeba, endolimax, and entameba). The San from Kade are reported to eat meat at levels of decay that would horrify a European, and such consump-tion is a likely source of intestinal infection. But the instance of diarrhea or stomachache associated with such consumption, as reported by Tanaka, is quite low. In fact, all observers of the San suggest that gastroenteritis, par-ticularly infantile and juvenile gastroenteritis, a common cause of infant and juvenile mortality elsewhere in the Third World, was rare among San popu-lations. Howell does report that "stomach troubles," presumably reflecting such infection, are implicated in a small number of childhood deaths among the Dobe !Kung.

Tuberculosis was found by Truswell and Hansen and by Howell to be common and a significant cause of death among the !Kung; it is reported as well among the San from Kade. But this is almost certainly a disease that, if not entirely new, is more severe in recent times than in the historic or prehistoric past.[41] In addition, both falciparum and vivax malaria occur and contribute significantly to mortality among the !Kung at Dobe. Neither was found at Kade (which is drier), and other studies have found that the incidence of malaria among San varies with proximity to standing water.[42] Confinement to drier portions of the desert may actually help reduce the risk and burden of malaria. The San do not display significant frequencies of the sickle cell trait or any other genetic adaptation to falciparum malaria. The San also have high frequencies of a blood variant of the Duffy blood group (another classification like the ABO classification) that is relatively susceptible to infection by vivax malaria. San genetics suggest, therefore, that neither falciparum nor vivax malaria have long been a significant factor in their environments.[43]

Recent epidemics of smallpox and measles were suspected among the !Kung at Dobe, and both colds and influenza were observed, presumably reflecting their contact with larger and more sedentary groups. Epidemics of rubella, mumps, and chicken pox had recently missed the Dobe population entirely. However, Silberbauer reported that, even in the central Kalahari, isolation was not sufficient to protect groups from all epidemics. He noted that a 1950 epidemic of smallpox did, in fact, reach the /Gwi, as did the influenza pandemic of 1918 and other waves of smallpox and measles of the nineteenth and twentieth centuries. At the same time he noted that the small group size and isolation tend to limit the spread of influenza, colds, and anthrax, and he reports that the 1950 smallpox epidemic did not reach all San groups. Pneumonia (as a result of infection by an unspecified agent) is reported among San groups.[44]

Gonorrhea, although present at Dobe, was considered by Truswell and Hansen to be a recent introduction; in fact, it was not found at Kade. Venereal syphilis also did not occur at Kade, but nonvenereal syphilis or yaws did occur in children of the population.[45]

PATTERNS OF BIRTH AND DEATH AMONG SAN POPULATIONS

By all accounts, San women produce relatively few babies (averaging a little more than 4 per woman) and produce them at relatively widely spaced intervals (averaging three to four years between children). Some observers attribute this pattern to widespread infanticide. Marshall, for example, says that !Kung women, who give birth in seclusion away from camp, may simply prevent a baby from ever drawing a breath.[46] And all observers agree that infanticide is an acceptable means of birth control among San that is practiced at least occasionally. In an economy that places a high premium on mobility and female economic contribution, and in which substitutes for mothers' milk, even if nutritious, are costly to prepare, a child that arrives too soon after the birth of a surviving older sibling poses a problem. It places a heavy burden on the mother and can endanger the survival of the older sibling.[47] It is clear from all accounts that infanticide plays some role in maintaining ideal spacing of children.

Yet, it now seems likely that early observers may have significantly overestimated the frequency and importance of infanticide because they noted the absence of other forms of birth control and presumed that natural primitive fertility would have been very high. We now know of several physiological mechanisms that may be capable of producing low fertility and wide birth spacing; in addition, a great deal of evidence indicates that the fertility of various San groups (as well as of some other hunter-gatherers) is relatively low, suggesting that infanticide may have been less common than once assumed.

Howell has conducted the most thorough research in San fertility, working with the !Kung of the Dobe area;[48] she reports very low fertility for the group, despite a relatively low rate of recorded infanticide (6 cases in 500 live births or 1.2 percent), the absence of other artificial means of birth control or abortion, and the avowed desire of the !Kung to make babies faster than they were able. Howell found that the Dobe !Kung women reached menarche at a relatively late average age of sixteen to seventeen and, despite early marriage and the absence of contraception, had their first child at an average age of nineteen. The average age of women at the birth of their last child was only thirty-four years; hence, a typical woman enjoyed a total period of fertility of only fourteen to fifteen years. During this period, women had births apparently naturally spaced at intervals of three to four years associated with frequent amenorrhea (absence of menstrual cycles). Older women appear to have had an average interval of 49 months between births; current patterns of births were somewhat more narrowly spaced, averaging 35.4 months between births. Howell estimated the completed or total fertility of women (that is, the average number of live births to a woman living long enough to complete her fertile period) to be about 4.7 live births. This figure can be compared to an average of more than 10 live births among women of the Hutterites of North America, who practice no contraception, and to an average of 7 for Third World populations without contraception.

Howell's relatively low figure for !Kung reproduction is not unique among San groups; if anything, it is high. Studying fertility in other groups of San, Harpending and Wandsnider saw even lower rates: 4.03 and 4.08 live births per mother in two groups, one sedentary and one mobile (although these figures are low partly because they counted children only from the third day of life, by which time some mortality, natural or cultural, would have reduced numbers somewhat). Hitchcock found that mobile Kua San women averaged 4.2 live births, whereas a more settled group of Nata San averaged 5.7 live births.

The reasons for this low fertility are in dispute. Howell notes that venereal disease recently introduced by contact with other African populations contributes to the low fertility at Dobe, but she argues that it does not account for the observed pattern. This is supported by Hitchcock, who reports venereal disease as more common in the settled Nata population that displays the higher fertility of his two samples. Howell herself argues in favor of the "critical fat" hypothesis proposed by Rose Frisch (discussed in chapter 5). She suggests that the leanness of !Kung women may account for late menarche and a relatively long interval between births. She notes that lean !Kung women did, in fact, have longer birth intervals than their relatively fatter counterparts. Hausman and Wilmsen provide supporting evidence for this view and argue that the !Kung living traditional lifestyles show a seasonal peak of births resulting from a tendency for conception to occur in periods of dietary abundance.[49] They note that the !Kung who become sedentary are fatter and show less seasonal weight fluctuation, which results in higher fertility and shorter birth intervals. Recent literature has suggested that seasonal fluctuations in caloric intake and fat level rather than low levels per se may restrict fertility.[50]

Lee, as well as Konner and Worthman, have suggested that prolonged nursing on demand, as practiced by the !Kung, accounts for low fertility.[51] Their studies suggest that !Kung women nurse their babies twenty-four hours a day on demand, the children nursing with a frequency that would horrify most breast-feeding Western women. The pattern continues until age four with relatively little supplementary food being provided. As possible support for this hypothesis, Hitchcock observed that the sedentary Nata San group he studied, which had relatively high fertility, nursed less often and weaned earlier than the more mobile Kua population.

A third possibility, recently suggested by Bentley, is that the workload of the women itself prevents conception, much in the manner that athletics seems to lower the fertility of Western females and cause irregular cycles.[52] Seemingly contradictory to all of these theories is the observation by Harpending and Wandsnider that San in their study who moved to cattle stations where they were more sedentary, more richly nourished, and fatter and had access to more readily available weaning foods did not become more fertile.

Howell also conducted a thorough analysis of the age structure and patterns of death in the Dobe population, which can be compared to more isolated observations by other workers. The !Kung do not measure age in our sense, so that the ages of individuals had to be estimated using the !Kung's memory of relative order of birth (which they remember with some care) and their memory of outside events that can be dated and placed in relation to the births of particular individuals. Howell's reconstruction of the age distribution of the living Dobe population contrasts with popular expectations about the shortness of primitive life. She found that 17 percent of the !Kung at Dobe were older than 50 and 8.2 percent were in their sixties or greater; a few individuals were in their eighties. Tanaka also encountered individuals at Kade that he considered to be in their sixties and seventies, all of whom were fairly fit. The fitness has two possible meanings. The group that Tanaka observed had moved its camp eleven times for a total distance of 250 kilometers in the seven months he followed them. It is not clear whether the fitness of the elderly he observed represented their athletic way of life or that any individuals less fit simply could not keep up. Silberbauer, in contrast, thought that he encountered few individuals more than 45 years of age.

Various attempts by Howell to estimate the life expectancy of the !Kung at birth—expectancy at age 0 or "e(0)," roughly the average number of years that a newborn baby will survive—resulted in estimates of life expectancy at birth ranging from 30 to 50 years. Of these she accepts a figure of e(0) = 35 as the most probable figure for the immediate past but of e(0) = 30 as the more likely figure for the earlier historic period. Her preference for the lower figure of life expectancy at birth is based on two lines of reasoning—

one convincing, one not so convincing. She makes the assumption that higher figures, which would make the !Kung compare favorably with their more civilized neighbors and with many historical populations, cannot be accurate for a group so removed from Western medicine—an assumption that is not necessarily tenable in light of evidence presented elsewhere in this book. More reasonably, she also argues that, given the observed distribution of deaths, $e(0) = 30$ would best balance observed fertility at levels to explain a nearly stable population. Higher life expectancies at birth would produce a population growing more rapidly than actually observed. Conversely, much lower life expectancy coupled with recorded fertility cannot have been a long-term pattern because it would have resulted in the complete elimination of the population. Working with a more limited sample at Kade, Tanaka estimated life expectancy at birth to be about 40 years.

Using Howell's data and combining them with statistical projections and observations developed by modern demographers in the form of "model life tables" (of Howell's own choosing), it is possible to make some further statements about patterns of !Kung life expectancy that will be helpful for comparison to other populations. Depending on whether one uses figures appropriate for life expectancy at birth of 30, 35, or 50, !Kung life expectancy at age 15 (the number of years on the average that a 15 year old can still expect to live) ranges from 37 to 54 years. Life expectancy at 20 ranges from 34 to 49 years. Life expectancy, of course, can actually be higher after birth than it is at birth itself and, in fact, commonly is. The expectancy statistic averages all deaths, and the relatively high proportion of individuals in all known populations who die as infants and young children means that life expectancy at age one or two, or even age ten, may be higher than that at birth.

Howell observed different rates of infant mortality (death of children before the age of one) in various samples of the Dobe population, ranging from 15 to 21 percent (more commonly expressed as 150 to 210 per 1,000). She noted that approximately 60 to 70 percent of children born survived to age 10 and that essentially the same 60 to 70 percent survived to age 20. She also observed that the frequency of infant deaths depended somewhat on the nutritional status of the mother, being more common for leaner mothers than for fatter mothers; she noted that the rate of infant mortality depended also on location, being more common among women living on the cattle posts than those living in the bush (that is, those living the more conservative hunter-gatherer lifestyle). Whereas thin cattle-post women had 24 percent infant mortality, fat cattle-post women had 15 percent; thin bush women had 13 percent infant mortality, whereas fatter bush women had none. She also reported that 550 pregnancies recorded ended in only 500 births, implying that about one pregnancy in 11 ended in miscarriage or stillbirth (or infanticide). She also noted that the death of the mother in childbirth was relatively rare, a pattern attributable in part to the absence of puerperal fever, an infection commonly complicating the process of birth in more civilized communities.

At Kade, Tanaka estimated that 15 percent of children died before the age of 5 and that of those reaching age 5 a further 15 percent died by age 10, such that 28 percent of those born were dead by age 10. Silberbauer observed an even lower rate (7 percent) of child mortality (defined as failure to reach marriageable age). Some anecdotal observations may suggest higher rates of infant or child mortality.

Like Howell, Hitchcock found that infant mortality rates were higher in a sedentary (Nata) San group than among a mobile (Kua) San population. Harpending and Wandsnider have, however, found the opposite pattern. Comparing nomadic and sedentary groups of !Kung relying on hunting and gathering and on cattle-post economy, respectively, they found that infant mortality rates were about 6 percent (60 per thousand) in the sedentary sample but about 12 percent (120 per thousand) in the sample with a higher proportion of mobile hunter-gatherers. They attribute the higher rate of infant mortality among the nomads in part to the problem of encountering new variants of disease organisms through travel discussed in chapter 4. Harpending has also suggested that the lower mortality of the San associated with sedentary cattle posts might relate to occasional availability of medical attention and antibiotics but is more likely to be a function of the regular availability of cows' milk in such settlements. Harpending and Wandsnider also suggest that, among the more nomadic of their samples, prereproductive mortality (the percentage of liveborn children who fail to reach reproductive age) was about 34 percent.[53]

All of these estimates of life expectancy figures must be considered in light of the fact that Howell considers 70 to 80 percent of observed deaths among the !Kung to be related to infectious disease, much of it to such diseases as tuberculosis and malaria, which are almost certainly more serious in the recent past than they were earlier in history, for the reasons outlined in chapter 4. Silberbauer also observed infectious disease, particularly smallpox, to be a major source of mortality. Howell points out, though, that the increasing risk of death by infection may be offset by the availability of cattle posts to relieve the stresses associated with more chronic diseases by providing respite from travel.

Howell suggests that an additional 10 to 15 percent of deaths among the

!Kung are caused by accidents, trauma, and violence. Lee argues that there is not a high risk of attack by wild animals and that women who do not hunt, in particular, are not at much risk of animal-related injuries. Falls from trees and fire can be causes of death, the latter particularly a danger to small children. Interpersonal violence contributes relatively little to the total death rate. Yet, the !Kung are not nonviolent. If the number of deaths by violence, as reported by Lee, is adjusted for the size of the populations in question, the !Kung rival civilized populations in the frequency with which they commit homicide. Howell also reports one individual at Dobe who would have died by exposure to his own arrow poison had the anthropologists not transported him rapidly to a regional hospital. Tanaka reported accidents and animal bites as significant causes of mortality at Kade and noted that fire was an important problem. Three of the deaths that he witnessed were associated with accidental burns to young children around campfires. Silberbauer also considered periodic drought and dehydration a cause of some mortality in the desert interior.

Howell suggests that only 8 to 10 percent of !Kung deaths are associated with cardiovascular diseases and cancers and suggests that these rates are low in comparison to Western populations, even when the comparisons are corrected for differences in age at death and for the relative importance of other causes of death.

Comparing the Health of the San to Other Band Societies and Other Modern and Historic Populations

DIETARY QUALITY

The dietary quality of the San (that is, balanced intake of protein, vitamins, and minerals) appears to be only average or below average among hunting and gathering populations, even though it is excellent by contemporary Third World standards. Descriptions of the diets of hunter-gatherers fairly uniformly report a relatively high intake of animal products. In fact, most appear to get substantially more meat than the San. Meat intakes of 100 to 200 grams or more (a quarter to a half pound) per person per day appear to be the rule among hunting and gathering groups whose dietary intake has been measured.[54]

Other desert-living populations, like the San, may obtain only moderate amounts of meat, particularly if large game are scarce.[55] In addition, tropical hunter-gatherers probably have a smaller proportion of meat in their diets than do their counterparts in temperate, subarctic, and arctic regions. As one moves away from the equator the relative proportions of edible plants and animals in the environment shifts, permitting—and ultimately forcing —human groups to rely more heavily on hunting.[56]

In addition, for unclear reasons (climate, depletion of game, legal restrictions, or their own poor technique) the San are comparatively inefficient as hunters, obtaining only a fraction as much meat per hour of hunting as many other groups.[57] But the San do not trade the meat they get. Many contemporary hunter-gatherers—the Birhor of India,[58] African pygmies,[59] or the Agta and Batek of the Philippines[60]—obtain comparatively large amounts of meat but then trade it away. In the Philippines, a population of eight hundred Agta hunters supplies several thousand farmers with meat (trading away about 80 percent of its catch) and consumes an average of only 6 grams of animal protein per person per day.[61]

The diet of the San (and of most other contemporary hunter-gatherers) almost certainly contains less meat than that of our historic and prehistoric forebears. The historic decline in large game, human movement into game-poor environments, and the resulting decline in hunting efficiency would have forced contemporary groups to place increased reliance on vegetable foods. Although proximity to farmers' fields where animals like to graze may occasionally help restore the population of game, in most cases there is little reason to believe that trade with other groups or the proximity of settlements helps hunter-gatherers obtain animal foods or protein.[62]

Such comparisons aside, the most important point is that, as a rule, levels of meat intake reported for most hunter-gatherer groups are comparable to intake by relatively affluent modern Western populations. They are substantially better than average Third World intake and dramatically better than that of the contemporary Third World poor, who may average only a few grams of animal foods per person per day.[63]

A wide range of reports about contemporary hunter-gatherers in various parts of the world suggests that they, like the San, eat eclectic diets of fresh vegetable foods that, along with their meat intake, tend to assure a good balance of vitamins and minerals.[64] These observations about dietary balance are largely confirmed by reports and observations on hunter-gatherer nutritional health. Most evaluations of serum levels of iron and protein (with measurement of the albumin fraction) in different populations suggest that levels are healthy, although it is common for these populations to display high levels of infection-fighting proteins (immunoglobulins) in proportion to serum albumin.[65]

Most casual descriptions of hunter-gatherer groups in tropical or temperate latitudes comment on their apparent vitality and the absence of obvious malnutrition.[66] There are some reports of vitamin A or C deficiencies and of anemia, but in most populations reported symptoms are mild and rare in comparison to those reported for many Third World populations.[67] In some instances authors infer slight qualitative malnutrition from marginal signs, and in some they report possible malnutrition on the basis of what now appears to be a misunderstanding of symptoms.[68] Reports of acute malnutrition or kwashiorkor are extremely rare. These descriptions present a striking contrast to descriptions and evaluations of many Third World populations and to descriptions of historic dietary quality for the lower classes in Europe.[69]

The major exception to the observations of dietary balance among tropical and temperate groups appear to be populations that suffer high rates of intestinal parasites, the Pygmies of the central African rain forest and (to a lesser extent) other rain forest populations, who often have good dietary intake but appear to lose large portions of their nutrients to their own parasites after ingestion.[70] But the risk of such loss appears to increase as the groups become larger and more sedentary, or more intimately associated with farming settlements.

It is fairly clear from almost all reports, moreover, that the quality of hunter-gatherer diets is eroded rather than supplemented by trade networks and outposts of civilization. Most descriptions of trade indicate that hunter-gatherers trade protein and variety for calories; most descriptions of attempts to force hunter-gatherers to settle suggest that dietary quality falls off markedly.[71]

Dietary analyses of isolated groups of subsistence farmers, such as those of the Amazon, who live at low population densities and maintain some mobility and ability to forage for wild resources, document that they often enjoy well-balanced diets. But many suffer from high rates of parasitism and secondary loss of nutrients.[72] Subsistence farmers like those of highland New Guinea, living at higher population densities and forced to rely heavily on such starchy crops as sweet potatoes for their subsistence, may suffer more malnutrition.[73]

The dietary regimes of such populations at high latitude as the Eskimos are necessarily far more restricted in their variety by the lack of edible plant foods, but even these groups can obtain appropriate vitamin and mineral balance in normal times by proper and sophisticated use of animal resources and the few vegetables available. Observers suggest that the quality of the Eskimo diet, once surprisingly well balanced, has declined since contact.[74] Surprisingly, for example, scurvy was not a common problem among Eskimos, even though it plagued early European arctic explorers. Calcium deficiency was a potential threat related to low calcium intake but also to lack of sunlight (and consequent poor production of vitamin D) for much of the year. Some anemia associated with low iron intake or secondary loss to parasites has been reported.[75] The biggest problem in the Arctic may have been that specific nutrients (like food itself) were not available at all times and places, so that loss of mobility could rapidly result in specific deficiencies.[76]

DIETARY QUANTITY

The adequacy of caloric intake among hunter-gatherers is somewhat more controversial. As noted in chapter 5, hunter-gather diets that are otherwise well balanced can be poor in calories because wild game is lean, wild vegetable foods often contain a very high proportion of bulk or roughage, and concentrated packages of calories—such as honey—are rare in the wild.

San caloric intake, particularly according to the more pessimistic estimates, is probably below average by hunter-gatherer standards and is certainly low by the standards of hunter-gatherers living in richer environments. The Hadza of Tanzania, who live in the kind of savanna that our ancestors preferred, are estimated to take in more than 3,000 kilocalories per person per day.[77] Other measures of caloric intake are usually on the order of about 2,000 kilocalories or more (often substantially more).[78] Where intake is not measured, most descriptions suggest that caloric intake is usually adequate, if not rich.[79] In some instances in which reported caloric intake appeared to be below the recommended daily allowance (RDA), the authors added disclaimers noting that people did not appear to be hungry and had passed up chances to obtain more food.[80]

The San, partly because of their inefficiency as hunters, display poor overall caloric returns for labor compared to other hunter-gatherers. Estimates of foraging efficiency for other hunting and gathering populations often suggest substantially higher returns for labor.[81] The only hunter-gatherer populations who do less well are populations that inhabit extremely dry desert conditions.[82]

It is not clear whether proximity to other societies and involvement in trade networks improve or reduce the caloric efficiency of most hunter-gatherers. Trading scarce meat for more plentiful agricultural produce may improve overall caloric returns, and some reports suggest that traded foods may help hunter-gatherers get through lean seasons.[83] Some observers have argued that, in locations like the central African rain forest, hunting and gathering might not be possible without caloric supplementation by traded foods. Some reports suggest that the proximity of farmed fields helps increase the supply of hunted game.[84] But the desire to trade for nonfood items and the disadvantageous terms of trade also appears to drain the food supply of some populations.[85] Perhaps most important, trade relationships

force hunter-gatherers to be relatively sedentary, leading to local depletion of larger game and a marked decline in the hunters' own efficiency.[86]
In addition, proximity to larger settlements reinforces legal restrictions on
hunting.

The lowest measured caloric intake I have seen for a hunter-gatherer
group, just over 1,500 kilocalories per person per day, was reported for
the Birhor of India, who hunted in an area recently depleted of game, in
which large game hunting was restricted and hunted produce was traded for
cultivated rice in village markets.[87]

As a group, contemporary hunting and gathering populations may not be
affluent in terms of caloric intake, but they are clearly average or better by
world standards. Estimates of average caloric intake for many contemporary
Third World countries, including India and China, hover around 2,000 kilocalories per person per day,[88] and estimated caloric intake among the poor
throughout the world even in normal times is often substantially below 2,000
kilocalories per day—sometimes substantially lower than 1,500 kilocalories
per person per day.[89]

In sum, hunter-gatherers, among whom the San are a relatively impoverished example, appear to be conspicuously well nourished in qualitative
terms and at least adequately nourished in quantitative terms by the standards of the contemporary Third World. At the same time, the caloric efficiency and intake of the San and other contemporary hunter-gatherers are
almost certainly low by historic and prehistoric standards for hunting and
gathering populations in choice environments where large game were still
plentiful (for reasons discussed in the last chapter).

THE RELIABILITY OF HUNTER-GATHERER DIETS

The likelihood of hunger and starvation appears to vary widely among
hunting and gathering groups, depending primarily on the environment they
inhabit. The Hadza of the African savannas—one hunter-gatherer group
that is not in a marginal environment—have never been observed to go
hungry in a serious way, except when they agree to go to the government
reservation and the food truck does not come. Otherwise, their concept of
hunger refers to days in which they must eat more vegetables and less meat
than they would like. A recent survey of their resources seems to suggest
that the simultaneous failure of all resources is very unlikely.[90] Most reports
of hunter-gatherer subsistence I have seen from other parts of the world also
indicate that food supplies are usually abundant and reliable.[91]

Many descriptions of hunting and gathering groups, however, do report
that seasonal hunger and food anxiety occur, as does occasional starva-

tion.[92] But hunter-gatherers may not be exceptional in this respect. There is little evidence that hunter-gatherers suffer disproportionate risk of hunger or starvation in comparison to more settled groups inhabiting similar environments. It is not clear, for example, whether weight loss was more common or more severe among the San than that widely reported among farmers elsewhere in Africa. (Seasonal weight loss is, in fact, fairly common elsewhere in Africa among more civilized groups.) The Herero herders neighboring the !Kung display a slightly smaller seasonal loss (500 grams). Other African populations display equal or larger losses (although weight loss may be less threatening to populations that are fatter to begin with).[93] Nurse and Jenkins suggest that seasonal hunger among the San is moderate compared to the more severe seasonal deprivation of many African farmers.[94] The Hadza have been observed to show smaller seasonal weight loss than their neighbors.[95] One cross-cultural survey of hunger and starvation found little difference in frequency between hunter-gatherers and farmers and suggested, if anything, that hunter-gatherers as a group had the advantage.[96]

Moreover, for most of the world civilized state apparatus has not protected populations significantly against hunger or even famine. The recent histories of India,[97] Russia,[98] China,[99] France, and much of the rest of Europe at least until the nineteenth century[100] display a record of frequent and severe famine that is not exceeded or even matched in simpler societies, much of the famine being attributed not to climate but to the failure of—and even burden imposed by—central administrative mechanisms.[101,102]

What does increase the risk of seasonal hunger and starvation—for both hunter-gatherers and farmers—is the presence of harsh environmental conditions. The risk of hunger is likely to increase with latitude, for example, because the growing season becomes shorter and the range of edible vegetation is reduced. In fact, distribution of hunger episodes reported among hunter-gatherers matches this expectation, increasing in extremely cold and extremely dry locations.[103]

Reports of actual starvation by hunter-gatherers are rare, except for those populations living in regimes so dry or cold that no other human communities (except heavily capitalized and specialized outposts of modern civilization) even attempt to compete for the space. In extreme northern latitudes where edible vegetation is extremely scarce, the problem is complicated by the scarcity or absence of sunlight by which to hunt for several months of the year, and arctic conditions may make foraging of any kind impossible. Under these conditions, famine can be a serious and frequent threat.[104]

In sum, although hunger and occasional starvation are reported among hunter-gatherers who, collectively, do not appear as affluent (or leisured) as once depicted, there is little to suggest that the hunting and gathering way of life (as opposed to the extreme environments in which many such groups find themselves) is more likely than other modes of subsistence to lead to hunger or starvation.

INFECTIOUS DISEASE

Comparative data suggest that the San are among the most fortunate of hunter-gatherers in terms of their parasite load. Desert conditions appear to discourage the transmission of most fecally transmitted parasites.[105] Like the San, other desert-living groups appear to suffer low rates of parasitization.[106] But even in moderately dry environments, such as the African savannas, rates of parasite infestation are higher. The Hadza, for example, seem to have a more cosmopolitan experience with parasites than the San;[107] among rain forest populations (whether in Africa, Southeast Asia, or South America) parasitization is commonly both varied and intense.[108]

Similar considerations appear to apply also to some vector-borne diseases. Malaria is discouraged in deserts because mosquitoes cannot survive, and hunter-gatherers in moister environments are likely to suffer in proportion. Schistosomiasis is an increasing problem in moister climates.

The general effect of increasing latitude is to reduce the parasite burden, at least for those parasites that spend part of their life cycles outside human or other mammalian hosts. Fewer pathogenic organisms and fewer vectors can survive outside a mammalian host in colder climates. Historically, the range of diseases experienced would have diminished as people moved north, just as the burden of disease is higher today in the tropics than in temperate latitudes.[109] But movement to high latitude also has a disadvantage: by focusing the human diet on animal foods, it may intensify infection by meat-borne parasites, particularly if the lack of fuel and other dietary needs require cooking to be minimized. Eskimos, for example, are likely to suffer heavily from trichinosis and tapeworms.[110]

But climatic factors are not the only variables involved. Small group size and mobility do help protect groups from intestinal and vector-born diseases, even in more permissive environments. The Hadza have lower rates of infestation of a number of parasites (including schistosomiasis) than their more sedentary neighbors.[111] Even in the rain forest, parasite transmission is encouraged when groups become larger and more sedentary.[112] Malaria is proportionate to population density and land clearance and has been observed to be less of a problem for hunter-gatherers than farmers in the same environment.[113,114] Among populations in Malaysia, Dunn suggests that farming reduces the range of parasites to which populations are exposed but intensifies the parasite load.[115] He also notes that the highest parasite rates occur among neither hunter-gatherers nor small-scale farmers but urban squatters. In fact, almost all observers throughout the world agree that the burden of infectious disease on hunting and gathering populations has increased since contact with settlements and is substantially increased by resettlement.

In short, hunter-gatherers display patterns of infection that vary markedly with environment, and most environments are more permissive of disease transmission than the Kalahari Desert, where the San live. But as a group, small and mobile hunter-gatherer bands do appear to experience lower rates of infection than their neighbors.

Experience of epidemic diseases among hunter-gatherers is hard to evaluate. Most modern hunter-gatherers are reported to have displayed epidemics of one or more of these diseases, and tests of blood serum for antibodies to reveal an individual's disease history usually suggest that even hunter-gatherer groups display fairly cosmopolitan experience with epidemic diseases.[116] All are in contact in some degree with outposts of civilization, however, so they do not provide a good test of the hypothesis that these diseases could not exist or spread among small isolated groups.

The best tests of isolation as a buffer against the spread of epidemics is probably the work of Francis Black among relatively (but never totally) isolated populations in South America, most of which are larger, horticultural populations. His tests suggest that the epidemic diseases have often appeared but that they do not reach all groups and that they apparently do not survive very long in any one group (since individuals of less than a certain age—born since the last epidemic—have never been exposed). His results suggest (but do not prove) that epidemic viruses (including influenza, parainfluenza, mumps, measles, polio, whooping cough, rubella, tuberculosis, and smallpox) could not have been transmitted continuously (and therefore could not have survived) in a world populated entirely by relatively small groups connected only by foot travelers without large urban systems to provide a reservoir of infection and civilized transportation to move them.[117] The best evidence demonstrating that isolated groups had no prior exposure to epidemic diseases is, however, the devastating effect that exposure to Western colonization appears to have had on those populations.

DEGENERATIVE DISEASES

Comparative study suggests that the relative absence of modern "degenerative" diseases (heart disease, cancers, hypertension, diabetes, bowel disorders) reported among the San is universal (or nearly so) among hunter-gatherers and subsistence farmers alike. Reports from a number of groups suggest that high serum cholesterol is extremely rare in such groups. Blood pressure is commonly low in such groups and does not increase with age,[118] and widespread reports suggest that such intestinal disorders as appendicitis, diverticulosis, and bowel cancer are rare until groups are introduced to civilized diets.[119] Diabetes mellitus is rarely observed—but becomes quite common among such populations introduced to civilized diets.[120] Coronary heart disease and most cancers have been observed to be comparatively rare.[121]

MORTALITY

Obtaining reliable mortality statistics for nonliterate populations that do not keep records or record ages is difficult. Painstaking records must be kept over long periods of time, and few studies rival Howell's in duration or detail. We know surprisingly little about what causes death in such societies, particularly among adults, partly because comparatively few deaths have been observed and partly because most observed deaths have been associated with such epidemic diseases as measles and smallpox, which we suspect are of modern origin.

If one discounts the recent effects of epidemic disease, it is possible to observe a changing distribution of causes of death with latitude. In the tropics, indigenous infections are a significant source of mortality, but by most accounts starvation is rarely a cause of death, and accidents are relatively unimportant. Malaria and other diseases of greater antiquity account for a significant fraction of deaths in some societies.[122] Hunting accidents appear surprisingly unimportant as causes of death. Such accidents as falls, burns, and (more rarely) snakebites are mentioned more frequently.[123] In high latitudes, in contrast, famine and accidental death are significant sources of mortality.[124]

Rates of mortality and life expectancy may be even harder to determine. I have found a number of reports—of varying quality—concerning rates of infant and child mortality in hunting and gathering groups. Infant mortality estimates range from a low of 6 percent (or 60 per 1,000) to a high of nearly 50 percent. But the majority of values cluster between 150 and 250 deaths per 1,000 infants and suggest that Howell's values for the San (200 per 1,000) are about average among hunting and gathering groups.[125] It seems likely that the lowest estimates are missing some births and deaths, because babies who die immediately after birth may never be observed. The highest estimates almost certainly err in the opposite direction. In one case, a high mortality rate is inferred from an extremely small observation,[126] and in one case high infant mortality is inferred from an impossibly high assumed birth rate.[127]

To put the value of 200 deaths per 1,000 infants in perspective it should be noted that contemporary infant mortality rates in affluent countries are on the order of 10 to 12 per 1,000 infants, but historical European and American values particularly in urban areas have commonly matched or exceeded the hunter-gatherer figures, often by substantial amounts. In the United States at the end of the nineteenth century, five major cities (including our national capitol) had official infant mortality rates of 300 per 1,000 or more, and many more exceeded 200 per 1,000.[128] In European history, average national values for infant mortality fell below 200 per 1,000 only late in the nineteenth century.[129] In the Third World, official rates still often hover between 100 and 200 per 1,000.[130] Moreover, such large-scale reports are at least as likely to underestimate mortality as are the more detailed observations anthropologists make on small societies.

In a similar manner, reports on other hunting and gathering populations suggest that the San have only average success if they rear 50 to 65 percent of all babies to adulthood.[131] Once again, though only average for hunter-gatherers, this value indicates reasonable survival by the standards of historic European and American populations and good survival by the standards of cities prior to the twentieth century.[132,133]

Adult ages at death are more difficult to estimate. Some casual observers of hunter-gatherer groups have sometimes reported that they see few elderly people,[134] and others have reported the presence of numbers of active, healthy elderly individuals.[135] In the nineteenth century, for example, Eyre reported that Australian aborigines commonly reached 65 years of age.[136]

But most estimates of adult life expectancy among hunter-gatherers (the average number of years that an individual can expect to live from age fifteen), averaging about 28 years,[137] are below those reported for the San and are very low by our standards. They are also low in proportion to the relative success of hunter-gatherers in rearing children.[138]

In some of these cases, adult life expectancy may benefit from the availability of modern medicine. On the other hand, the available sample is heavily skewed toward populations (such as Eskimo) in extreme environments. In addition, few studies have been as carefully done as Howell's work was. Given the difficulties of age estimation, the studies may be biased by expectations of low life expectancy. More important, some studies may have been done under conditions in which the populations in question were in negative balance between reproduction and death and were becoming extinct. Most studies clearly have been done under conditions where a large proportion of deaths reflect epidemic diseases recently introduced. Such epidemics in virgin populations would have precisely the disproportionate effects on adult mortality that the life expectancy figures suggest. In one instance where records of adult life expectancy have been recorded for a hunting and gathering group (the Aleuts) for more than a century, a clear and dramatic recent reduction of adult life expectancy associated with epidemic diseases has been observed.[139]

Published estimates of life expectancy at birth for hunter-gatherers range from as low as 20 years to as high as 50 years.[140] The Hadza, who may be the best model we have of prehistoric groups, have been estimated like the San to have a life expectancy at birth of about 30 years. If we combine average observed survival of children to age 15 and average life expectancy at age 15 for the various groups, we can estimate an average life expectancy at birth for such groups of 25 to 30 years.[141]

Life expectancy at birth of 20 (which for demographic reasons is the lowest reasonable estimate of average prehistoric hunter-gatherer life expectancy),[142] given the most probable estimates of fertility, would equal or exceed that for some European cities of the eighteenth century and for the poorer portions of other cities of Europe as late as the nineteenth century.[143]

It would also equal life expectancy for all of India as late as 1920 (after more than a century of British colonial rule).[144] Life expectancy at birth of 25 years (a more reasonable long-term estimate of hunter-gatherer survivorship)[145] would approach that for much of Europe as late as the eighteenth and early nineteenth centuries and for many urban European communities well into the nineteenth.[146]

FERTILITY

One of the most controversial questions is whether San fertility of 4 to 5 live births per woman who completes her reproductive period (well below the Third World average for populations not using contraception of 6 to 8)[147] is typical of hunter-gatherers.

Part of the controversy is about whether any or all of the physiological mechanisms thought to limit San fertility naturally are truly effective and whether any or all can be shown to apply to hunter-gatherers as a rule. Observations of hormone levels or the regularity of menstruation in some other hunter-gatherer groups suggest that they also may experience naturally low fertility. Some additional evidence suggesting a physiological limit on fertility among hunter-gatherers is afforded by the widespread observation that mobile groups commonly enjoy increased fertility when they settle down,[148] although whether physiology or birth control choices change is not always clear.

Actual reports on hunter-gatherer fertility in a number of populations most often suggest that 4 to 6 children is the average number ever born or at least the number, living or dead, that can be accounted for. But not all of these reports appear to have been as carefully done as Howell's; not all clearly distinguish physiological and intentional birth spacing or even natural deaths of infants too young to be counted. Some studies, moreover, may be complicated by the recent complication of venereal disease limiting fertility.[149] Many of the studies have been criticized for these reasons.[150]

Several recent reports suggest that hunter-gatherers in some areas can enjoy substantially higher fertility, approaching Third World averages.[151] Particularly of note are the values of 7.8 live births reported for the Ache of the Paraguay[152] (a value that represents at least a 10 percent increase in the recent past, associated with sedentism) and of 6.5 live births for the Agta of the Philippines,[153] a society in which women engage in the same range of hunting activities as men, often even when pregnant. These figures raise questions about the assumption that inherent physiological mechanisms common to the hunter-gatherer way of life automatically curtail fertility, but they leave open the possibility that some combination of circumstances may tend to reduce average fertility in such groups. Whether hunter-gatherer fertility is naturally low, and if so why, is still widely debated.[154]

Whether hunter-gatherers of the past—who were active and mobile, who must have nursed their young intensively, who experienced seasonal weight fluctuations, but who otherwise were probably better nourished than their modern counterparts—were also relatively infertile is unresolved.[155]

These studies of contemporary groups suggest that hunter-gatherers enjoy low or at best average fertility among human groups and that average rates of observed child production in these groups are low. The assumption that primitive people are more fertile than civilized ones is a popular one, but it is completely unsupported by scientific observation even though it occasionally sneaks into the scientific literature.[156] The data suggest that, whether or not hunter-gatherer fertility is restrained in part or whole by physiological mechanisms, members of these groups are quite capable of limiting family size by cultural means (birth control, abortion, and infanticide) and are apparently motivated to do so. Some pattern of natural or cultural birth spacing to limit family size to four to six children is a common, though not universal, hunter-gatherer practice and could well have been the practice of prehistoric groups.

Summary

Contemporary hunter-gatherers appear to be relatively well-nourished by current Third World standards, in qualitative terms enjoying high protein intake and good dietary variety and displaying only relatively rare and mild signs of qualitative malnutrition. The adequacy of their caloric intake is less certain. Caloric intake is low by affluent modern standards but usually at least average by modern Third World standards. Hunger and food anxiety occur, but extreme hunger and starvation are common only in extreme environments. There is reason to believe, moreover, that prehistoric hunter-gatherers in choice environments with more game available would have fared better than their modern counterparts.

Rates of infection vary markedly from place to place among hunter-gatherers, but small group size and mobility appear to mitigate parasite burdens. Contemporary groups are partially though not wholly isolated from epidemics, but there are indications that relatively small and isolated prehistoric communities alone could not have maintained epidemic diseases.

Hunter-gatherers appear to be reasonably successful by historical standards in rearing their infants and children to adulthood. Adult life expectancies appear very low in proportion but may be distorted by problems of age estimation and by the conditions of recent contact with civilization. Overall life expectancies, although low by our standards, do not compare as unfavorably with historic and Third World populations as we commonly believe. Observed family size clearly refutes assumptions about high primitive fertility and suggests, if anything, that some combination of natural and cultural birth spacing keeps reproductive rates below modern Third World averages.

Chapter 7

The Evidence of Prehistoric Skeletons

Human skeletal remains from archaeological sites provide additional, direct evidence about health and disease in ancient populations. For our purposes, in fact, using skeletal samples has several advantages over the analysis of contemporary hunting and gathering populations. The skeletons testify directly about the state of health of actual prehistoric groups, rather than about the health of small-scale contemporary societies in which health may be significantly altered by interaction with modern civilizations. In addition, skeletal evidence is available from many parts of the world that hunting and gathering societies no longer inhabit. In particular, archaeological evidence of prehistoric hunter-gatherers is available in temperate latitudes and in areas of rich soil and organic growth from which contemporary hunter-gatherers have almost entirely been displaced. It is hard to compare contemporary hunter-gatherers and other groups because they occupy different environments; but the use of skeletal materials from archaeological sites permits us to make fairly direct comparison of populations that differ in size and economy but have occupied the same or similar environments at different times—sometimes even living one after the other at the same village site.

Archaeological evidence also has its drawbacks, however. Like all archaeological evidence, skeletons may be scattered and hard to find. Like all prehistoric organic remains, they may be poorly preserved and incompletely recovered. In fact, the farther back one goes in time (or the smaller and more mobile the group being studied), the poorer preservation and recovery are likely to be. Most hunter-gatherers discussed in this chapter—especially those for which large sample sizes are reported—are larger, more settled populations than those described in chapter 6, even though they are commonly smaller and more mobile than their more civilized successors.[1] The best samples are from sedentary hunter-gatherers in large, socially complex aggregates who were manipulating staple plant species and may even have been involved in incipient cultivation.

There is also a geographical bias to the distribution of archaeological populations. Good series of archaeological skeletons spanning either the transition from hunting and gathering to fully developed intensive agriculture or the emergence of large political units are available for several regions of North America, particularly in the American Midwest and the southeastern states. Fewer good sequences are available from Europe and the Middle East, and fewer still from Asia, Africa, and South America.[2] To some extent, these biases represent differences in the quality of natural preservation, but they primarily represent differences in the attention paid to skeletal materials by archaeologists. Unfortunately, well-studied samples are often lacking from some of the earliest and best-known centers of civilization, many of which were excavated before there was serious interest in the analysis of comparative health.

Like all archaeological evidence, skeletons may provide only a selected sample of the population they represent—a sample biased by the rules of a given society about the proper treatment of the dead. A society may omit or underrepresent individuals of a certain age or sex in a cemetery. Infants are often left out; warriors may die at a distant place. One social class, but not another, may be represented in the cemetery.

A further drawback in using skeletal material is that, unlike a mummy, which may provide a fairly complete record of health, the skeleton—which is all that is usually recovered—provides only a limited and selected view of the health of the individual. The skeleton records only a fraction of the stresses and illnesses affecting the living individual, as most illness affects only the perishable soft tissues. Other than fractures and wounds to the bone itself, the skeleton primarily reflects chronic or long-term illness, rather than short-term illness. The skeleton rarely displays the immediate cause of death, for example, unless death followed fairly directly from a wound. Skeletal samples may also underrepresent the incidence of certain illnesses in a population because only prolonged or severe cases affect bone. As a result, estimates of the incidence of disease in skeletal populations are more useful for comparison to one another than for direct comparison to rates reported in living groups.[3]

In addition, bones can only respond to illness in a limited number of ways. Different diseases tend to look alike in the skeleton. Diagnosis often has to be inferred from the pattern of bones affected. Specific diagnoses may be impossible, forcing paleopathologists to refer only to broad categories of manifest pathology with uncertain relationships to specific modern diseases.

These problems aside, skeletal samples of reasonable size permit us to draw statistical profiles of health, nutrition, and mortality in different societies that can readily be compared with one another.

The Potential of Skeletal Analysis

1. A number of techniques by which the constituents of prehistoric diets can be identified using only the skeleton are now in use.[4] These techniques supplement more traditional methods of dietary analysis in archaeology, such as the study of food refuse and tools for food preparation. Identification of macroscopic and microscopic patterns of wear on teeth and the analysis of dental caries provide clues to the texture of the diet. High rates of dental caries, for example, are almost invariably associated with soft, sticky diets usually associated with agricultural diets. Rates of caries go up so uniformly with the adoption of agriculture that several scholars have inferred agricultural diets from high caries rates in the absence of confirming food refuse.[5]

In addition, bones and teeth are now fairly routinely analyzed to determine the proportions of such constituent trace elements as strontium, zinc, magnesium, and copper and to determine the proportions of various isotopes of common elements (carbon, nitrogen, strontium) that are thought to act as signatures of the foods eaten.[6] These techniques are becoming instrumental in identifying changes in the proportions of foods consumed—the proportion of meat and vegetable foods in the diet, the proportion of terrestrial and aquatic resources consumed, the relative importance of maize in the diet, and even the proportion of mother's milk to cereal in the diet of a child. The latter may make it possible to identify the average age of weaning in children.[7]

2. A number of techniques now permit us to evaluate the nutritional status of individuals. Several specific dietary deficiencies can be assessed.[8] For example, iron deficiency, which may be primary or secondary to various kinds of infection and parasites, results in anemia. Anemia, in turn, produces characteristic changes in the thin bones of the skull vault and eye sockets. The central marrow cavity filled with porous bone expands, and the outer layers of dense cortical bone become porous, giving a thick and spongy appearance to bone that is normally thin and smooth. The condition is known as porotic hyperostosis when it affects the skull vault and as cribra orbitalia when it affects the eye sockets.[9] As will be evident below, porotic hyper-

ostosis and cribra orbitalia are among the most visible and widely discussed pathologies in prehistoric populations.

Vitamin D deficiency results in rickets, a disease in which bone remains soft while growing. The legs, which bear the weight of the body, commonly grow bent. Perhaps more important, the pelvis, which carries the weight of the upper body, may be distorted, affecting the size and shape of the birth canal.[10] More controversially, vitamin C deficiency or scurvy may be identifiable in the form of tooth loss combined with anemia-like symptoms and scars of subperiosteal hemorrhage (bleeding of the bone surface) resulting from the inability of the body to repair damaged tissues.[11]

Malnutrition and undernutrition in prehistoric skeletons of a more general sort have been identified using a number of measures. Reductions in adult stature or other measurements of the adult skeleton have been used as indicators of declining nutrition in much the same way (and with the same controversies) that the stature of historic populations has been used to indicate nutritional status.[12] In addition, reductions in the thickness and density of cortical bone (the dense ring of bone observed in cross section of long bones)[13] and in the size of teeth (particularly deciduous teeth, the growth of which are known to be sensitive to nutrition)[14] have been used as indicators of poor nutrition. Poor nutrition can also be inferred from patterns of growth in childhood. Malnourished children may display long bones that are short and/or thin for their age and dental development, when compared either to published modern standards or to other prehistoric populations.[15] These techniques permit us to identify malnutrition and to discuss the frequency of malnutrition and its distribution by age and sex in a given population.

3. We can identify certain kinds of infection in prehistoric skeletons and can therefore describe the frequency and distribution by age and sex of infection in various prehistoric groups. Some individual diseases of considerable historical importance can be identified because they leave diagnostic traces on the skeleton. Tuberculosis, for example, leaves characteristic traces on ribs and tends to destroy the bodies of lower (lumbar) vertebrae, producing a characteristic angle in the lower spine.[16] Treponemal infection (venereal syphilis and its more common nonvenereal relatives, yaws and endemic syphilis) characteristically attacks bone closest to the skin surface and therefore usually appears on the anterior or front surface of tibia (shin) and on the frontal bone of the skull or forehead. When passed on to a child in utero, it can result in a characteristic malformation of teeth.[17] Leprosy is characterized by damage to the bones of the face, fingers, and toes.[18] More controversially, smallpox may be identifiable from patterns of inflammation on the ulna (forearm).[19] As Allison and others have shown, a far broader

range of specific infections can be identified when mummies are preserved. In fact, specific disease-causing microorganisms can often be isolated and identified.[20] Unfortunately, skeletons do not permit specific identification of most diseases, including most of the major epidemic diseases.

Perhaps more important from the anthropological point of view—because they are far more common—we can identify low-grade or chronic infections or inflammations in the skeleton, even when the specific disease or pathogenic agent cannot be identified. Such lesions are referred to as periostitis or periosteal reactions when they involve only bone surfaces or as osteitis or osteomyelitis when they involve progressively deeper penetration of bone. Infections resulting from wounds can be distinguished from systemic infections by their distribution in the skeleton. The former tend to be limited to a single bone or limb, and the wound itself may be obvious; the latter are distributed throughout the body, their distribution determined by patterns of blood flow, local body temperature, or other local predisposing factors.[21]

4. Various cancers are identifiable in the skeleton. Primary bone cancer is rare, but the skeleton is a common site for the secondary spread of cancerous growth from other tissues. The skeleton therefore provides a rough (although reduced) reflection of the frequency of advanced cancer in other tissues. Studies of rates of bone cancers in prehistoric populations suggest, however, that they are extremely rare—even when the relative scarcity of elderly people is taken into account.[22]

5. We can identify trauma (fractures and dislocations of the skeletons) and analyze a population in terms of the frequency and distribution of trauma by age and sex.[23] Individual traumatic injuries often tell us something about what caused them. It is often possible to distinguish between traumas resulting from a fall and a blow and to distinguish accidents from violence. For example, a fracture of the forearm resulting from a fall appears different from a fracture of the same bones resulting from a blow the individual received while protecting his head.

6. We can tell something about individual workload. High rates of physical labor are recorded in the skeleton in the form of degenerative joint disease, a kind of arthritis that appears as striation and polishing of the articular surfaces of bones at the joints and the growth of extra spicules and ribbons of bone around the joint. In addition, muscular development associated with repeated use of limbs results in increasing size of muscle-attachment areas on bone. For example, women who spend a lot of time grinding corn develop large areas for attachments of the deltoid muscles of the arm (so-called deltoid tuberosities) similar to those that develop among modern bodybuilders. Since different activities affect different joints and limbs it is possible to infer

changing patterns of activity as well as changes in the overall workload. We can also assess changes in the division of labor by age, sex, or social class.[24]

7. We can identify and count the occurrence of specific episodes of growth-disrupting and growth-retarding stresses during childhood. Harris lines or transverse lines of dense bone visible in radiographs (x-rays) of long bones of the body are thought to indicate disruptions in bone growth and the subsequent acceleration or rebound in growth when health is restored.[25] The formation of tooth enamel is also sensitive to stress. Defects in tooth enamel related to stress are referred to as enamel hypoplasia when they are visible to the naked eye and as Wilson bands when visible only in microscopic cross section.[26]

These markers—hypoplasia, Wilson bands, and Harris lines—can be produced in the skeleton by a variety of stressors, including starvation, severe malnutrition, and severe infection. As a result, they do not permit us to make a specific diagnosis of disease. Their importance is that they record the frequency of stress in individuals (and therefore in populations or sub-populations) and permit us to make crude quantitative comparisons of the degree to which particular lifestyles exposed individuals to stressful episodes. Because bones and teeth grow on fairly precisely determined schedules, moreover, it is possible to use the position of the defect to identify the age at which a particular event occurred and the intervals between successive episodes. We can get a sense of a pattern of stress through an individual's childhood. We can tell whether children were commonly stressed before birth, whether stress commonly occurred at the age of weaning or later, and whether stress occurred annually (suggesting regular seasonal hardship) or at irregular intervals.

8. We can determine the age of individuals at death and describe patterns of death in a society. Children's ages at the time of death can be assessed based on the development and eruption of their deciduous and permanent teeth, which provide a fairly precise indicator of age until about age fifteen. Age can also be determined from the growth and formation of bones, some of which do not assume their final form until the early twenties, although this method is less precise because bone growth is more sensitive than tooth eruption to the individual's health and nutritional status.[27] Adult ages at death are much harder to determine because they are calculated using rates of degeneration, which are far more sensitive to individual (and group) differences in activities than biologically programmed patterns of development in children. Signs of degeneration include patterns of wear and other changes to the teeth; changes in the sutures, or joints between the bones of

the skull; changes in the articular surfaces of the pelvis; and changes in the microscopic structure of bone.[28]

Such degenerative changes can give us a reliable, if rough, idea of the relative ages of adult individuals at death because patterns of degeneration are progressive. But assigning specific ages at death has proved difficult. Many osteologists only attempt to determine the decade of life in which an adult died; many only describe adults as younger, middle, or older. It appears to be particularly difficult to recognize older adults since few techniques to assign ages appear to be reliable for individuals older than about forty years of age. Determining the age of older adults is also complicated by the deceptiveness of contemporary experience with the elderly. We are used to very sedentary elderly people whose skeletons reflect not just their age but their lack of physical activity. Moreover, many of the modern skeletal collections on which comparative analysis is based are composed of poor and often vagrant individuals whose own life histories may not be accurately known. We may not recognize the skeletons of elderly individuals who are fit and athletic, the type described in the last chapter.

With some caution, age assessments can be turned into statistical descriptions of patterns of death in the population for comparison with the descriptions provided for historic and modern populations. We can refer to the percent dying as infants or children, the average age at death for adults, the percent dying as older adults, and the life expectancy at birth, age 15, or other ages. In a few instances, cemetery samples are considered sufficiently complete that standard demographic life tables can be set up.

Controversy about this method arises for several reasons, some of which are obvious. Although children's skeletons may be aged with considerable precision, they may not be included or fully represented in cemeteries. Adult skeletons may be more fully represented, but estimates of age using them may be inaccurate. The elderly may be missed, either because they, like children, are excluded or because we fail to recognize them. As suggested above with reference to the incidence of disease, mortality profiles for prehistoric populations are primarily valuable for comparison to one another rather than for comparison to demographic studies of living populations. We have a better sense of the relative ages at death of adult individuals (and of whole populations) in prehistory than we have of absolute ages. In addition, a number of more subtle biases in cemetery samples need to be considered.[29]

In short, paleopathological data provide clues to a number of significant aspects of prehistoric human experience—patterns of work; diet and dietary shortcomings; risk of violence, accident, or disease; cultural protection (or lack of protection) against episodes of stress; survivorship and death. These data enable us to provide a reasonable profile of life and health in a prehistoric group. Comparing two or more populations permits us to evaluate the real human impact of economic, political, and social changes that scholars have otherwise evaluated on indirect and often strictly ideological grounds.

A number of paleopathological descriptions of prehistoric populations that use these signs and symptoms now exist. Direct comparison between populations often involves large differences in time, geography, and climate —and perhaps in genetics—as well as differences in human activities. If we are to evaluate the impact of changing human technology and society on health and nutrition, we need to compare sequential populations in the same environment, and ideally we should compare populations that follow one another in relatively rapid succession and can be shown to be culturally and genetically similar. Equally important, because not all scientists use precisely the same standards in determining age or assessing health and disease, the best comparisons are those in which the same individual (or team) has undertaken comparative analysis of several populations.[30]

Health Changes Associated with the Broad Spectrum Revolution

Although existing remains of the earliest hunter-gatherers are primarily scattered and fragmentary, a few studies permit us to assess changes in their health through time. In the Old World it is possible to document changes in the skeleton from early (Paleolithic) to later (Mesolithic) hunter-gatherer economies[31]—changes that roughly parallel the disappearance of large game animals and the consequent adoption of broad spectrum foraging patterns aimed at a wider array of small animals, seeds, and aquatic foods. Because of the scattered, fragmentary nature of remains, however, most of these comparisons are based on collections of all known human specimens from a particular period in a particular region rather than from remains of a single cemetery representing a natural population.

Several studies in different parts of the Old World—Greece and the Northern Mediterranean basin, Israel, India, and western and northern Europe (in fact, all areas of the Old World where measurements have been reported)—report that adult stature for both sexes declined at the time of the broad spectrum revolution during the Mesolithic period of prehistory. The average reduction in stature reported is about five centimeters (or two inches).[32]

The significance of this decline is in dispute. The decline accompanies the disappearance of large game animals in the environment as well as changes in climate associated with the end of the last glaciation. Angel[33] and Kennedy[34] attribute the trend to declining nutrition, an interpretation in keeping with the observation that protein and calorie returns for effort probably declined as big game disappeared.[35] In support of this hypothesis, Angel noted that two other skeletal dimensions he believed to be sensitive to nutrition—the height of the base of the skull and the diameter of the pelvic inlet—also declined. This hypothesis is also supported by evidence of bone chemistry suggesting that the proportion of meat in human diets in the Middle East declined during the same timespan.[36] An alternative explanation has been offered by Frayer, who suggests that with the decline of big game hunting there was less need—less "selection"—for human beings to maintain a large body size.[37]

In addition, Kennedy maintains that adult ages at death in India declined over the same timespan; Angel concludes that adult male ages at death declined slightly in the northern Mediterranean, although female ages rose slightly—conclusions that in both cases need to be tempered with caution because of the small and eclectic nature of the samples involved.[38]

Two studies have been undertaken to compare rates of enamel hypoplasia (that is, the frequency of episodes of childhood stress) between Paleolithic and Mesolithic groups. In a pioneering study undertaken twenty-five years ago, Brothwell found that hypoplasia rates were higher—suggesting more frequent episodes of biological stress—in later Mesolithic period samples than in earlier Paleolithic samples from Western Europe.[39] Patricia Smith and associates found no change in hypoplasia rates between Paleolithic (including Neanderthals) and Mesolithic Natufian populations in Israel; both groups displayed very low rates in comparison to later populations.[40]

Although existing information is spotty and interpretations uncertain, the evidence points to a decline in human health and nutrition from Paleolithic to Mesolithic periods in the Old World. The interpretation of some of this evidence is controversial, but there is no countering evidence to suggest progress in nutrition or an improvement in health.[41]

Prehistoric hunting and gathering populations in Australia were once thought to be models of ecological and demographic stability whose populations and food economies had remained essentially unchanged for thousands of years.[42] But recent archaeological investigations have suggested that prehistoric Australians went through a sequence of economic changes very much like the Paleolithic-Mesolithic transition in Europe and Asia during the broad spectrum revolution.[43] Webb has compared rates of pathology among prehistoric groups of Australian aborigines, and his results suggest a decline rather than an improvement in health through time. The only well-defined sample from early in the archaeological sequence (at the end of the Pleistocene period) exhibited comparatively low rates of enamel hypoplasia and porotic hyporostosis (anemia) compared to more recent groups. Webb also reported that rates of pathology indicative of old infections, anemia (porotic hyperostosis), and stress (enamel hypoplasias) are relatively common in those recent populations that were thought to have lived in large permanent settlements, which were supposedly more civilized and affluent.[44]

In the New World no significant skeletal samples are available to represent the earliest (Paleoindian) period of human occupation. But relatively early hunter-gatherers (Archaic period) can be compared with later hunter-gatherers (Woodland period) in several locations. The samples available are often substantially larger than those reported in the Old World, and the analyses, in consequence, are often more complete.

In the American Midwest, Mensforth has undertaken a comparative analysis of two large skeletal samples representing relatively sedentary hunting and gathering populations at two distinct periods of time. The earlier population (354 individuals) is from the Carlston Annis site in Kentucky, a late Archaic period site inhabited between 1500 and 3000 B.C. The later population (1,327 individuals) is from the late Woodland period Libben site dated between A.D. 800 and 1100. Mensforth's study provides one of the few instances in which two hunter-gatherer populations of such size have been compared; it is one of the few studies in which comparison can be made between two arguably complete hunter-gatherer cemetery samples. He found that the later (Woodland) population displayed more frequent growth retardation, shorter bone-shaft lengths in children of comparable ages, higher infection rates, and higher rates of porotic hyperostosis than the earlier (Archaic) group. He suggests that the main difference between the groups was not primarily their diets but the greater burden of infectious disease on the later group. Mensforth also reported that although the earlier population displayed slightly higher infant mortality than the later it also reared a larger proportion of its infants to maturity and had slightly higher life expectancy at birth and at age 15. Both groups exhibited rates of infant and childhood survival comparable to the average of ethnographically reported hunting and gathering groups described in the last chapter.[45]

In Illinois, Cook has found that the earliest hunter-gatherers in her sample (Archaic period) display lower rates of porotic hyperostosis than later hunter-gatherers (Woodland period), in fact lower than all subsequent populations. Similarly, the Archaic period group displays lower rates of infection than any subsequent population. In addition, the Archaic population is the only one in the Illinois sequence that displays no hypoplasia of deciduous teeth.[46] The chances of an infant surviving to adulthood, apparently fairly good by historic standards in both Archaic and Woodland groups, appeared to improve somewhat in the later group. But adult life expectancy [e(15)] declined slightly in the later group.[47]

In California, where American Indians ultimately developed large and complex societies based on intense exploitation of fish and nuts without ever farming, the data on changing health and nutrition through time are mixed, at best. McHenry reported some years ago that the frequency of Harris lines declined through time among central California Indian populations, suggesting an improvement in the reliability of their diets and confirming the then widely accepted assumption that progress meant improved nutrition.[48] But more recent study of enamel hypoplasia in these same populations suggests the opposite trend.[49] Moreover, using one of the nutritional indicators developed by Angel (the height of the base of the skull), Dickel found a gradual decline in nutritional quality through time, although he and his coworkers have found no significant change in adult stature over the same timespan.[50] In southern California, Walker has also reported that the frequency of enamel hypoplasia increased through time, although he argues that background nutrition appeared to be improving.[51]

In Peru, Benfer has described a sequence of preagricultural populations from the Paloma site (one of the few such sequences available in South America and one of the few instances in which sequential populations actually occupied the same site).[52] He reports an increase in stature through time and a decrease in the frequency of Harris lines, both of which appear to suggest an improvement in nutrition, but he also reports an increase in rates of enamel hypoplasia. Survivorship appears to have improved over time at the site.

Although the data are mixed, the preponderance of existing evidence suggests that nutrition and health were declining, not improving, among hunter-gatherer groups during the broad spectrum revolution prior to the adoption of agriculture (and declining through time in those areas of the world like California and Australia in which agriculture was never adopted). In most locations studied so far, stature was declining or other measures of the skeleton were becoming smaller, rates of enamel hypoplasia were increasing, and rates of porotic hyperostosis and signs of infection were increasing. These data seem to support the contention that the decline in big game hunting and the intensification of foraging activities characterizing re-

cent hunter-gatherer populations represents diminishing returns, not technological progress. Increasing rates of infection also suggest that increased
community size and sedentism had negative effects on health.

The Health of Hunter-Gatherers Compared
to Subsequent Farmers

Comparisons between hunter-gatherers and subsequent farmers are
more numerous and are usually based on larger samples. Most comparisons
reported here are based on natural cemetery populations (usually of 50 to
200 individuals, occasionally far more). Several points of interest emerge
from the comparisons.

TRAUMA

As a group, these comparisons do not yet yield any clear trend in
the frequency of trauma and violence. Trauma rates appear to increase in
some regions with the adoption of agriculture[53] but to decrease in others.[54]
For example, Rathbun reports that the frequency of trauma was relatively
high among hunting and gathering populations in Iran but subsequently declined.[55] In contrast, Kennedy reports that the frequency of trauma was low
among early hunter-gatherers in India but seems to have gone up after the
adoption of agriculture.[56] Describing a chronological series of populations
from a single site, Goodman et al. report that the frequency of trauma increased with the adoption and intensification of maize-based farming at the
Dickson Mounds site in Illinois (a late Woodland and Mississippian period
site, ca. A.D. 900 to 1350).[57]

Trauma associated with violence also shows no clear pattern through
time, although we can speak about peaks of violence surrounding specific
cultural episodes in specific locations. Cook suggests, for example, that there
may have been an increase in violence in Illinois in the late Woodland period
during the transition from hunting and gathering to agriculture.[58]

In general, the skeletal evidence provides little support for the Hobbesian
notion that the hunter-gatherer life is particularly violent or for the assumption that hunting is particularly dangerous. But there is also no support for
the proposition recently debated in anthropology that hunter-gatherers are
particularly nonviolent people.

ARTHRITIS AND MUSCULAR DEVELOPMENT

Comparisons also yield no clear trend in rates of arthritis and skeletal
robustness indicative of workload, so it is not clear whether the adoption

of agriculture eased workloads as once thought or increased workloads as some of us have argued.[59] The size of muscle attachments and the level of degenerative arthritis seem to go up with the adoption of farming in some regions[60] and to decline in others.[61] For example, Indians on the Georgia coast who adopted agriculture at around A.D. 1150 underwent not only a decline in size but also a decrease in robustness and arthritis, suggesting a reduction in workload.[62] Indians in Alabama seem to have become more robust as a consequence of the greater labor demands of an agricultural economy.[63]

Sometimes, changing patterns of arthritis point not to a rise or decline in overall workload but to a changing pattern of activities or a changing distribution of labor by sex. Cook reports that among Indians in Illinois the adoption of agriculture seem to have resulted in increasing arthritic degeneration for women, suggesting that their workload increased; men displayed an altered pattern of arthritis but no overall increase, suggesting that their workload changed but did not become heavier.[64]

Skeletal evidence of physical stresses (arthritis and trauma) does not show clear trends through time. In several other respects, however, comparisons of prehistoric hunter-gatherer and farming populations reveal clear trends.

INFECTION

Signs of infection observable on bone usually seem to increase as human settlements increase in size and permanence. Nonspecific skeletal lesions—periostitis and osteomyelitis—increase through time in most cases.[65] For example, at the Dickson Mounds site in Illinois, the percentage of individuals displaying signs of infection doubled in the transition from hunting and gathering to intensive maize agriculture.[66] Infection in the later group is also much more likely to be severe.

Working with populations from Arkansas, dated between 400 B.C. and A.D. 1800, Rose et al. demonstrated that rates of infection were positively correlated with the size and permanence of communities, although not necessarily with an agriculturally based diet.[67]

Treponemal infection also commonly appears to increase in frequency and severity with increased population size.[68] In addition, tuberculosis appears to be more frequent after the adoption of agriculture. Contrary to what was once thought, tuberculosis was clearly present in the New World before Columbus, and it has been reported at least occasionally among hunter-gatherers.[69] But descriptions almost always focus on large and sedentary agricultural groups. In Illinois, for example, Cook and Buikstra suggest that tuberculosis—or tuberculosis-like pathology—is evident only in the latest, fully agricultural groups in the archaeological sequence, sometime later than A.D. 1000.[70]

Working with mummies from Peru, Allison has been able to provide a much more refined breakdown of infectious disease involving varying tissues of the body, often identifying specific pathogenic agents. In the only quantitative comparison of mummies of which I am aware, he has been able to show that there is an increase in a particular intestinal parasite (salmonella) associated with sedentism (after ca. 500 B.C.). In contrast, rates of respiratory infection do not appear to increase with the adoption of sedentary habits. (Allison suggests that respiratory infections provided the most common probable cause of death in all of the populations he studied.)[71]

Working with preserved human feces from archaeological sites on the Colorado Plateau, Reinhard has been able to document an increase in the range and intensity of intestinal parasites as groups became sedentary.[72]

It is worth noting, incidentally, that few, if any, reports of skeletons or mummies suggest signs of infection of a previously unknown kind or suggest that any specific type of infection regularly disappears as people become more civilized.

NUTRITION

A second common trend is that farmers often appear to have been less well nourished than the hunter-gatherers that preceded them, rarely the reverse. For example, rates of porotic hyperostosis (suggestive of anemia) are almost universally higher among farmers in a region than in earlier hunter-gatherers from the same region.[73] At Dickson Mounds, for example, Goodman et al. report a progressive increase in rates of porotic hyperostosis through the three successive phases of the archaeological sequence spanning the adoption and intensification of maize agriculture.[74]

This increase in porotic hyperostosis with the adoption of agriculture was once commonly thought to represent a decline in the quality of diet associated with cereal—particularly maize-based agriculture.[75] The observation at Dickson Mounds that later maize-eating populations display reduced traces of zinc in bone supports this hypothesis. This may suggest reduced meat intake or greater interference with mineral absorption by the cereal-based diet.[76] But porotic hyperostosis is increasingly thought to represent anemia secondary to parasite infestation, either alone or in combination with cereal-based diets, because the same trend sometimes accompanies increasing community size and permanence, whether or not agriculture is practiced. The trend may even be related to changes in techniques of food preparation in some instances.[77]

Other independent measures of nutrition are less widely reported but most often seem to suggest a decline in the quality of nutrition associated with the adoption and intensification of agriculture. Several studies report that bone cortical area (the cross-sectional area of bone minus the area of the central medullary cavity) is reduced among farmers in comparison to earlier hunter-gatherers in the same region.[78] In addition, both Cook[79] and Goodman et al.[80] report that childhood growth is retarded among early farmers in comparison to earlier hunter-gatherers in Illinois. In Georgia, Larsen notes that deciduous teeth (whose growth is sensitive to nutritional intake) decline in size with the advent of agriculture.[81]

In several areas, the stature, size, and robustness of adult individuals declines with the adoption of farming.[82] Angel reports, for example, that, in the Mediterranean, early Neolithic men on the average are 3 centimeters shorter than their Mesolithic counterparts; the women about 4 centimeters shorter. He also suggests that a decline in dimensions of the skull base and pelvis that began in the Mesolithic period continued through most of the Neolithic period.[83] Meiklejohn and associates also report a slight decrease in average stature below the already reduced Mesolithic levels in western Europe.[84] There are some counterexamples. Smith and associates, working with populations in Israel, for example, note that there is a slight temporary rebound from low Mesolithic levels in adult stature associated with animal domestication early in the Neolithic period. The trend is accompanied by evidence from trace element analysis suggesting a temporary increase in animal foods in the diet—one of the few clear indications that the domestication of animals at least temporarily reversed the long-term decline in the availability of animal foods.[85]

It is worth noting, incidentally, that hunter-gatherers and early farmers rarely displayed signs of scurvy or rickets, which became more common in the civilized world, especially during medieval times. (Rickets was still a problem for early twentieth-century Americans.) And early prehistoric populations rarely match rates of porotic hyperostosis reported for more civilized populations.[86]

EPISODIC STRESSES

Although the overall quality of nutrition seems most often to have declined with the adoption of agriculture, one class of skeletal pathology may suggest that food supplies became more reliable and episodes of hunger became less common. Most studies comparing rates of Harris lines in hunting and gathering and subsequent populations have found the lines to be more common in the earlier groups.[87] For example, Cassidy reports Harris lines to be more common in the hunting and gathering population from Indian Knoll, an Archaic period site in Kentucky (ca. 2500 B.C.), than in the population from Hardin Village, a later, Mississippian period population of farmers from the same region (after ca. A.D. 950).[88] Goodman et al. report that Harris lines gradually become less common through the transition to agriculture at Dickson Mounds.[89] These data appear to indicate that, despite superior background nutrition, hunter-gatherers were more exposed to such episodes of stress as seasonal hunger than were later farmers.

But enamel hypoplasias and microscopic enamel defects (Wilson bands) of teeth—more often studied and more commonly relied on as markers of stress—tell a different story. They are almost invariably reported to have become more frequent and/or more severe as farming replaced hunting and gathering in different parts of the world.[90] For example, Cassidy found severe enamel hypoplasias less common in her Archaic period hunter-gatherer sample in Kentucky than in the subsequent farming population. Similarly, Goodman et al. found hypoplasia to be twice as frequent in later agricultural populations at Dickson Mounds as in the earlier hunter-gatherers.[91]

The apparent contradiction between trends in hypoplasias and Harris line can be explained in one of several ways. One possibility is that the two indicators of stress represent events of different cause, severity, and duration. Perhaps hunter-gatherers traded frequent mild stresses (recorded as Harris lines) for less frequent but severe stresses (recorded as hypoplasia) when they adopted sedentary agriculture. Cassidy has suggested, for example, that seasonal hunger may have been more frequent for prehistoric hunter-gatherers, starvation and epidemics more frequent for later farmers.[92]

A second possibility is that the different trends reflect the different age of development of teeth and long bones. Teeth seem to be particularly sensitive to stress in the early childhood years, and rates of hypoplasia may be particularly reflective of weaning-age stress; Harris lines, in contrast, present a broader picture of childhood growth. We may, therefore, be seeing a difference in the age distribution of stress episodes, with hunter-gatherers commonly providing better protection for weanlings but buffering older children less successfully.

A third possibility is that one of the two indicators, most probably Harris lines, are a misleading indicator of episodic stress. Several questions have been raised about the validity of Harris lines, and most skeletal pathologists seem to consider hypoplasia a more reliable index of stress.[93]

Various interpretations of these contradictory data are possible, but none suggests that the adoption of agriculture was marked by a significant decline in episodic stress. The more reliable indicator seems to suggest that stress episodes became more frequent and/or more serious in later populations.

Hypoplasias of deciduous or baby teeth represent stress in utero or immediately after birth and therefore tend to reflect maternal health and nutrition. At least three studies explicitly compare rates of deciduous tooth hypoplasia between hunter-gatherers and later farmers in the same region. Cassidy found no deciduous tooth hypoplasia in her sample of hunter-gatherers from Kentucky but found hypoplasia on a significant fraction of deciduous teeth of individuals from the later, Mississippian period farming population.[94] Sciulli also found higher rates among farmers than among hunter-gatherers in Ohio;[95] Cook and Buikstra found no difference between hunter-gatherers and farmers in Illinois but did suggest that the infants with hypoplasia had a higher mortality rate in the later group.[96]

MORTALITY

It is hard to draw reliable conclusions about relative mortality and life expectancy because skeletal samples are so easily distorted and so often incomplete. But the available evidence suggests that prehistoric hunter-gatherers often fared relatively well in comparison to later populations, particularly with reference to the survival of children. At the very least, the data fail to confirm our naive expectation that the earliest, least civilized groups had the highest mortality.

For example, at Dickson Mounds where recovery of skeletons was sufficiently complete to permit construction of detailed life tables, the hunting and gathering population and transitional populations displayed a higher life expectancy at birth (and at all ages) than the later agricultural populations.[97]

On the basis of relatively large samples, Cook concludes that, elsewhere in the Illinois Valley, mortality rates increased at least temporarily with the adoption of farming;[98] life tables for other Illinois populations (despite caveats about their interpretation) appear to confirm that hunter-gatherer life expectancies matched or exceeded those of later groups.[99]

In a comparison of large hunter-gatherer and farmer populations from Indian Knoll and Hardin Village in Kentucky, Cassidy concludes that the earlier group reared a higher percentage of its children to adulthood and enjoyed higher adult life expectancy than the later agricultural group.[100]

Some other studies involving smaller and less complete samples also appear to suggest that hunter-gatherers lost smaller proportions of their infants and children than later farmers in the same region; several other studies of hunting and gathering populations (some but not all involving large and apparently complete samples) suggest rates of infant and child mortality comparable to the historically modest rates of contemporary hunter-gatherer populations.[101] These data, although potentially clouded by biased cemetery samples and by poor preservation and recovery of children's skeletons, nonetheless imply that infant and childhood mortality were relatively low in these early populations. At least, they provide no evidence of particularly high childhood mortality in hunting and gathering groups. None of the available samples, many of them fairly large, suggests infant or child mortality levels among hunter-gatherers that are particularly high by historic standards.

Most other comparisons of mortality are based on smaller samples and far more fragmentary material, which make estimates of childhood mortality rates impossible and that of adult mortality rates suspect. But reported average adult ages at death and estimates of life expectancy at age 15 are, in fact, higher in hunting and gathering groups than among early farmers in many parts of the world.[102] For example, Larsen reports that a sample of 272 hunter-gatherers found in Georgia (prior to A.D. 1150) had substantially higher average ages at death than a sample of 344 farmers from a later time (whether or not children's deaths are averaged in).[103] Welinder reports a very substantial decline in life expectancy among adults with the adoption of farming in Scandinavia after ca. 3500 B.C.[104] Kobayashi suggests that there was a two-to-five-year drop in average age at death for men and a three-year drop for women between hunter-gatherer populations of the late Jomon period and populations of rice cultivators of the Yayoi period in Japan.[105]

Fragmentary as they are, the data are bolstered somewhat by replication in various parts of the world. At the very least, the data offer no support for the assumption that adult ages at death increased with the adoption of farming.[106]

Most comparisons between hunter-gatherers and later farmers in the same locale suggest that the farmers usually suffered higher rates of infection and parasitization and poorer nutrition. Farmers may have suffered less from mild seasonal hunger (represented by Harris lines), but they almost invariably suffered more severe episodes of stress (represented by enamel hypoplasia). Poor as it is, the data also suggest that hunter-gatherers reared a good proportion of their children to adulthood—a proportion commonly equal to or greater than that of later prehistoric populations. The data also suggest that average adult ages at death among prehistoric hunter-gatherers, though low by historic standards, were often higher than those of early farmers.

The Intensification of Farming and the Rise of Urban Civilizations

If the adoption of agriculture seems commonly to have had negative effects on health and nutrition—and perhaps even survivorship—the later intensification of agriculture and the rise of civilization appear to have had only mixed results. Some populations clearly rebounded to levels of health, nutrition, and survival equaling and exceeding those of prehistoric hunters, but others just as clearly did not.

Among Old World populations, for example, Angel argues that Bronze Age populations of Greece rebounded substantially from low Neolithic levels of health and nutrition; stature increased, and rates of porotic hyperostosis appear to have declined after the Neolithic period.[107] Angel also notes, however, that Bronze Age royalty (visible as a distinct class for the first time) enjoyed much more of the rebound than commoners. Moreover, he observes that enamel hypoplasia rates increased markedly in the Bronze Age and associates the increase with the appearance of density-dependent epidemic diseases. He further notes that tuberculosis was identifiable for the first time in the Iron Age.

Angel reports that average ages at death for adults in Greece rebounded from low Neolithic levels and rose above Paleolithic and Mesolithic levels for the first time in the Bronze Age. Adult ages at death were generally higher thereafter. But average male ages at death fell back to Paleolithic levels between A.D. 1400 and 1800, and according to his reconstruction, the average age at death for women fell to Paleolithic levels or lower during the same period.[108]

Moreover, Mediterranean cities do not appear to have shared in the rebound in health and life expectancy. Judging by one archaeological sample, adult life expectancy in ancient Athens was not much more than that of the Paleolithic;[109] life expectancy in ancient Rome has been estimated to have been lower than that of Stone Age groups—in fact, so low that it could not have sustained an isolated population in prehistory.[110]

Western European populations display increasing rates of pathology beginning in the Bronze Age. Porotic hyperostosis is not common in European populations until the Bronze Age or later; the early historic cities of Europe during medieval times and later display types and degrees of malnutrition (including scurvy and rickets) not matched in earlier populations. Calvin Wells argued some years ago that infection, relatively rare in European skeletons as late as the Bronze Age, became widespread in European cities only in the last few centuries and were associated with widespread and severe malnutrition. Leprosy, usually considered an ancient scourge, does not appear in European skeletons until after A.D. 500 and reaches its peak around A.D. 1200. Tuberculosis, which appears in isolated examples in the Neolithic period in Germany and Denmark, does not become common in Britain until Roman times and may have become a significant disease burden only in the Middle Ages. Enamel hypoplasia was more common in populations of medieval towns and cities than ever before.[111] According to Bennike, adult stature, which generally increased after the Neolithic in Scandinavia, fell back below Neolithic levels in the nineteenth century.[112] Fogel has suggested that British statures in the eighteenth century were among the lowest of ethnographically or historically recorded populations, which would make them among the lowest recorded anywhere.[113] Wurm points out that diet and stature, which dropped with the adoption of cereal agriculture in Germany, declined again between the Middle Ages and the nineteenth century.[114]

European populations appear to have enjoyed a rebound in adult life expectancy after the Neolithic period. Acsadi and Nemeskeri suggest that scattered populations in central Europe show a gradual, although by no means universal, improvement in adult life expectancy from the Neolithic period through the Iron Age.[115] Figures collected by Weiss tell a similar story.[116] Welinder suggests that adult life expectancy in Scandinavia rebounded from Neolithic lows in the Iron Age;[117] Bennike suggests that adult longevity generally increased after the Neolithic period in Scandinavia.[118] But Sellevold reports that average adult ages at death in Denmark during the Iron Age were not substantially different from those reported elsewhere for Paleolithic populations.[119]

Some medieval populations from Scandinavia appear to have experienced extremely high rates of infant and child mortality. Gejvall reports that individuals in the large Westerhus cemetery (ca. A.D. 1200 to 1550) had an average life span of 17 to 18 years.[120] According to Bennike, 50 to 80 percent of individuals in some populations died as children.

In other parts of the Old World, health trends are equally mixed. Martin et al. argue that populations in Sudanese Nubia, south of Egypt and alternately satellite to civilizations in Egypt and Meroë (the Sudan), suffered declining nutrition with the intensification of agriculture and, more particularly, displayed worsened health during episodes of civilized political unification.[121] Apparently, early trade networks sometimes siphoned nutrients away from the Nubians and resulted in high rates of enamel hypoplasia and retarded growth, rather than contributing to Nubian well-being.[122]

In Israel, average age at death among adults appears to rise from the Mesolithic period through the Hellenistic and Roman periods but to drop back to levels comparable to those of the Mesolithic in the early period of Arab influence. In this region, the rates of several types of pathology are higher in the more recent groups. Enamel hypoplasia, comparatively rare in preagricultural populations, increases in later periods of prehistory and history. Cribra orbitalia (indicative of anemia) also increases significantly in frequency in later phases of the archaeological sequence. Pathological thinning of bone cortices, which is rare in individuals from preagricultural populations, increases slightly in the Bronze Age and again in the Iron Age and increases more substantially in the period of Arab expansion.[123]

Rathbun argues that Bronze Age and Iron Age populations in Iran suffered surprisingly low rates of infection but high rates of enamel hypoplasia and cribra orbitalia.[124] The average age at death for adults during these periods shows no advance over Paleolithic levels, and Rathbun is led to conclude that civilized state apparatus did not significantly improve the reliability of the dietary base.

In India, studies suggest a decline in deciduous tooth size from the Neolithic period to the present. Porotic hyperostosis and rickets are more prevalent in the cities of Harappan civilization than in preagriculture populations, although rates of hypoplasia that increased during the Neolithic period decreased thereafter.[125]

Among populations in the New World, trends in health in the most recent sites (and often the largest political units) are mixed at best. In North America there is a sharp partitioning of health among the most recent prehistoric societies (Mississippian period). Powell describes the Mississippian period Moundville site in Alabama as a relatively healthy community.[126] At Moundville, porotic hyperostosis and severe infection were rare, and tuberculosis was uncommon. Severe enamel hypoplasia was also comparatively rare, although mild infection was fairly common. The Mississippian period population of the Etowah Mounds site in Georgia also appears to have been comparatively healthy and long-lived—but there is substantial difference between classes. Male adults given privileged mound burial had a relatively high average age at death. In the surrounding village the average age at death was much lower. The Etowah population also displays relatively low rates of porotic hyperostosis and infection. But Etowah itself appears to display generally poorer health and nutrition than its own satellite King site, an outlying community still subsisting primarily by hunting and gathering whose inhabitants were taller and more robust, had greater cortical thickness to their long bones, lower rates of infection, and lower rates of arthritis.[127]

Buikstra and Cook suggest that despite the appearance of tuberculosis (and relatively high rates of treponemal infection, porotic hyperostosis, and enamel hypoplasia) Mississippian period farming populations in Illinois clearly rebounded from the low levels of health and nutrition endured during the transition to maize agriculture.[128] Adult stature and patterns of childhood growth improved, and adult life expectancy appears to have rebounded, although there is no clear rebound in survivorship among infants and children.

But several other Mississippian sites tell a different story. At the Dickson

Mounds site in Illinois, the decline in almost all measures of health, nutrition, and longevity that began with the transition to agriculture continues into the Mississippian period. Goodman et al. suggest that this decline may reflect the marginal, satellite status of Dickson Mounds in Illinois trade networks of the period.[129] The Mississippian period site of Averbuch in Tennessee (ca. A.D. 1275 to 1375) displays high rates of nutritional and infectious pathology that have been associated with crowding and singularly high rates of trauma suggestive of interpersonal violence—the latter possibly reflecting its position on a political frontier.[130] And the Mississippian period Hiwassee Dallas site in Tennessee has left a record of high levels of biological stress and low life expectancy unmatched by any earlier North American group. Life expectancy for both children and adults was extremely low, below that of any known, reasonably complete hunter-gatherer sample.[131] Palkovich has provided an analysis of ages at death for two late agricultural Pueblo settlements from the American Southwest during the thirteenth and fourteenth centuries that suggest life expectancies at or below those of hunter-gatherer groups reported elsewhere in North America.[132]

In Mesoamerica (prehistoric Mexico and central America), populations show a steady decline in stature accompanied by an increase in rates of porotic hyperostosis and other signs of malnutrition through the flowering of early civilization. Preclassic Maya are taller than classic and postclassic Maya.[133] At prehistoric Teotihuacan, the major urban metropolis of Mexico and arguably the largest city of the world in its day (ca. 150 B.C. to A.D. 750), rates of malnutrition, delayed or stunted growth, deciduous tooth hypoplasia, and infant and child mortality (in a single ward that has been studied) are higher than in any known earlier or less civilized group.[134] Storey suggests that this ward at Teotihuacan had higher rates of juvenile mortality than any other known New World site except that of (Mississippian period) Hiwassee Dallas.

In Peru, working with a small sample of mummies, Allison suggests that the people in the later urban periods and the period of Inca domination were smaller and displayed higher rates of infection and enamel hypoplasia than earlier populations.[135]

It is worth noting, finally, that extremely high levels of stress among the less privileged citizens of complex societies can even be traced archaeologically into the late nineteenth and twentieth centuries. Several descriptions of skeletal samples of black American populations—both slave and free and as late as the 1920s in the United States—suggest rates of malnutrition, infection, and death that equal or exceed those of most prehistoric groups.[136]

In sum, the archaeological record of civilizations, ancient and recent, provide a very mixed record of changing health. Skeletal indicators of infection and malnutrition increased in some sites or regions and declined in others. What we seem to be seeing is not an improvement in human health and nutrition but rather a partitioning of stress such that some privileged classes or successful communities enjoyed good health and nutrition but others suffered unprecedented degrees of stress associated with low social status, unfavorable trade balance, and the parasite loads of dense settled communities engaged in trade. In some instances, major settlements or cities seem to have experienced economic privileges, as recorded in the health of skeletons; in other instances, urban environments displayed extremely poor health and short life expectancy. Outlying communities appear in some cases to have enjoyed good health because they were less crowded or had better diets; in other cases outlying communities seem to have suffered declining nutrition and health associated with their weak and marginal status in trade networks. We have yet to map the distribution or partitioning of health and illness during these later periods with sufficient precision, but the overall picture clearly does not conform to our simple expectations of progress in health and longevity.

Early civilizations may also have partitioned stress in another sense, rather than reducing it. Many measures and estimates of adult life expectancy, such as those just reported, suggest that after a nadir at the adoption of agriculture, average adult age at death and adult life expectancy gradually improved. At the same time I can find no actual evidence of regular improvement in child survivorship anywhere in the world until the late nineteenth century (and for much of the world the mid–twentieth century). If anything, the reverse is the case. For most of history, civilized societies may have lost a higher proportion of their children than their primitive forebears. Perhaps, as Lovejoy and his colleagues argued some years ago, the two trends are related: average adult longevity improves with civilization in part because children are being more selectively weeded out before maturity.[137] Civilized individuals who make it to adulthood are already a relatively select sample.

The Paradox of Accelerating Population Growth

We are left with something of a paradox. Most reconstructions of the history of the human species suggest that the total human population grew very slowly prior to the adoption of farming but grew more rapidly thereafter. In the most recent major synthesis of prehistoric demography, Hassan suggests that Paleolithic and Mesolithic populations in the Old World grew at an average rate of only 0.01 percent and 0.003 percent per year, respectively, but that population grew at an average rate of 0.1 percent per year during the Neolithic and about 0.12 percent during the formation of the early empires (with occasional brief periods of more rapid growth averaging 0.5 percent per year or more).[138]

The traditional and popularly held assumption has been that high mortality restrained the growth of human populations before the adoption of agriculture. This could have been the case—despite the apparent good health of preagricultural populations—if zoonotic diseases from wild animals had pronounced effects on mortality, particularly mortality among adults, with indirect consequences for children.[139] High mortality might also have been common despite good health and nutrition if group mobility placed severe stress on those individuals who were even mildly incapacitated. There is evidence that settling down improves survivorship for at least some groups in the twentieth century.[140]

Both the ethnographic evidence of mobile bands and the archaeological evidence, usually of comparatively sedentary hunter-gatherers, however, suggest that infant and childhood mortality among hunter-gatherers is comparatively low or at worst moderate by historic standards. The archaeological evidence suggests that adult life expectancy among hunter-gatherers, though apparently low by historic standards, was probably higher than that of early farmers. The evidence from ethnography and archaeology does not appear to suggest that rates of mortality were sufficiently high (by themselves) to explain the relatively slow growth of hunting and gathering populations.

Another possible explanation has been proposed by Ammerman, who suggests that normally rapid population growth among prehistoric hunter-gatherers was curtailed by frequent population crashes resulting from starvation and epidemics.[141] But models of epidemic disease transmission make it appear extremely unlikely that epidemics were a more serious threat to population growth prior to the origins of agriculture and cities than thereafter; there is little evidence from either skeletons or ethnographic groups to suggest that food crises were more pronounced for hunter-gatherers than for later farmers. Ammerman's proposal does gain some credence when it is realized that preagricultural populations commonly inhabited an Ice Age world in which a greater proportion of the globe had arctic or subarctic environments with the attendant risks. Prehistoric populations might have grown slowly not because their technology was primitive but because a larger part of their natural world posed severe challenges to human survival. The Ice Age world was, however, also one relatively rich in efficiently exploited large game, and in many parts of the world this rich fauna was available without the perils of extreme cold or the absence of backup resources.

The alternative hypothesis suggests that a combination of low rates of natural or controlled reproduction and moderate rates of mortality restrained the growth of prehistoric hunting and gathering groups and that population growth rates accelerated after the adoption of sedentary lifestyles and farming because fertility increased or birth control was relaxed (perhaps in spite of the fact that mortality also increased). Howell's analysis of the San suggests that their low fertility combined with moderate infant and child mortality and moderate life expectancy (30 years at birth) combine to produce a rate of population growth very close to zero.[142] In contrast, the more fertile Agta could maintain themselves with a life expectancy at birth of only 20 years, and the Hadza (who enjoy a life expectancy of about 30 years) could maintain themselves with a life expectancy at birth in the low twenties. The average rate of child production among observed hunter-gatherers, somewhere in between these groups, suggests that a life expectancy in the midtwenties, on the average, would produce rates of population growth near zero. If prehistoric hunter-gatherers commonly spaced their children widely (whether by natural or cultural means), they would have had to maintain a life expectancy at birth of 25 years or more just to break even or expand very slowly. (If we assume that Ammerman was partly correct and that Ice Age population growth was marred by episodic crashes, then life expectancy at birth under normal conditions may have been slightly higher.) Life expectancy of 25 years is about the average observed in contemporary hunter-gatherers, and it is in keeping with archaeologically documented hunting and gathering groups (especially if we keep in mind that adult ages at death are probably underestimated in archaeological samples but often appear to be *relatively* high in hunter-gatherer groups compared to the earliest farmers).

If we also recall ethnographic evidence that child production increases when groups become sedentary and paleodemographic analyses suggesting that fertility did increase during the adoption and intensification of farming, then it seems likely that low rates of prehistoric population growth were maintained at least in part by restricted fertility. I suggest that this scenario—comparatively low rates of child production balanced by historically moderate mortality and relatively rare population crashes—although not yet provable, fits the various fragments of ethnographic and archaeological evidence better than any alternative assumption.[143] The growth rate of the human population increased after the adoption of sedentism and agriculture not because survival improved but because human populations—for natural or cultural reasons—produced more children.

Chapter 8

Conclusions

I began by calling attention to two conflicting images of the primitive and the civilized—conflicting images that appear both in popular beliefs about progress and in professional reconstructions of history. Perhaps the best way to begin a summation of the evidence is to suggest that neither image appears to be accurate, at least if health and physical well-being are used as measures.

The smallest human societies that we can identify, either among living groups or among the populations of prehistory, do not appear to live up to the more romantic images we sometimes paint of them in popular literature. Nor do they live up to the image of primitive "affluence" that has become popular among anthropologists in the past twenty years. Hunger has clearly been at least a seasonal problem for many historic and contemporary groups, and starvation is not unknown. Contemporary hunter-gatherers appear to be chronically lean, as well as at least occasionally hungry. Their low caloric intake results in part from the sparse distribution of most wild foods, both plant and animal, and in part from the low caloric content of their foods in proportion to bulk compared to more extensively processed domestic foods. The problem also exists because many contemporary small-scale societies live in impoverished environments—those that are particularly dry or cold —to which they have been relegated by competition with more powerful neighbors. It has been suggested that the low caloric intake of contemporary hunter-gatherers may be related to their small body size.

Parasite infestation is common and varied among contemporary foragers, and occasionally infections are intense, particularly in rain forest environments. Infectious diseases often appear to be the most common cause of death. Such degenerative diseases as heart problems and cancers, although relatively rare, are not entirely unknown. Although accidents are not as common as we might naively expect, the risk of death by accident is uncommonly high; surprisingly, the risk of death associated with hunting dangerous animals apparently is not.

These societies typically lose a large fraction of their children to death by natural causes prior to adulthood. In the ethnographic groups reviewed, an average of approximately 20 percent of infants die natural deaths in their first year of life; an average of 35 to 50 percent die from natural causes before they reach 15 years of age. The average age at death among adults is also relatively low by our standard. Relatively few individuals reach their sixties or seventies. Life expectancy at age 15 averages only an additional 25 to 30 years (a figure that may have been depressed in the recent past by the impact of exogenous epidemic diseases on inexperienced populations, since most observed adult deaths appear to result from such diseases). Life expectancy at birth is also relatively low, apparently averaging between 25 and 30 years in most contemporary hunting and gathering groups, in contrast to our own expectations of 70 years or more.

The more limited evidence provided by skeletons suggests that prehistoric hunting and gathering groups experienced frequent bouts of growth disruption representing episodes of hunger or disease, displayed significant rates of infection, lost at least as many of their children as their modern counterparts, and endured as low or lower adult life expectancies, although the short life expectancy of prehistoric populations appears to be exaggerated by the tendency to underestimate the age of adult skeletons at death.

In addition, the well-being of living members of contemporary small-scale societies (and presumably those of the prehistoric past, as well) is clearly maintained at least in part by selective elimination of unwanted individuals. Infanticide may represent either an occasional trimming of already modest birth rates or the outcome of a substantial fraction of all live births (depending on controversial reconstructions of fertility patterns). Small-scale societies may also write off the elderly, the handicapped, or the severely injured when they can no longer fend for themselves or keep up with group movements; other forms of social mortality may also be relatively common. Even in groups without patterns of formal warfare, such as the San, homicide may be surprisingly common when measured on a per capita basis.

Having made these points, however, one must then conclude that the smallest contemporary human societies and the earliest visible populations of prehistory nonetheless do surprisingly well if we compare them to the actual record of human history rather than to our romantic images of civilized progress. Civilization has not been as successful in guaranteeing human well-being as we like to believe, at least for most of our history. Apparently, improvements in technology and organization have not entirely offset the demands of increasing population; too many of the patterns and activities of civilized lifestyles have generated costs as well as benefits.

There is no evidence either from ethnographic accounts or archaeological excavations to suggest that rates of accidental trauma or interpersonal violence declined substantially with the adoption of more civilized forms of political organization. In fact, some evidence from archaeological sites and from historical sources suggests the opposite.

Evidence from both ethnographic descriptions of contemporary hunters and the archaeological record suggests that the major trend in the quality and quantity of human diets has been downward. Contemporary hunter-gatherers, although lean and occasionally hungry, enjoy levels of caloric intake that compare favorably with national averages for many major countries of the Third World and that are generally above those of the poor in the modern world. Even the poorest recorded hunter-gatherer group enjoys a caloric intake superior to that of impoverished contemporary urban populations. Prehistoric hunter-gatherers appear to have enjoyed richer environments and to have been better nourished than most subsequent populations (primitive and civilized alike). Whenever we can glimpse the remains of anatomically modern human beings who lived in early prehistoric environments still rich in large game, they are often relatively large people displaying comparatively few signs of qualitative malnutrition. The subsequent trend in human size and stature is irregular but is more often downward than upward in most parts of the world until the nineteenth or twentieth century.

The diets of hunter-gatherers appear to be comparatively well balanced, even when they are lean. Ethnographic accounts of contemporary groups suggest that protein intakes are commonly quite high, comparable to those of affluent modern groups and substantially above world averages. Protein deficiency is almost unknown in these groups, and vitamin and mineral deficiencies are rare and usually mild in comparison to rates reported from many Third World populations. Archaeological evidence suggests that specific deficiencies, including that of iron (anemia), vitamin D (rickets), and, more controversially, vitamin C (scurvy)—as well such general signs of protein-calorie malnutrition as childhood growth retardation—have generally become more common in history rather than declining.

This decline in the quality and quantity of human nutrition appears to have had several causes. The growth of the human population and the decimation of now-extinct large mammalian prey forced human groups to gather more plentiful small game and small seeds and then to focus on the production of calorically-productive, storable staple crops. Dietary quality and variety were sacrificed for quantity. In addition, the shift from big game hunting to small game foraging, small seed harvesting, and finally subsistence agriculture seems to have represented a sequence of diminishing caloric returns for labor never fully offset by improved technology, although subsistence farming does seem to represent an improvement on the most impoverished of foraging economies.

Among farmers, increasing population required more and more frequent cropping of land and the use of more and more marginal soils, both of which further diminished returns for labor. This trend may or may not have been offset by such technological improvements in farming as the use of metal tools, specialization of labor, and efficiencies associated with large-scale production that tend to increase individual productivity as well as total production.

But whether the efficiency of farming increased or declined, the nutrition of individuals appears often to have declined for any of several reasons: because increasingly complex society placed new barriers between individuals and flexible access to resources, because trade often siphoned resources away, because some segments of the society increasingly had only indirect access to food, because investments in new technology to improve production focused power in the hands of elites so that their benefits were not widely shared, and perhaps because of the outright exploitation and deprivation of some segments of society. In addition, more complex societies have had to devote an increasing amount of their productive energy to intergroup competition, the maintenance of intragroup order, the celebration of the community itself, and the privilege of the elite, rather than focusing on the biological maintenance of individuals.

In any case, the popular impression that nutrition has improved through history reflects twentieth-century affluence and seems to have as much to do with class privilege as with an overall increase in productivity. Neither the lower classes of prehistoric and classical empires nor the contemporary Third World have shared in the improvement in caloric intake; consumption of animal protein seems to have declined for all but privileged groups.

There is no clear evidence that the evolution of civilization has reduced the risk of resource failure and starvation as successfully as we like to believe. Episodes of starvation occur among hunter-gatherer bands because natural resources fail and because they have limited ability either to store or to transport food. The risk of starvation is offset, in part, by the relative freedom of hunter-gatherers to move around and find new resources, but it is clear that with limited technology of transport they can move neither far nor fast enough to escape severe fluctuations in natural resources. But each of the strategies that sedentary and civilized populations use to reduce or eliminate food crises generate costs and risks as well as benefits. The supplementation of foraging economies by small-scale cultivation may help to reduce the risk of seasonal hunger, particularly in crowded and depleted environments. The manipulation and protection of species involved in farming may help to reduce the risk of crop failure. The storage of food in sedentary communities may also help protect the population against seasonal shortages or crop failure. But these advantages may be outweighed by the greater vulnerability that domestic crop species often display toward climatic fluctuations or other natural hazards, a vulnerability that is then exacerbated by the specialized nature or narrow focus of many agricultural systems. The advantages are also offset by the loss of mobility that results from agriculture and storage, the limits and failures of primitive storage systems, and the vulnerability of sedentary communities to political expropriation of their stored resources.

Although the intensification of agriculture expanded production, it may have increased risk in both natural and cultural terms by increasing the risk of soil exhaustion in central growing areas and of crop failure in marginal areas. Such investments as irrigation to maintain or increase productivity may have helped to protect the food supply, but they generated new risks of their own and introduced new kinds of instability by making production more vulnerable to economic and political forces that could disrupt or distort the pattern of investment. Similarly, specialization of production increased the range of products that could be made and increased the overall efficiency of production, but it also placed large segments of the population at the mercy of fickle systems of exchange or equally fickle social and political entitlements.

Modern storage and transport may reduce vulnerability to natural crises, but they increase vulnerability to disruption of the technological—or political and economic—basis of the storage and transport systems themselves. Transport and storage systems are difficult and expensive to maintain. Governments that have the power to move large amounts of food long distances to offset famine and the power to stimulate investment in protective systems of storage and transport also have and can exercise the power to withhold aid and divert investment. The same market mechanisms that facilitate the rapid movement of produce on a large scale, potentially helping to prevent starvation, also set up patterns of international competition in production and consumption that may threaten starvation to those individuals who depend on world markets to provide their food, an ever-increasing proportion of the world population.

It is therefore not clear, in theory, that civilization improves the reliability of the individual diet. As the data summarized in earlier chapters suggest, neither the record of ethnography and history nor that of archaeology pro·· vide any clear indication of progressive increase in the reliability (as opposed to the total size) of human food supplies with the evolution of civilization.

Similar points can be made with reference to the natural history of infectious disease. The data reviewed in preceding chapters suggest that prehistoric hunting and gathering populations would have been visited by fewer infections and suffered lower overall rates of parasitization than most other world populations, except for those of the last century, during which antibiotics have begun to offer serious protection against infection.

The major infectious diseases experienced by isolated hunting and gathering bands are likely to have been of two types: zoonotic diseases, caused by organisms whose life cycles were largely independent of human habits; and chronic diseases, handed directly from person to person, the transmission of which were unlikely to have been discouraged by small group size. Of the two categories, the zoonotic infections are undoubtedly the more important. They are likely to have been severe or even rapidly fatal because they were poorly adapted to human hosts. Moreover, zoonotic diseases may have had a substantial impact on small populations by eliminating productive adults. But in another respect their impact would have been limited because they did not pass from person to person.

By virtue of mobility and the handling of animal carcasses, hunter-gatherers are likely to have been exposed to a wider range of zoonotic infections than are more civilized populations. Mobility may also have exposed hunter-gatherers to the traveler's diarrhea phenomenon in which local microvariants of any parasite (including zoonoses) placed repeated stress on the body's immune response.

The chronic diseases, which can spread among small isolated groups, appear to have been relatively unimportant, although they undoubtedly pose a burden of disease that can often be rapidly eliminated by twentieth-century medicine. First, such chronic diseases appear to provoke relatively little morbidity in those chronically exposed. Moreover, the skeletal evidence suggests that even yaws and other common low-grade infections (periostitis) associated with infections by organisms now common to the human environment were usually less frequent and less severe among small, early mobile populations than among more sedentary and dense human groups. Similar arguments appear to apply to tuberculosis and leprosy, judging from the record of the skeletons. Even though epidemiologists now concede that tuberculosis could have spread and persisted in small groups, the evidence suggests overwhelmingly that it is primarily a disease of dense urban populations.

Similarly, chronic intestinal infestation by bacterial, protozoan, and helminth parasites, although displaying significant variation in occurrence according to the natural environment, generally appears to be minimized by small group size and mobility. At least, the prevalence of specific parasites and the parasite load, or size of the individual dose, is minimized, although in some environments mobility actually appears to have increased the variety of parasites encountered. Ethnographic observations suggest that parasite loads are often relatively low in mobile bands and commonly increase as sedentary lifestyles are adopted. Similar observations imply that intestinal infestations are commonly more severe in sedentary populations than in their more mobile neighbors. The data also indicate that primitive populations often display better accommodation to their indigenous parasites (that is, fewer symptoms of disease in proportion to their parasite load) than we might otherwise expect. The archaeological evidence suggests that, insofar as intestinal parasite loads can be measured by their effects on overall nutrition (for example, on rates of anemia), these infections were relatively mild in early human populations but became increasingly severe as populations grew larger and more sedentary. In one case where comparative analysis of archaeological mummies from different periods has been undertaken, there is direct evidence of an increase in pathological intestinal bacteria with the adoption of sedentism. In another case, analysis of feces has documented an increase in intestinal parasites with sedentism.

Many major vector-borne infections may also have been less important among prehistoric hunter-gatherers than they are in the modern world. The habits of vectors of such major diseases as malaria, schistosomiasis, and bubonic plague suggest that among relatively small human groups without transportation other than walking these diseases are unlikely to have provided anything like the burden of morbidity and mortality that they inflicted on historic and contemporary populations.

Epidemiological theory further predicts the failure of most epidemic diseases ever to spread in small isolated populations or in groups of moderate size connected only by transportation on foot. Moreover, studies on the blood sera of contemporary isolated groups suggest that, although small size and isolation is not a complete guarantee against the transmission of such diseases in the vicinity, the spread from group to group is at best haphazard and irregular. The pattern suggests that contemporary isolates are at risk to epidemics once the diseases are maintained by civilized populations, but it seems to confirm predictions that such diseases would and could not have flourished and spread—because they would not reliably have been transmitted—in a world inhabited entirely by small and isolated groups in which there were no civilized reservoirs of diseases and all transportation of diseases could occur only at the speed of walking human beings.

In addition, overwhelming historical evidence suggests that the greatest rates of morbidity and death from infection are associated with the introduction of new diseases from one region of the world to another by processes associated with civilized transport of goods at speeds and over distances outside the range of movements common to hunting and gathering groups. Small-scale societies move people among groups and enjoy periodic aggregation and dispersal, but they do not move the distances associated with historic and modern religious pilgrimages or military campaigns, nor do they move at the speed associated with rapid modern forms of transportation. The increase in the transportation of people and exogenous diseases seems likely to have had far more profound effects on health than the small burden of traveler's diarrhea imposed by the small-scale movements of hunter-gatherers.

Prehistoric hunting and gathering populations may also have had one other important advantage over many more civilized groups. Given the widely recognized (and generally positive or synergistic) association of malnutrition and disease, the relatively good nutrition of hunter-gatherers may further have buffered them against the infections they did encounter.

In any case, the record of the skeletons appears to suggest that severe episodes of stress that disrupted the growth of children (acute episodes of infection or epidemics and/or episodes of resource failure and starvation) did not decline—and if anything became increasingly common—with the evolution of civilization in prehistory.

Aside from some freedom from exotic diseases associated with handling wild animals and living in "wild" environments—and aside from modern medicine, which has dramatically reduced infection rates in the twentieth century when and where it was applied—the major advantage of civilization, with reference to infectious disease, appears to be precisely that it ultimately permitted epidemic diseases to become both cosmopolitan and endemic in most world regions. This transformation meant that exposed populations had a history of recent prior exposure. Such prior exposure may have resulted in populations genetically selected for resistance to these diseases, although specific evidence of such evolved immunity is controversial and hard to pinpoint. More clearly, prior exposure has meant that in each community at least some portion of the adult population is likely to have been infected already. Repeat epidemics are therefore likely to hit new individuals in childhood, when individual cases tend to be mild. More important, these repeated waves of disease tend to incapacitate only a fraction of the population. Because family and community services are not disrupted and the relatively small proportion who become sick can be tended, the epidemic may have only relatively mild effects. Civilizations have therefore come to enjoy an advantage in dealing with infectious disease that results paradoxically because their social organization is so permissive of disease transmission; this has proved to be a major political advantage that civilizations have not been loathe to exploit in displacing and decimating their less civilized competitors.

There is also evidence, primarily from ethnographic sources, that primitive populations suffer relatively low rates of many degenerative diseases compared, at least, to the more affluent of modern societies, even after corrections are made for the different distribution of adult ages. Primitive populations (hunter-gatherers, subsistence farmers, and all groups who do not subsist on modern refined foods) appear to enjoy several nutritional advantages over more affluent modern societies that protect them from many of the diseases that now afflict us. High bulk diets, diets with relatively few calories in proportion to other nutrients, diets low in total fat (and particularly low in saturated fat), and diets high in potassium and low in sodium, which are common to such groups, appear to help protect them against a series of degenerative conditions that plague the more affluent of modern populations, often in proportion to their affluence. Diabetes mellitus appears to be extremely rare in primitive groups (both hunter-gatherers and farmers) as are circulatory problems, including high blood pressure, heart disease, and strokes. Similarly, disorders associated with poor bowel function, such as appendicitis, diverticulosis, hiatal hernia, varicose veins, hemorrhoids, and bowel cancers, appear rare. Rates of many other types of cancer—particularly breast and lung—appear to be low in most small-scale societies, even when corrected for the small proportion of elderly often observed; even those cancers that we now consider to be diseases of underdevelopment, such as Burkitt's lymphoma and cancer of the liver, may be the historical product of changes in human behavior involving food storage or the human-assisted spread of vector-borne infections. The record of the skeletons suggests, through the scarcity of metastases in bone, that cancers were comparatively rare in prehistory.

The history of human life expectancy is much harder to describe or summarize with any precision because the evidence is so fragmentary and so many controversies are involved in its interpretation. But once we look beyond the very high life expectancies of mid–twentieth century affluent nations, the existing data also appear to suggest a pattern that is both more complex and less progressive than we are accustomed to believe.

Contrary to assumptions once widely held, the slow growth of prehistoric populations need not imply exceedingly high rates of mortality. Evidence of low fertility and/or the use of birth control by small-scale groups suggests (if we use modern life tables) that average rates of population growth very near zero could have been maintained by groups suffering only historically moderate mortality (life expectancy of 25 to 30 years at birth with 50 to 60 percent of infants reaching adulthood—figures that appear to match those observed in ethnographic and archaeological samples) that would have balanced fertility, which was probably below the averages of more sedentary modern populations. The prehistoric acceleration of population growth after the adoption of sedentism and farming, if it is not an artifact of archaeological reconstruction, could be explained by an increase in fertility or altered birth control decisions that appear to accompany sedentism and agriculture. This explanation fits the available data better than any competing hypothesis.

It is not clear whether the adoption of sedentism or farming would have increased or decreased the proportion of individuals dying as infants or children. The advantages of sedentism may have been offset by risks associated with increased infection, closer spacing of children, or the substitution of starchy gruels for mother's milk and other more nutritious weaning foods. The intensification of agriculture and the adoption of more civilized lifestyles may not have improved the probability of surviving childhood until quite recently. Rates of infant and child mortality observed in the smallest contemporary groups (or reconstructed with less certainty among prehistoric groups) would not have embarrassed most European countries until sometime in the nineteenth century and were, in fact, superior to urban rates of child mortality through most of the nineteenth century (and much of the twentieth century in many Third World cities).

There is no evidence from archaeological samples to suggest that adult life expectancy increased with the adoption of sedentism or farming; there is some evidence (complicated by the effects of a probable acceleration of population growth on cemetery samples) to suggest that adult life expectancy may actually have declined as farming was adopted. In later stages of the intensification of agriculture and the development of civilization, adult life expectancy most often increased—and often increased substantially—but the trend was spottier than we sometimes realize. Archaeological populations from the Iron Age or even the Medieval period in Europe and the Middle East or from the Mississippian period in North America often suggest average adult ages at death in the middle or upper thirties, not substantially different from (and sometimes lower than) those of the earliest visible populations in the same regions. Moreover, the historic improvement in adult life expectancy may have resulted at least in part from increasing infant and child mortality and the consequent "select" nature of those entering adulthood as epidemic diseases shifted their focus from adults to chidren.

Until the nineteenth or even twentieth centuries, the improvement in overall life expectancy appears to have been fairly small in any case. Life expectancy at birth was still in the high twenties or low thirties in much of Europe in the eighteenth and early nineteenth centuries. Moreover, the pattern of life expectancy was highly irregular or, perhaps one should say, socially partitioned. The experience of India suggests that some Third World populations may have had life expectancies at birth as low as or lower than those of most prehistoric and primitive groups well into the twentieth century. Many urban centers even in Europe may not have exceeded or even matched primitive life expectancies until the mid–nineteenth or even the twentieth century; the world's poor clearly did not share in the recent improvements in life expectancy until the past 150 years or less and still share only to a substantially reduced degree.

These data clearly imply that we need to rethink both scholarly and popular images of human progress and cultural evolution. We have built our images of human history too exclusively from the experiences of privileged classes and populations, and we have assumed too close a fit between technological advances and progress for individual lives.

In scholarly terms, these data—which often suggest diminishing returns to health and nutrition—tend to undermine models of cultural evolution based on technological advances. They add weight to theories of cultural evolution that emphasize environmental constraints, demographic pressure, and competition and social exploitation, rather than technological or social progress, as the primary instigators of social change. In particular, the demonstrable diminishing returns of the intensification of hunting and gathering, measured both in studies of efficiency and skeletal indicators of health, strongly support the argument that farming was more often a response to the deterioration of the hunting and gathering lifestyle or the increasing demand of growing population size or complex social organization than a technological breakthrough. Similarly, the archaeological evidence that outlying populations often suffered reduced health as a consequence of their inclusion in larger political units, the clear class stratification of health in early and modern civilizations, and the general failure of either early or modern civilizations to promote clear improvements in health, nutrition, or economic homeostasis for large segments of their populations until the very recent past all reinforce competitive and exploitative models of the origins and function of civilized states.

In popular terms, I think that we must substantially revise our traditional sense that civilization represents progress in human well-being—or at least that it did so for most people for most of history prior to the twentieth century. The comparative data simply do not support that image. At best, we see what might be called a partitioning of stress by class and location, in which the well-to-do are progressively freed from nutritional stress (although even they did not escape the ravages of epidemics until recently) but under which the poor and urban populations, particularly the urban poor, are subjected to levels of biological stress that are rarely matched in the most primitive of human societies. The undeniable successes of the late nineteenth and twentieth centuries have been of briefer duration, and are perhaps more fragile, than we usually assume. In fact, some of our sense of progress comes from comparing ourselves not to primitives but to urban European populations of the fourteenth to eighteenth centuries. We measure the progress that has occurred since then and extrapolate the trend back into history. But a good case can be made that urban European populations of that period may have been among the nutritionally most impoverished, the most disease-ridden, and the shortest-lived populations in human history. A Hobbesian view of primitive life makes sense from the perspective of the affluent twentieth century. But Hobbes was probably wrong, by almost any measure, when he characterized primitive life as ". . . poor, nasty, brutish, and short" while speaking from the perspective of urban centers of seventeenth-century Europe. At best, he was speaking only for his own social class.[1]

For most of history, the successes of civilization have been of rather a different sort. There can be no doubt, given the number of individuals for whom they must provide, that civilized states in some form are an essential mode of organization. Given the increasing numbers of human beings (whether as cause or effect of new technology and organization), states clearly cope in a manner that societies with simpler technologies and modes of organization could not. There is not enough room—nor are there enough natural resources—for modern numbers of human beings to hunt and gather their own food; nor could they individually grow anything like a sufficient quantity and variety of crops to promise adequate nutrition. Modern civilizations are clearly successful in the sense that they provide for increasing numbers of people, even if they have added little to the health and nutrition of the individuals involved until quite recently.

Civilized states have also been successful in another, and I think historically more important, sense: Historically, they have been successful as systems competitively displacing simpler systems in the political arena. In this sense more than any other, the superiority of civilized state systems is clearly manifest; they control those portions of the globe that they wish to control and absorb or destroy such other populations as they wish to absorb or destroy. But it is the systems, not always the people (or all of the people) that they represent, that succeed.

There is a practical implication to all of this—at least, if we are to maintain the ideal that civilization is about individual well-being and not just about numbers, competition, and power. We tend to assume that progress is inevitable, and we tend to promote membership in civilization as if the mere fact of being civilized were itself a worthy goal. The data presented here suggest, in fact, that the organization and style of civilization are at least as much the cause of biological stress as they are the cure. The one clear blessing of civilization from the point of view of the individual is the potential for investment. It is only by generating investment in solutions to human problems that civilizations offset the problems generated by increasing human numbers and the problems that their own organizations create; only by permitting the benefits of these investments to be shared can we truly be said to share the blessings of civilization.

Notes

Chapter 1

1. More detailed description of the three revolutions will be found in chapter 3.

2. Morgan 1877; White 1959; Steward 1955; Childe 1950.

3. Alexander Alland (1967) has cogently equated cultural and biological adaptation using population growth as a measure of success for both animals and people. He effectively reminded us that people, too, are subject to Darwinian principles. More recently, sociobiologists and ethologists have explicitly argued for measuring success in terms of the reproductive success of individuals (see, for example, Wilson 1975; Blurton Jones and Sibley 1978). I accept these as statements of Darwinian principles and as alternative meaningful grounds on which the success of social systems can be evaluated; but these are not the grounds on which commonly held beliefs about the success of civilization are based, nor are they the grounds on which most contemporary political choices are made.

4. Acsadi and Nemeskeri 1970; Weiss 1984. Petersen 1975. Petersen suggests, for example, that life expectancy has doubled twice—from approximately 20 years at birth in prehistory to about 40 in early preindustrial states to 70–80 in the modern world.

5. Lee and DeVore 1968; Sahlins 1968, 1972.

6. Boserup 1965.

7. Black et al. 1974; Black 1980; Bartlett 1960; Polgar 1964; Boyden 1970; Smith 1972.

8. See, for example, Truswell and Hansen 1976; Black 1975; CIBA 1977. See also chapter 6. There is considerable debate about the degree to which any of these societies is a "pristine" example of ancient life (Schrire 1984; Myers 1988).

9. Buikstra and Cook 1980; Cohen and Armelagos 1984; Gilbert and Mielke 1985; Ortner and Putschar 1981; Steinbock 1976. See also chapter 7.

10. For a discussion of these shortcomings, see chapters 6 and 7.

Chapter 2

1. Top and Wehrle 1976; Hubbert et al. 1975.

2. Gangarosa 1976; Overturf and Mathies 1976.

3. Hudson 1965; Hackett 1963; Rosebury 1971; Rudolf 1976.

4. Top and Wehrle 1976.

5. Benenson 1976.

6. Richard 1975; Selby 1975a, 1975b, 1975c; Smith 1975.

7. Norman 1985; Quinn et al. 1986. Blattner et al. 1988; Duesberg 1988; Piot et al. 1988.

8. Kleeburg 1975.

9. Alland 1967, 1970; Desowitz 1980; Livingstone 1958, 1984.

10. Brunell 1976.

11. Epstein-Barr (EB) virus is apparently ubiquitous among human groups, infecting almost every human group that has ever been studied, regardless of group habits and the degree of contact between the group and the rest of the world (see Black et al. 1974 and Black 1975, which are discussed more fully in chapter 4). But the most serious pathological consequences of the virus, including the disease mononucleosis and particular forms of cancer, appear to be more limited in their distribution and associated with particular lifestyles. Mononucleosis is most commonly associated with modern Western populations, apparently because of the relatively late age (adolescence or adulthood) at which individuals are likely to be infected in such societies (Miller 1976). But the virus is thought to be more likely to produce cancer (either Burkitt's lymphoma or nasopharyngeal carcinoma) when it attacks early in life. The latter are cancers more common in "developing" countries than in the Western world (Marx 1986). Such other factors as diet or the presence of other infections may be necessary to trigger carcinogenesis. Learmonth (1988) suggests that EB virus and malaria together may be needed to produce Burkitt's lymphoma.

12. Polio ("infantile paralysis"), normally a fairly mild infection of the intestine, is more likely to produce paralysis when it attacks an individual comparatively late in life. Infectious hepatitis is also a disease that increases in severity with improving sanitation, presumably because the organism acts differently when it infects human hosts of different ages (Mosley 1976a, 1976b; McCollum 1976). Multiple sclerosis (MS) is clearly associated with affluent Western lifestyles (see, for example, Leibowitz et al. 1971; Whitaker 1983). If it is an infectious disease, as many believe, a similar age-dependent infectious agent may be involved, since rates of MS are related to where individuals lived as adolescents. One theory of MS has implicated the virus associated with canine distemper, thereby also implicating the Western habit of keeping dogs as house pets.

13. Hudson 1965; Hackett 1963; Rosebury 1971; Rudolf 1976.

14. Scrimshaw et al. 1968; Beisel 1982.

15. Taylor 1983.

16. The latter, until recently a relatively controversial point, can be demonstrated by studies of the epidemiological patterns of human disease that demonstrate association with certain social and psychological conditions (Cassell 1976). It can also be demonstrated by analysis of the actual chemical pathways by which the body fights infection. It is possible to show that both people and laboratory animals have spe-

cific chemical pathways connecting the perceptions of their senses and their social interactions to the production of disease-fighting antibodies (Christian 1980). The principle is one that Western medicine, fascinated with germ theory, has missed until recently; but it seems to be one that many primitive medical systems grasped intuitively. The analysis of the work of traditional curers (whom we are prone to write off as witch doctors) often suggests that they are rather good psychotherapists (Robbins 1973; Turner 1967). See also House et al. 1988.

17. Cassell 1976.

18. Alfin-Slater and Kritchevsky 1980; Winick 1980; Bogert, Briggs, and Calloway 1973. The human body is rather well designed to avoid the toxic (which tends to taste bitter or sour), to be attracted to the calorically rich (which commonly tastes sweet), to store the scarce, and to excrete the excess. But one of the flaws or anachronisms in human design resulting from our evolutionary heritage is that our mechanisms of ingestion, storage, and excretion are often not set appropriately for the concentrations of nutrient substances that occur in the world we now inhabit (or, more particularly, for the concentrations of those substances that occur in the packaged food created by civilization). We and other primates are almost the only mammals unable to synthesize their own ascorbic acid (vitamin C), a trait that reflects our evolution in fruit-rich (and hence rich in ascorbic acid) tropical rain forests but that creates the danger of scurvy in any other environment (Stone 1965). We absorb only about 5 to 10 percent of the iron in our dietary intake (White 1980) but absorb fat readily (about 95 percent of intake) (Alfin-Slater and Aftergood 1980). We excrete sodium poorly and store calories readily but expend excess calories only with great difficulty. All of these may be adaptations to a past in which meat, vitamins, and minerals, such as potassium, were relatively abundant, but fats, calories, and sodium were relatively scarce.

Most human beings (at least most nonwhite human beings) also digest milk poorly as adults (despite the advertising of the Dairy Council) because, like most other adult mammals, adult human beings do not produce the enzyme lactase necessary for the digestion of milk sugar (Harrison 1975; Simoons 1970; Friedl 1981).

19. Animal protein enhances iron absorption, whereas its absorption from vegetable foods is more difficult. In fact, absorption is strongly inhibited by particular substances in vegetable foods, such as the phytates and phosphates found in cereals and the oxalates found in some leafy vegetables. Iron absorption is facilitated by such reducing agents as ascorbic acid (vitamin C). Ultimately, iron sufficiency is a function of diet and the presence or absence of parasites that compete with the body for available iron, either by directly consuming the iron freed by human digestion in the intestine or by consuming such iron-rich body parts as red blood cells (Winick 1980; NAS NRC 1973; White 1980; Alfin Slater and Kritchevsky 1980; Weinberg 1974).

20. Groups that travel or trade for food or salt over a range of soil zones or that exploit marine resources should rarely be deficient in iodine. Those populations spatially confined to iodine-poor regions will suffer, especially if they further deplete soils through intensive farming. Where iodine intake is marginal, other dietary choices affect the nutritional status of individuals. Certain classes of plants, including cabbages, contain chemicals that inhibit the successful use of iodine and may thus render an otherwise marginal intake pathological. Ultimately, of course, we can and do solve the problem by adding iodine chemically to salt. We can (and do)

occasionally create the problem, as we have in parts of New Guinea, by forcing or enticing other populations to buy noniodized salt in place of naturally iodized salt once supplied by indigenous trade networks. (See Gajdusek and Garruto 1975; Alfin Slater and Kritchevsky 1980; Winick 1980.)

A third example is provided by vitamin D, which is essential to human use of calcium and hence to the formation of strong, correctly shaped bones (and also to normal functioning of the nervous system). Vitamin D in the diet is most commonly obtained from the oils of fish; hence it is rarely lacking in the diets of populations heavily dependent on aquatic resources. And it is now added intentionally to milk. Vitamin D is also a hormone that the human body itself produces in the skin, in response to bombardment by ultraviolet light from the sun (or from some artificial light sources). Populations exposing skin to sufficient sunlight will rarely be deficient, but such cultural variables as clothing, shelter, and air pollution can all affect vitamin D production adversely, as can occupational specializations or rules of privacy and modesty that confine some people to secluded indoor locations. Rickets, or bone deformities associated with lack of the vitamin, is predominantly an urban disease or a disease of people so confined (Winick 1980; Loomis 1967).

21. Several types of cancer, including those of the lung, breast, and colon, are more common in Western-style societies than in other human groups. Stomach cancer is more common in Japan than in the United States (Marx 1986). How much of the current burden of cancer in the industrial world is associated with industrial processes, occupational hazards, or air pollution —as opposed to smoking and diet— is a matter of some debate. (See Ames 1983; Letters to *Science* in response to Ames, *Science* 224:658ff. [1984]; Learmonth 1988; Marx 1986; Trowell and Burkitt 1982; Alfin Slater and Kritchevsky 1980.)

Some cancers, including virally induced cervical cancer, bladder cancer, liver cancer, and also Burkitt's lymphoma and nasopharyngeal carcinoma (associated with Epstein-Barr virus; see note 11) are more common in developing countries. Bladder cancer may be associated with schistosomiasis infection; liver cancer may be associated with infection by liver flukes (parasitic worms; see Higginson 1980). Liver cancer may also be associated with aflatoxins that grow on maize or groundnuts stored in the tropics (Learmonth 1988).

22. Winick 1980; Marx 1986; Kolata 1987b.

23. We know, for example, that, just as short-term color variation (tanning) in human skin is protective against solar rays, inborne, genetically determined variations in human skin color are adaptations to differing degrees of ultraviolet radiation received by inhabitants of different latitudes on earth. Dark skin tends to filter out ultraviolet light, protecting equatorial populations where ultraviolet radiation is intense from sunburn and skin cancer. And, indeed, black or dark-skinned populations are commonly less at risk for these diseases than light- or white-skinned groups. But dark skin also minimizes the ability to generate vitamin D from ultraviolet light, such that dark-skinned people are relatively at risk for rickets, especially when moved to northern latitudes poor in ultraviolet light. Black skin is also apparently relatively susceptible to frostbite (Loomis 1967, 1970; Post et al. 1975).

We also believe that human beings have evolved to drink milk as adults in only a few parts of the world (mostly in Europe)—those where dairying has historically been important. The concentration of adult milk drinking among people of European ancestry may be related to the evolution of white skin. Light skin maximizes the production of vitamin D and the utilization of calcium in an environment with limited solar radiation. Drinking milk fresh (as opposed to making cheese or yogurt) is a way to maximize calcium absorption (Simoons 1970; Kretchmer 1972; Friedl 1981; Harrison 1975).

Variations in the chemistry of hemoglobin (including the sickle cell trait, hemoglobin C, and thalassemia) are genetic traits common in tropical and subtropical populations that help individuals resist malaria, although the traits can be dangerous, sometimes lethal, in their own rights. (Livingstone 1958, 1964; Allison 1954). We now believe that variations in the Duffy blood group (a lesser-known equivalent of the ABO group) affect susceptibility to malaria as well (Livingstone 1984). We know that glucose-6-phosphate dehydrogenase (G6PD) deficiency, a common genetic trait in southern Europe, defends against malaria but produces favism in people who eat broadbeans and related legumes (Katz 1986).

We know that there is genetic variation in ability to taste phenylthiourea (PTC), as many students have experienced in high school biology labs. Phenylthiourea is similar to natural iodine-inhibiting compounds found in vegetables (see note 20). The variable ability to taste PTC and iodine-inhibiting compounds explains why some but not all individuals find certain vegetables bitter and, more significantly, may assist or hinder individuals in avoiding iodine deficiency in iodine-poor environments (Van Etten and Wolf 1973; Boyce et al. 1976).

Furthermore, human tissue antigens (proteins called histocompatibility antigens, because they determine the ability of individuals to receive tissue grafts from others whose tissues are either compatible or incompatible) and blood antigens (proteins that determine blood types and control our ability to receive blood transfusions from others) may represent evolved adaptations by particular human populations to particular biological risks or insults. Types B and O blood, for example, appear to confer more immunity to smallpox than type A blood (Vogel and Chakravartti 1971). Individuals with type B blood, however, appear in some studies to be more than normally susceptible to tuberculosis (Overfield and Klauber 1980), just as individuals with type O blood appear more susceptible to cholera (Levine et al. 1979; Barua and Paguio 1977). Variations in ABO blood type may even affect the biting habits of certain classes of mosquitos, affecting, in turn, the susceptibility of human hosts to the diseases they transmit (Wood 1979). In fact, such patterns of genetic variation provide one kind of evidence that can be used, albeit with considerable caution, to trace the history of certain diseases. For example, the presence of the sickle cell trait is commonly used as evidence that a population has a history of exposure to malaria; the absence of the trait or of other known genetic adaptations to malaria among Amerindians is one kind of evidence suggesting that malaria was not present in the New World prior to the age of Columbus.

Of more serious moment in the modern Western world, we are finding that there are important and apparently inborn (genetic) variations between groups in the incidences of such diseases as obesity, diabetes, and hypertension. Blacks, for example, seem somewhat more prone to obesity, diabetes, and hypertension than are whites under similar conditions (Lieberman 1985), and American Indians are also more susceptible than whites to these diseases, as well as to cholesterol gallstones and cancer of the middle intestinal tract, when they are fed comparable diets (Knowler et al. 1983; Weiss et al. 1984). In these instances the traits of whites, blacks, and Amerindians seem to be adapted not so much to different ancestral climates as to different historic dietary regimes. We are finding, too, that human groups display variations in the incidences of specific cancers and of functional problems that are not entirely explained by their lifestyles but do appear to be related, for unknown reasons, to otherwise minor genetic variations in body composition.

24. Winick 1980; Alfin-Slater and Kritchevsky 1980; Bogert, Briggs, and Calloway 1973.

25. Alland 1967, 1971; Rappaport 1968; Leeds and Vayda 1965; Desowitz 1980; Durham 1976, 1982; Harris 1974. Some of these adaptive behaviors are simple matters of ritual or style that would be trivial if they did not have profound effects on health. For example, building houses on stilts can minimize malaria if, as a consequence, people live and sleep at elevations slightly above the normal flying height of the local mosquito vector. Conversely, building houses of clay can have negative effects, because the borrow pits from which the clay is taken from the ground often fill with water, making ideal breeding ground for mosquitos. Ceremonial slaughtering of animals in accordance with ritual cycles often appears to serve the function of optimizing the distribution of scarce animal protein.

How adaptive strategies emerge in the history of each population is not entirely clear. What is clear is that many if not most such strategies are developed without conscious knowledge—or at least without scientific explication—of the ecological rules that are involved. Presumably, people proceed by trial and error, and learn to associate certain behaviors with relative freedom from disease, and then repeat the successful actions.

For example, many societies appear to recognize the symptoms of kwashiorkor (severe protein deficiency), even though they have no knowledge of protein or daily protein requirements. Moreover, many groups have enough sense of the pattern of the disease to develop reasonably effective avoidance strategies (such as spacing babies far enough apart so that a mother is not pregnant and nursing at the same time), even though they do not understand the physiological mechanisms by which pregnancy and lactation compete for the mother's protein supply (Whiting 1969).

Even in our own society, much of our successful adjustment to disease has developed independent of our scientific theories. For example, a classic piece of epidemiological research was done on the distribution of cholera in England in the nineteenth century, and effective corrective action was taken involving abandonment of a particular water supply—long before the organism responsible for cholera was identified (Snow 1849). Similarly, we now recognize the pattern of distribution of various cancers and recognize factors that appear to increase their risk, even though we do not fully understand the mechanisms of carcinogenesis.

But consciously perceived or not, the existence of patterns in nature and the explicit or intuitive recognition of those patterns by human beings presumably underlie the existence of reasonably successful, if unscientific, human adaptation. The diets of the vast majority of free-living human groups, though hardly perfect, are on balance strikingly successful at meeting qualitative nutritional needs (the needs for proteins, vitamins, minerals, and the like) in the absence of scientific knowledge. Indeed, this success is particularly striking in the face of the concern we express and the need we seem to feel to obtain these substances from artificial sources.

26. We might expect that it is commonly newly introduced diseases and deficiencies that are most stressful to a population—a point made aptly by Desowitz (1981) in a charming essay entitled "New Guinea Tapeworms and Jewish Grandmothers." Desowitz pointed out that New Guinea tribesmen and Jewish grandmothers in New York (both living in the twentieth century and possessed of unscientific patterns of hygiene and behavior appropriate to avoiding their traditional parasites) were equally helpless in the face of newly introduced infections. In each case the victims were newly exposed to disease risk as a result of behavior that facilitated the persistence of parasites by people in very different places.

The New Guineans displayed what Desowitz called "Stone Age toilet habits"—a lack of hygienic concern in their toilet habits—as well as the habit of eating meat only partly cooked. Even in combination, however, those habits did not generate a health problem until after Balinese pigs, infected with tapeworms, were introduced by a colonial government. The tapeworms were then able to take advantage of cooking and toilet habits to complete their life cycle between people and pigs and, incidentally, to wreak profound health stresses on the population. The Jewish grandmothers, whose own toilet habits were probably impeccable (at least by Western Judeo-Christian standards) and whose dietary laws protected them from some parasites to which their ancestors were historically exposed, were done in by their habit of sampling undercooked fish from the pot. This habit exposed them to the risk of ingesting tapeworms from fish, but only because they began to eat imported fish. The imported fish, in turn, were contaminated by the poor sanitary habits of fishermen many hundreds of miles away who, by defecating in the lakes where they fished, permitted the tapeworm to complete its life cycle.

There are, in fact, three very practical lessons to be learned here: first, that change itself is risky; second, that patterns of human behavior are most likely to appear unclean and to be risky in the face of newly introduced health risks to which cultural habits have not yet had a chance to adjust; third, that risk is generated in a cosmopolitan world when a people's exposure to infection is complicated by the behavior of other groups of people whose behavior they can neither observe nor control.

27. Eating raw meat, a strategy by which the Eskimos obtain vitamin C (otherwise scarce in the Arctic) and conserve precious fuel, greatly increases the risk of infection by the worms that cause trichinosis (Draper 1977). Cooking in iron pots, which enhances the availability of iron in the diet, tends to eliminate vitamin C from foods. Although some types of tsetse flies that carry sleeping sickness prefer the uncleared bush, mosquitoes that carry malaria prefer landscape that human beings have cleared to natural bush or forest. Dubos (1965) has pointed out that some of the organisms inhabiting our intestines are our major defense against others. Killing off one kind may invite further invasion.

Moreover, not all human behaviors that affect insect vectors are trivial. Some, such as the clearance of forest for farming, the building of dams, and the creation of irrigation systems (all of which promote mosquito breeding—see chapter 4), may be important and hard to correct, because they are inextricably linked with the development of civilization (Livingstone 1958, 1984; Desowitz 1980).

As Alexander Alland (1967, 1970) has cogently argued, much of the structure of human adaptive strategy is a balancing act in which different behavioral strategies are selected and maintained not because they are ideal but because they make a relatively positive overall or average contribution to the health, well-being, and success of the population that employs them. That is, they attempt to optimize the balance of benefits and risks. Each cultural choice embodies a tradeoff, and each human culture is a collection of such choices honed through prior experience and handed down as tradition.

28. Hussain and Ahmad 1977.

29. One does not tell one's Jewish grandmother that she can no longer cook as she has always done (see note 26). Her good will is too important; the threat to her ego and the threat of her displeasure may loom larger than the health benefits involved. Similarly, Desowitz (1981) could not convince the New Guinea tribesmen to cook their meat more thoroughly. Their response was that adhering to certain traditional eating patterns was more important than risks to health. Nor do modern Americans abandon their eating habits or, as Desowitz himself points out, their smoking habits simply because associated detriments to health are pointed out to them.

Chapter 3

1. Fried 1967; Harris 1977, 1987; Childe 1950; Johnson and Earle 1987. Like all classifications, this sequence is necessarily simplified for ease of presentation and will appear too orderly, the implied correlations too neat, to individuals with detailed knowledge of individual cultures.

2. Neither trend is uniform, of course; individual populations occasionally decline and disappear, and large political units occasionally disintegrate into smaller ones, as when an empire collapses. Apparently, some very ancient human groups, such as those inhabiting Europe late in the Pleistocene Ice Age, blessed with a particularly rich resource base, managed to maintain larger communities than some of their descendants (Price and Brown 1985). What is primitive or small scale is not always ancient, nor does it always come before larger or more civilized forms. At least some contemporary small-scale societies may be the recent creation of adjoining large-scale societies—in effect, rebels rather than remnants (Schrire 1984). But for the human species as a whole, the overall trend is clear (Carneiro 1981).

I am intentionally presenting a relatively simple, idealized summary of the trend in size so that logical links between behavior and disease can be pursued in later chapters. That the historical reality was more complicated need not destroy the broad patterns suggested, although it does suggest caution in the interpretation of individual cases.

In presenting this simplified and generalized outline, I am aware that I am acting in explicit opposition to recent fashion in anthropology, and particularly in hunter-gatherer studies, which favors the exploration of variety and abhors what it perceives as the overgeneralization of data from one case, the Kalahari San, to all of human history (Lee and DeVore 1968; cf. Lewin 1988b; Myers 1988). My own survey of the ethnographic literature (chapter 6) suggests that broad parallels described in the text do, indeed, reasonably characterize hunting and gathering bands in a variety of contexts. These parallels were visible to anthropologists before the publication of the San data, and many are contained in subsequent work even by those who are critical of the San model.

3. Why the human population gets larger is not as obvious as it may seem. The traditional answer of both anthropologists and historians, at least since Malthus (1830), has been to say that natural tendencies toward population growth are held in check by limited resources until fortuitous technological inventions increase "carrying capacity." A more modern version has been to assume that human populations are self-regulating below the ceiling set by resources but that self-regulation is relaxed when resources are abundant or technology opens new doors (Hayden 1981a). An alternative answer offered by Boserup (1965) and by me (Cohen 1977) has been that natural human population growth is a common if not ubiquitous force in human history, necessitating economic and social change. I have argued that, even though human groups may seek to regulate their own population, true zero population growth is hard to maintain: so population creeps upward, at least in the long run. If Boserup and I are correct, technology is not so much an independent variable as others have assumed but more often an elastic response to increasing demand.

4. Lee and DeVore 1968; Bicchieri 1969; Cohen 1977; Service 1966. Such groups have occasionally been observed to plant, fertilize, cultivate, and even irrigate selected species of plants; they often raise pet animals but rarely if ever do they appear to manage the whole life cycle of any species used for food or to obtain more than a small fraction of their subsistence from the plants or animals they help to grow. Johnson and Earle (1987) have pointed out that some band societies are horticultural. Schrire (1984) has emphasized the degree to which contemporary hunter-gatherers are often trading partners with farmers.

This pattern of dependence on wild foods can be identified in the archaeological record. Domesticated or cultivated plants and animals are commonly different in shape from their natural or wild relatives, and the differences can often be seen in parts preserved in archaeological garbage. Preserved organic remains at human sites generally do not display such signs of domestication or modification from the natural state once we move back more than a few thousand years in the prehistory of any region. Hence, it is clear that the hunting and gathering mode was the rule for essentially all human societies more than about ten thousand years ago.

5. Foraging for food need not be entirely synonymous with immediate consumption, although the two tend to go together. Binford (1983) has distinguished two types of foraging, one of which involves a more complex division of labor with some delay in consumption (see note 18).

6. Lee and DeVore 1968; cf. Suttles 1968; Koyama and Thomas 1981; Price and Brown 1985.

7. Lee and DeVore 1968; Lee 1972a. It is clear that the foragers themselves perceive the increased labor costs associated with large villages; they commonly split the community, forming two or more new ones, if band size begins to become unwieldy. The newly separated communities often retain ties of friendship and kinship and often continue to exchange members, forming networks of intermarriage, occasional trade, and mutual dependence in times of economic crisis. It is presumably by this process of growth and fission that hunter-gatherer populations spread over the earth.

8. Lee 1972; Cohen 1977, 1985; Turnbull 1968; Woodburn 1968b. Mobility is a means of maintaining sanitation: groups commonly move on when a particular campsite begins to get dirty or to smell, when the huts they have built become infested with vermin, when a given water supply has become polluted, when individuals are sick,

or when a death occurs. Mobility is also used simply to obtain a change of scene or neighbors or as a means of staying in touch with information about changing patterns of available resources in neighboring locations. Hunter-gatherers also commonly use their mobility as a means of resolving social disputes, simply parting company with others whose behavior is insufferable. It is characteristic of such groups that they are often very fluid in composition and membership, with groups splitting and realigning frequently. Individuals or families (who are largely self-sufficient and are not committed to remaining in one place because, unlike farmers, they have made little or no investment in future food supplies) are relatively free to come and go from the group and regularly use this freedom to satisfy social as well as dietary whims.

Although it is difficult to get precise quantitative estimates of group size, population density, or group movement from archaeological data, archaeology can confirm, at least in a general way, that similar behavior characterized prehistoric groups; early archaeological sites are typically small in area and few in number, indicating small local populations and low overall population densities. Moreover, the pattern of frequent movement can be confirmed by observation of the relatively thin layer of refuse that accumulates at any one location, in combination with the general absence of permanent house foundations and the scarcity of immovable objects. (In contrast, the presence of larger, denser areas of refuse, as well as signs of more complex social organization, lead us to conclude that some very ancient hunting and gathering populations did not fit the "band" model.) It may even be possible to verify the occurrence of frequent splitting and reforming of groups. Archaeologists rely on the style and form of tools and other artifacts to identify social boundaries; it is typical of such early campsites that their tool styles are often far less distinctive from site to site than are the tools and other paraphernalia of later, more permanent, and apparently socially more tightly bounded, communities (Isaac 1972; Cohen 1977).

As a result of such movement, hunter-gatherers typically have a very different pattern of interaction with plants and animals than do more sedentary and civilized human groups. Whereas sedentary communities may coexist continuously with certain species of plants and animals, their lives intertwined, mobile hunter-gatherers tend to interact with other species at discrete intervals that represent only a small fraction of the life cycles of the people or the plants and animals themselves. This principle applies not only to the plants and animals that people use as food but also to plants and animals that might live as parasites or cause disease among human hosts. This means, in turn, that hunter-gatherers typically encounter a very different array of plants and animals (and parasites) than those that sedentary populations experience. Sedentary populations encounter and create a very high proportion of "weeds" —plants (but also animals and parasites) that have become adapted to living in the presence of human groups and in the landscapes that human activities create. The plant and animal species that hunter-gatherers encounter will generally be species adapted for life in natural landscapes without human interference that commonly carry out the better part of their life cycles without human company and without exposure to human products and waste products. Even simple, temporary human camps tend to gather some weeds, however, and they accumulate animal pests and parasites as well, although to a lesser degree than more permanent settlements do.

9. Fried 1967; Service 1966; Lee and DeVore 1968. However, in the modern world the group as a whole may act as economic specialists vis-à-vis another society (Schrire 1984; Bird 1983).

10. Cohen 1985.

11. Fried 1967; Woodburn 1982. Specialization, rank, and formal leadership can be identified or verified in prehistory. In contemporary populations, economic specialization, formal membership in clubs and classes, and formally defined leadership or political rank are all commonly marked by badges of style and status and by the spatial distribution of activities within the community. The absence of such indications in small, early archaeological sites and the relatively homogeneous distribution of artifacts in such hunter-gatherer campsites are clues to their economic and social simplicity. Conversely, the presence of such paraphernalia at some large early sites is a clue to their social complexity.

12. Fried 1967; Polanyi 1953.

13. Woodburn (1968a), for example, states fairly explicitly that East African Hadza who are injured too seriously to keep up with the group are in jeopardy of not being cared for. Hill and Kaplan (1988) document a high rate of infant and child mortality among Ache whose parents die. There is evidence that the accidental loss of parents and providers may have an exceptionally serious effect on their individual dependents in such communities.

14. Cohen 1985; Johnson 1982.

15. Lee 1972a, 1972b; Carneiro 1967. Complex organization may emerge temporarily as a means of maintaining social order when bands aggregate seasonally into larger groups, as Carneiro points out.

16. Judging from the distribution of their archaeological remains, for example, the earliest biologically modern human inhabitants of each of the major continents (*Homo sapiens*) appear to have preferred open grasslands, savannas, mixed savanna/forest, or open forest. They appear to have avoided dense forest, particularly tropical forest or jungle, on the one hand, and extremely arid environments, on the other. Tropical rain forests may have been avoided as much because of their parasites as because of any limits on available food. Not surprisingly, early populations also avoided extremes of high latitude and high altitude. Later expansion into these secondary zones was accompanied, generally, by signs of the increasing size and number of campsites, suggesting an overall increase in population density, as well as by signs of economic intensification (Cohen 1977; Butzer 1971).

17. Cohen 1977; Flannery 1973; Binford 1983. Big game hunting is unlikely ever to have provided the bulk of the diet for most populations (except in high latitudes). Judging from modern hunter-gatherers, it may have only rarely provided as much as half the diet. Vegetable foods may commonly have been more reliably, if less efficiently, obtained in most environments, and human palates, digestion, and nutrition are clearly geared to a mixed diet.

But early prehistoric hunter-gatherers on each continent appear to have focused more heavily on hunting big game than did their descendants. (The initial choice of open grasslands, which are rich zones for hunting, also suggests that these economies were heavily focused on hunting, as do archaeological food remains and the proportions of different tools found.) Vegetable foods (particularly small seeds), small game, and aquatic foods—and the tools to process them, such as grindstones—all became proportionally more important in later hunting and gathering sites.

The interpretation of this pattern of intensification has been the subject of some controversy in recent years. Some prehistorians have argued that the apparent movement away from big game hunting toward the eclectic gathering of various other resources simply reflects a pattern of archaeological preservation—the relatively durable bones of large animals being all that is well preserved in early sites and the apparent broad spectrum exploitation of recent sites being simply a product of their more complete preservation of organic refuse. It has also been argued that the apparent increase in use of aquatic resources might reflect either differences in preservation or changes in sea level that made these resources more available, rather than changes in human habits or preferences. But several lines of evidence now suggest that the apparent trend represents a real sequence of human choice.

Studies of the relative efficiency of various foraging techniques (which will be discussed more fully in chapter 5) commonly suggest that hunting and gathering groups ought, as a matter of efficiency, to pursue resources in the sequence that the archaeological record indicates, taking big game as long as it is available and relying on smaller animals, birds, aquatic resources, and many vegetable foods, particularly small seeds, only when supplies of large game are inadequate or particularly unreliable. The data suggest that, with the tools available in prehistory, large game would have been by far the most efficient resource to exploit. Various studies of contemporary groups confirm that hunter-gatherers are sensitive to what is efficient and commonly pursue an exploitative sequence similar to that just described, preferring to take large mammals when they are available and moving on to progressively smaller animal species and other resources as the large animal populations are exhausted (Hames and Vickers 1983; Werner 1979).

Furthermore, as the archaeological record is expanded it becomes increasingly clear that a similar sequence of changes can be identified repeatedly, even in places where the effects of changing sea level can be ruled out and where differences in preservation are likely to be unimportant. Athol Anderson (1983) has shown, for example, that early colonizers of New Zealand, who were in fact quite recent by the scale of archaeological time, quickly exhausted the supplies of vulnerable large animals (in this case, birds) and rapidly repeated the same economic sequence that other human populations had played out over longer periods on other continents. Moreover, some aspects of the archaeological record, such as the late appearance of grindstones independently in many parts of the world, cannot be explained by poor preservation. Finally, as documented more fully in chapter 7, the record of human skeletons itself suggests that real changes in human food economies and in the quality of human nutrition commonly occurred in different parts of the world during the periods in question. I will argue therefore that, although our perception of prehistory may be—undoubtedly is—distorted in some ways by imperfect preservation, the general pattern of these economic trends almost certainly represents real prehistoric shifts in human adaptation. Whether the trend primarily reflects the growth of human populations or primarily represents the decline of resources may still be disputed, and the balance of the two may differ in different regions.

18. The archaeological record displays two alterations in human food economy that pertain not so much to the choice of foods as to the logistics used in their handling. First, we can witness a quantitative shift over time away from the use of resources for immediate consumption and toward the collecting of resources for future consumption after a period of storage—a new technology most readily applied to the small seeds newly added to the menu. Second, we can witness a shift in the style of movement of groups—away from the simple movement of the band

as a whole from resource to resource, toward a more complex pattern involving the gathering of resources from several localities toward a central location where the main group resides (Binford 1980; Cohen 1985). Both of these trends imply increasing sedentism, and both foreshadow or parallel agricultural economies in the sense that they are based on the storage of main crops and the bringing home of subsidiary resources.

In recent years there has been a significant change in our perception of the archaeological record. We now realize that comparatively high population densities, moderate group size, and complex social organization appropriate to such groups occurred fairly often in prehistory without the adoption of agriculture. Apparently, large groups occasionally assembled, at least temporarily, very early in prehistory when such favored resources as game were plentiful or when there was a need for collective hunting. However, large sedentary groups become a more significant and more permanent part of the archaeological record when people began to rely on intensive harvesting and storage of certain wild plant resources, such as acorns. These nuts and seeds paralleled cereals and other domestic crops in their contribution to the human economy, although they were never domesticated. Apparently, it was the choice of appropriate food plant staples, not their domestication, that was most directly linked to group size, population density, and complex social organization (Price and Brown 1985; see also Johnson and Earle 1987).

19. The new economy appears to have been "invented" repeatedly in different parts of the world by populations that had reached highly intensified forms of hunting and gathering. It also seems to have spread from such early centers to neighboring populations. It is a matter of some dispute whether the adoption of farming results from the invention of a new and advantageous technology or diminishing returns from the old hunter-gatherer lifestyle (see chapter 5; Reed 1977; Megaw 1977; Cohen 1977; Childe 1950).

20. Bronson 1977; Anderson 1952; Cohen 1977. The staples were not chosen for their palatability, since they are rarely among the foods for which people express preference or that people choose to eat when they are sufficiently affluent to have a choice. Moreover, as the archaeological record itself makes clear, they were not foods that hunter-gatherers first chose to exploit. Nor (as will be elaborated in chapter 5) is it likely that they were chosen for their nutritional value, since they often compare unfavorably with wild plant foods available to hunter-gatherers.

In a few parts of the world this intensified focus on a few staple resources occurred without actual domestication of the species in question. For example, the Indians of California did not practice agriculture at the time that they were first contacted by Europeans, and they were thus, technically, hunter-gatherers. Many did, however, have a dependence on stored acorns comparable to the dependence of other populations on corn or wheat. Like other staples, acorns seem to have been chosen for their prolific production and their potential for storage but hardly for their palatability or nutritional value. They are highly unpalatable, in fact toxic, unless extensively processed. The major difference between this pattern and agriculture is simply that —in contrast to wheat, which could be altered genetically by selection of preferred types—the life cycles of oak trees largely defied human control; hence, acorns were never modified genetically to meet human needs. In terms of effects on the human community, this economy was essentially equivalent to agriculture, although, in the long run, perhaps not quite as capable of sustained economic growth because the resources could not respond as readily as agricultural crops to increased human attention.

21. Cohen 1977; Isaac 1970; Heiser 1973; Anderson 1952; Flannery 1965.

22. Anderson 1952; Helbaek 1969; Isaac 1970; Harlan 1971, 1977; Schwanitz 1966. Quite characteristically, for example, the natural mechanisms by which wild plants disperse their seeds and the mechanisms by which both wild plants and animals protected themselves from predation were altered to make the species more tractable to human management. Mutant seed-retaining specimens of plants (that is, plants that failed to disperse their seeds successfully, a lethal characteristic in the wild) appear to have been selected, probably inadvertantly, because these seed-retaining specimens lent themselves naturally to human planting. Simultaneously, such protective mechanisms as toxic chemicals or thorns of plants and horns of cattle were altered. And individual plants and animals that were particularly "meaty"—that is, those that provided the largest proportion of edible parts to inedible "waste"— were favored. These changes are commonly identifiable archaeologically in preserved portions of the plants and animals themselves and recognized by archaeologists as the hallmark of the new economy.

One of the major consequences of the change in the composition of the natural environment would have been an increase in plant and animal species dependent on human habits for survival. By shifting the competitive balance in favor of their preferred species, human beings would have created communities of plants and animals (and their dependent species) that were increasingly dependent on continuing human inputs.

Another sequel is that hunter-gatherers and farmers live in very different environments. Hunter-gatherer bands tend to live in relatively diverse ecosystems—in natural animal and plant communities with large numbers of different species but with relatively low population densities of any particular species. Natural environments, of course, vary enormously in the number of kinds of plants and animals that occur.

The consequence of farming will usually be a reduction in species diversity. Although the initial increase in investment in particular crops may have enriched the natural fauna and flora of a region, the emphasis on removing competitors and the increasing focus on specific staples would ultimately have resulted in an overall reduction in species diversity and an increase in the numbers of individuals of each selected species. These effects would again have extended not only to the crops themselves but also to their parasites and dependents. At the same time, it should be pointed out that modern Americans and Europeans probably have an exaggerated sense of this trend because they envision contemporary wheat fields. The latter are particularly pure stands of one crop with minimal diversity, partly because wheat, unlike such other crops as maize, tends to grow most efficiently in pure stands and partly because such purity is artifically maintained for the sake of efficiency in the use of modern farm machinery. The gardens of subsistence cultivators in maize- or manioc-growing regions tend to be far more varied in their composition (see, for example, Anderson 1952).

Human alteration of the natural fauna and flora probably also contributed to an overall increase in the seasonality of growing crops. As specific crops assumed increasing importance, the whole annual cycle of food production would be geared increasingly to their growth patterns. Human labor requirements would become increasingly seasonal, and more important, harvests would have tended increasingly to peak as major crops became ripe and to fall near zero at other times, necessitating increasing investment in storage. Again, although this is a common trend, its importance may be exaggerated in the minds of Westerners accustomed to highly specialized fields of wheat ripening simultaneously and to highly seasonal temperate climates. Tropical gardens, which perhaps show greater seasonality than eclectic gathering economies, are far less seasonal than modern temperate fields (Anderson 1952).

In addition, since growing organisms exert an impact on the chemical composition of the soil on which they grow, on the physical surface of the ground, and even on the climate, changes in the composition of fauna and flora are likely to have had an effect on the physical environment. Most obviously, the reduction in diversity and the concentration of particular species is likely to have focused and enhanced specific physical processes. For example, since each species of plant has its own typical but specialized nutrient requirements from soil, concentrating members of a single species is likely to have increased the drain on particular soil nutrients; since animals have preferred foods, concentrated animal populations are likely to have strained the regenerating capacity of their select plant foods. Such patterns can and have led to soil exhaustion, as key nutrients are eliminated by specialized crops, or to soil erosion, as concentrations of grazing animals strip away ground cover.

23. Rindos 1984. The relationship is a symbiotic one in which human habits are domesticated just as much as those of our crops, in which the crops benefit just as much as the human populations, and in which the crops are as much the choosers as the chosen. Our domesticates are all, in a sense, weeds and pests—plants and animals that "enjoy" human company and that more or less voluntarily live with human groups. We eat beef rather than zebra not because beef is tastier or more nutritious but because cattle and not zebra will live with people. Similarly, we chose wheat or corn more for their positive response to human attention than for their food qualities.

There is even some evidence that human beings have evolved genetically as part of the symbiosis. Some genetic traits, such as the sickle cell trait, apparently became common among human populations only after the adoption of farming and as a fairly direct result of altered human habits (see Livingstone 1958, 1984).

24. To the extent that they become large permanent groups, hunter-gatherer societies will be subject to most of the same economic and social requirements as farmers, even though their food supplies are not domesticated (see Price and Brown 1985).

25. Harris 1985; Harner 1970. It is common in such societies for rights to specific pieces of land to be assigned to individual members of the group for the duration of the cycle of cultivation. It is also common for particular permanent resources, such as trees or choice pieces of land, increasingly to be associated with particular groups of kin. Moreover, the community as a whole is commonly more concerned with asserting exclusive control over land in its vicinity than is true of most hunter-gatherer groups. On the other hand, it is rare in the simplest of farming groups for any individual to be excluded totally from access to that land or to other essential resources. Any member of the group has the right to claim unused land for cultivation.

26. Why human communities get larger is also not as obvious as it may seem.

Population growth, even if it occurs, does not necessarily mean larger community size. It could simply mean the creation of more small bands or villages. For some reason, however, as the human population gets larger and denser overall, people also become increasingly attracted to living in large communities. It has been traditional to assume that communities get larger simply because they can—whenever enough food is available in one place. Human beings clearly enjoy the social benefits of large groups. Large aggregations of population, like country fairs, are clearly attractive, and even hunter-gatherers appear to enjoy temporary large gatherings in seasons of plenty. And there are some practical benefits to large size, even in societies without specialists.

However there are also disincentives to aggregation, even for farmers. It is not clear why farmers would aggregate in larger clusters just because they are economically capable of doing so. After all, even for farmers, large community size means that at least some individuals will have to walk farther to their fields each day or will have to settle for land that is less desirable than what they might obtain by striking out on their own. In addition, the same social strains that rupture hunter-gatherer groups should affect farmers (Cohen 1985; Lee 1972a, 1972b; see discussion in text). Overcoming those strains and maintaining the unity of the larger group apparently implies acceptance of certain limitations to personal freedom that most hunter-gatherers are unwilling to accept. The implication is that some stronger motivation underlies the change in community size.

One reason for aggregation may be the arms race in its earliest form: as the environment gets crowded, large communities can compete successfully with small ones (Hassan 1981). In addition, agriculture and sedentism imply a degree of political vulnerability not experienced by hunter-gatherers. Stored resources, and to a lesser extent cultivated fields themselves, encourage raiding because they are vulnerable to expropriation in a way that the wild resources of hunter-gatherers are not. One can displace a hunting and gathering group from a particularly rich patch of wild resources, but one cannot obtain the fruits of their previous labor because they are commonly consumed almost immediately. Moreover, because farmers are tied to their own past investments for future consumption, they are vulnerable to political coercion to a degree not experienced by hunter-gatherers. Unlike hunter-gatherers, they cannot simply leave when threatened.

Marvin Harris (1985) has suggested that the creation of agricultural villages contributed significantly to an increase in warfare affecting human societies. If he is correct, the combination of hostility and vulnerability may go a long way toward explaining not only why the size of local population aggregates increased after the adoption of farming but also why the settlements of early agriculturalists (and those of large-scale populations of hunter-gatherers that exploit and store staple foods intensively) are often fortified in a manner almost never witnessed among small hunting and gathering bands.

27. Cohen 1985; Johnson 1982. We begin to see signs in the archaeological record that informal aggregates, presumably made of friends and loosely defined kin (as described above), give way to increasingly formally defined groups in which membership is limited and is carefully marked by badges of group affiliation. As hinted above, one of the striking patterns in prehistory is that the early bands inhabiting each continent are strikingly homogeneous in their tools and display few other

forms of nonfunctional decoration. Later groups are, in contrast, increasingly distinct in the style of their tools and are also increasingly given to paraphernalia that seems to be decorative and stylistic, without other function. We see similar signs that subdivisions within local groups are also more formally symbolized by stylistic markers.

28. Johnson 1982; Cohen 1985. The appearance in archaeological sites of fancier homes, tombs, and artistic items not available to everyone suggests that special status was accorded to particular individuals. To judge from contemporary examples, such differentiation appears to imply that privileged individuals enjoyed high status and prestige that were "ascribed"—that is, enjoyed independent of skill or prowess and therefore less limited and ephemeral than the status of leaders in earlier bands. It probably also implies relatively fixed, unchanging political authority and centralized decision making by those individuals. But to judge by contemporary examples, such differentiation did not initially imply true coercive power on the part of the privileged; nor did it yet imply a monopoly of such major economic resources as land or water as much as a more limited monopoly of luxury items.

29. So-called big men, who act as centers of redistribution in relatively small sedentary groups, still commonly lack the monopoly of force and resources that characterize the leaders of more civilized groups. Their pivotal position in both trade and decision making is often maintained only as long as they are perceived as acting in the interests of their followers. Even the chiefs of larger, more formally organized groups often cannot use force to get their way, although their authority is commonly reinforced by established customs of respect and obedience and by ritual or religious sanctions.

30. Early civilizations begin to appear in the archaeological record only after about five thousand years ago. Pristine states—civilizations developing independently of earlier civilizations—appeared in only a few scattered locations: Egypt and Mesopotamia, India and China, and Mexico and Peru. These early civilizations seem to have acted as catalysts, transforming the landscape around them toward civilization such that, secondary to the appearance of these early centers, civilization gradually spread at the expense of smaller social units to cover the globe (see Fried 1967; Service 1975; Cohen and Service 1975; Claessen and Skalnick 1978; Jones and Kautz 1981).

Early archaeological analyses of the origins of civilization, such as that offered by Childe (1950), were fascinated by its visible trappings: the building of great monuments, the display of monumental forms of art, the display of such newly sophisticated technologies as metallurgy, and, at least in some parts of the world, the adoption of written forms of communication and the appearance of the first permanently recorded written laws and forms of art. Such trappings continue to fascinate because many are beautiful and because they do indeed represent singular accomplishment; as such, these trappings often form the core of the descriptions that civilizations themselves make in celebration of their own historic roots. The focus on such trappings, as well as contemporary use of the word *civilized* as a synonym for *polite, fair, advanced,* and *sophisticated,* has provided us with a one-sided image of civilization that some of these more recent sources—focused on the social structure of civilized society—can help to balance.

31. Boserup 1965.

32. See, for example, Wittfogel 1957. In addition, such improvements in agricultural land would have increasingly become the focus of economic and political competition at two levels. As improvements made some land more valuable than others, rights to use land may have become more exclusive, either in the sense that community membership became more exclusive or in the sense that individuals or families came to exert increasingly "private" control of particular parcels of land. For example, land that lay fallow until it reverted to natural bush or forest might become part of the common land pool in between harvests, even though it was the "property" of one individual or family while a crop was growing; but land cropped repeatedly might well tend to become more or less permanently associated with the farmers who worked it. In any case, the free access to land that had hitherto prevailed was undermined. In addition, as a limited resource, improved or improvable land may have increasingly become the focus of conflict between groups.

33. Fried 1967; Service 1975; It is a moot point whether social stratification is necessary to civilization in a structural sense—whether it is probable or inevitable as the most efficient way of carrying out group purposes or whether it is simply a historical pattern that states taught one another.

34. Cf. Wittfogel 1957; Fried 1967; Service 1975; Claessen and Skalnik 1978; Cohen and Service 1978; Carneiro 1970.

35. Carneiro 1981.

Chapter 4

1. Haldane 1932; Polgar 1964; Burnet and White 1972; Fenner 1970; Smith 1972; Cockburn 1967, 1971; Black 1975, 1980. J. B. S. Haldane was, to my knowledge, the first person to argue that prior to the adoption of agriculture infectious disease would have played only a small role in our evolution because there would have been relatively little natural selection of human populations for resistance to most of the diseases that we now recognize.

2. The survival of a disease organism depends on an unbroken chain of generations. If human behavior lowers the probability of successful transmission even slightly, the odds favor eventual elimination of the parasite. If, for the sake of illustration, we say that a single parasite has a 90 percent chance of successful transmission of its offspring from one host to the next (an extremely optimistic assumption), it will still only have a 50 percent chance of completing seven successful transmissions and a 4 percent chance of completing thirty-two transmissions. Thirty-two generations of any parasite in question is a trivial period in terms of human history. The more common the parasite, the higher the probability that some will succeed. But the smaller the human group, the smaller the number of parasites attempting to reproduce and the greater the odds against continued success.

3. In addition to visible chronic diseases there is a class of hidden or latent viruses —slow viruses—that remain dormant in the body for a number of years before producing any symptoms (Brody and Gibbs 1976; Eklund and Hadlow 1975).

4. Hatwick 1976; Sikes 1975; Andrewes and Walton 1977. Rabies is an interesting example of a disease that appears to produce a behavioral modification in its hosts to serve its own ends: it stimulates "mad-dog" aggressiveness, which tends to assure that a new host is bitten.

5. Olsen 1975; Poland 1976; Andrewes and Walton 1977. A few years ago, my students and I attempted to collect fur-bearing animals from upstate New York for experiments in bone chemistry. Our efforts were thwarted by an outbreak of tularemia among wild mammals of the region. Biologists on our campus were afraid that the disease might spread to laboratory rodents then under study.

6. Feldman 1976.

7. Johnson and Webb 1975.

8. Deisch and Ellinghausen 1975; Ellinghausen and Top 1976; Andrewes and Walton 1977.

9. Borts and Hendricks 1976; Andrewes and Walton 1977.

10. Brachman 1976; Andrewes and Walton 1977.

11. Overturf and Mathies 1976; Andrewes and Walton 1977.

12. Hubbert et al. 1975; Andrews and Walton 1977; Burnet and White 1972; Downs 1976. Diseases that primarily live in other animals or in the soil and for which human beings are only incidental hosts will be relatively unaffected by human population density, except insofar as that density disturbs their normal host species. Increasing human population might destroy these diseases by eliminating their natural hosts. But increasing human population density may also encourage some such diseases to evolve forms that become adapted to human populations as their primary hosts. The latter appears to be the case, for example, in the evolution of human sleeping sickness and of human typhus, both diseases in which a modern form that affects humans appears to be the evolutionary offspring of a disease once circulating primarily among wild animals (Lambrecht 1964, 1967; Burgdorfer 1975).

13. Geist 1978; Ledger 1976; Andrewes and Walton 1977.

14. Mathies and Macdonald 1976; Zimmerman 1975.

15. Geist 1978; Marks 1977; Rausch 1975; Turner 1975.

16. Geist 1978.

17. Davis et al. 1975.

18. Burgdorfer 1975; Andrewes and Walton 1977.

19. McIntosh and Gear 1975: McLean 1975; Parkin 1975; Downs 1976.

20. Scholtens 1975; Desowitz 1980.

21. Neva 1975; Lambrecht 1967.

22. Work 1975; Andrewes and Walton 1977.

23. Burgdorfer 1975; Wisseman 1976; Andrewes and Walton 1977.

24. Smith 1975.

25. Selby 1975b; Pappagainis 1976.

26. Dubos 1965. Parasites which depend on particular hosts to complete their life cycles commonly tend to evolve strains that are milder in their effects on that host. A mild strain contributes to its own dissemination by permitting its host to live and move; a severe strain tends to be self-defeating because it prevents a host from disseminating it. Long-standing interactions between parasites and hosts are likely to produce only mild symptoms; conversely, zoonotic infections, though relatively rare, are likely to be severe, even life-threatening in a way that many infections housed in the human population are not. One of the best known examples of evolution of milder forms of a parasite involves myxomytosis, a disease purposefully introduced in Australia to kill rabbits, that stopped killing them after several generations.

27. Goodman et al. 1975.

28. Sikes 1975.

29. Davis et al. 1975; McNeill 1980.

30. Hudson 1965; Hackett 1963; Rosebury 1971; Rudolf 1976. Such treponemal diseases as yaws or syphilis, which are handed directly from person to person by touch, may be less affected by population density because successful transmission depends more on such intimacy and less on the laws of chance, which are density dependent. Even treponemal infections, however, appears to show some density-related effects, as will be discussed in chapter 7.

31. Fiennes 1978; Dunn 1966; Kuntz 1982.

32. Dunn 1966; Fiennes 1978.

33. Norden and Ruben 1976.

34. Dunn 1966; Fiennes 1978.

35. Consideration of these two classes of diseases likely to afflict small-scale or primitive groups (zoonoses and chronic infections) incidentally raises an interesting point about the awareness or lack of awareness of contagion—that is, the emergence of germ theory, or the awareness that one "catches" a disease. It is no coincidence that such an awareness emerges in civilization; nor is it a reflection of greater sophistication. Rather, it is a reflection of the reality of the diseases that different groups experience. Contagion is most obvious in the spread of epidemic diseases common to civilizations but hard to perceive in either the very slow movement of chronic infection more common in small and isolated groups or the rather random pattern of zoonotic infections that they are likely to encounter.

36. Archaeological skeletons also show few signs of unprecedented or clearly unusual ancient diseases, although the skeletal record often does not permit specific diagnosis and might mask unknown infections (see chapter 7).

37. Crosby 1972; Black 1980.

38. Kamien 1980; Cleland 1928; Joske 1980; Packer 1961–62.

39. Black 1975, 1980.

40. Black 1980; Truswell and Hansen 1976; Bennett et al. 1973; Barnicot et al. 1972.

41. Eklund and Hadlow 1975; Brody and Gibbs 1976.

42. The origin of the AIDS virus (HIV or human immunodeficiency virus) remains something of a mystery. A related virus (SIV or simian immunodeficiency virus) has been found in populations of wild monkeys in Africa, suggesting that AIDS could be a recent mutant form of a zoonotic disease much in the same way that influenza and measles are thought to be mutant forms of animal diseases.

But HIV is also one of a family of retroviruses (HTLV, human T-cell leukemia/lymphoma viruses) able to persist for long periods of time in the individual human being. AIDS itself appears to have a long period of dormancy, and it seems closely related to another virus, HIV2, which appears able to persist in the human body and is endemic in groups in Africa. Retroviruses, as a group, tend to replicate themselves inaccurately. They change form relatively rapidly, frustrating the body's attempts to develop immunity and incidentally making the task of developing a vaccine more difficult.

In short, AIDS could be a zoonosis, but, alternatively, it could be derived from an ancient human infection that had persisted in small and isolated groups. The deadly form known to us is, however, apparently quite modern. (It has not been identified in blood samples dating from before 1959.) Moreover, it appears to be largely an urban disease, even in Africa; it is spread by a combination of circumstances peculiar to civilized lifestyles: promiscuous commercial sex among large groups of people, long-distance travel, availability of syringes, and increased use of blood transfusions. If AIDS or a similar disease ever appeared earlier in history by mutation of a virus of monkeys or people, it has apparently long since burned itself out (Essex and Kanki article and others in *Scientific American*, August 1988 [whole issue]; Marx 1988; Norman 1985; Quinn 1986; Piot et al. 1988).

43. See note 26.

44. Harpending and Wandsnider 1982. Local antigenic variants of an organism produce subtly different immune responses and prevent the body from reaching a stable adjustment to its parasites. Conversely, sedentary populations may enjoy some adaptive advantages.

45. Neel 1970, 1977.

46. Dubos 1965.

47. Dubos 1965. Large doses of antibiotics may actually threaten health because they eliminate this protective community.

48. Johnson 1975; Desowitz 1980.

49. Mogabgab 1976; McKenzie 1980.

50. The worms can presumably be carried by small mobile groups because they produce a debilitating, chronic challenge to health rather than an acute one and thus persist in individuals for prolonged periods, requiring only occasional transmission for survival; the buildup of these infections should, however, still be minimized by movement away from accumulated feces. Sedentism should tend to increase both the frequency and severity of infection.

51. Macdonald 1976.

52. Busvine 1980. Murine typhus was originally a zoonosis transmitted by rodents and fleas but was a fairly mild disease. The mutant form associated with large human populations and transmitted by body lice is the dangerous form. The recent origin of the latter is attested to by the lethality of the disease to its louse vector.

53. Nelson 1975.

54. Livingstone 1984; Warren 1975.

55. de Zulueta 1956; Livingstone 1958, 1984.

56. Desowitz 1980; Scholtens 1975; Busvine 1980.

57. Burgdorfer 1975; Work 1975.

58. Nelson 1975; Grove 1980.

59. Livingstone 1958, 1984.

60. Livingstone 1958, 1984.

61. See note 23 of chapter 2.

62. Livingstone 1984; cf. de Zulueta 1980.

63. In recent history, at least in some parts of the world, the intensification of agriculture and the investments that it entails probably have helped human populations to eliminate malaria. Irrigation systems undoubtedly increase mosquito breeding, but two other aspects of agricultural intensification probably help destroy mosquito populations. First, as cropping becomes more frequent and land becomes converted permanently rather than temporarily from forest or bush to field, the increasing proportion of sunlight to shade destroys mosquito breeding habitats; second, since water

control often means drainage of swamps as well as irrigation, breeding places for mosquitos may further be eliminated. Malaria, which was a serious disease hazard in parts of North America and much of Europe within the past century, has been almost completely eliminated in temperate climates, largely as a result of changes in the landscape associated with intensified farming (see Learmonth 1988). The disease posed a serious health risk in Britain as late as the eighteenth century, after which it was eliminated as the result of the draining of low-lying, swampy fen land. But such elimination of the disease is predominantly limited to climates in which the ecology of the mosquitos is fairly fragile because temperatures and humidity values are marginal to their survival; it is limited also to regions where wealth is sufficient to undertake the massive construction that such improvements imply and where population density is sufficiently high to undertake and warrant permanent conversion of land to farming.

64. Burnet and White 1972.

65. Desowitz 1980.

66. Intentional hearths appear in several sites associated with ancestral human beings of Homo erectus grade.

67. See Marks (1977) for a description of the Bisa of Zambia.

68. Brothwell and Brothwell 1969.

69. Overturf and Mathies 1976; Cohen and Tauxe 1986. More recently, animal salmonella that is resistant to antibiotics has become more common, as domestic animals are routinely dosed with antibiotics.

70. Wilson and Hayes 1973.

71. Keith and Armelagos 1983; Brenton and Keith 1986; Bassett et al. 1980. These researchers have identified the antibiotic tetracycline as an apparently natural contaminant of stored grain in ancient Nubia. Armelagos and his archaeological coworkers in Nubia have suggested that tetracycline ingestion may actually have reduced infection rates in those populations eating the contaminated grain.

72. Bassett et al. 1980.

73. Reinhard in press; Reinhard et al. 1987; McNeill 1979.

74. Dunn 1972.

75. Sikes 1975; Hattwick 1976.

76. Feldman 1976.

77. Rosen 1975; Spaeth 1976.

78. Rausch 1975.

79. Turner 1975.

80. Zimmerman 1975.

81. Rausch 1975.

82. Cockburn 1967, 1971; Hare 1967; Brothwell and Sandison 1967; Mims 1980.

83. Kleeburg 1975; Dubos 1965.

84. Livingstone 1958, 1984.

85. Epidemic diseases are commonly viral diseases, as the human body characteristically develops a more efficient, permanent immunity to viral diseases as a class than to other classes of infection (bacterial, protozoan, or helminth). These also tend to be diseases for which long-lasting vaccines are available or being actively sought, since vaccines work by stimulating the same sort of long-term immunity that the diseases themselves generate.

86. Top and Wehrle 1976; Morley 1980. The survival of the measles virus de-

pends on a supply of victims arriving as rapidly as the old ones are used up. In this sense, a measles epidemic is very much like a forest fire that requires a constant supply of new fuel to continue burning; in the absence of such a fresh supply, the disease, like a fire, will burn itself out. The supply of new hosts, of course, depends on the number of births in the population, the number of immigrants, and the speed with which emigrants from an infected population can reach new potential host populations. Measles virus may persist in the body, and there has even been speculation that its persistence is related to the emergence of multiple sclerosis in later years; apparently, the stored virus does not retain its ability to reinfect other individuals with measles.

Francis Black (1975, 1980) in particular has collected documentation of the failure of measles epidemics to persist on various islands historically isolated by long sea voyages before the era of air travel. He has also documented its failure to thrive and persist in such populations on larger continents as the Eskimos in the Canadian Arctic and Indian populations in the Amazon basin of South America, which are isolates in the sense that small group size, wide geographical dispersal, and the absence of transport separate them from their neighbors. Black has also noted that, after Columbus, even relatively populous parts of the New World commonly failed to sustain measles, a disease newly introduced to American Indians by European explorers. He points out that the disease had to be reintroduced repeatedly from the Old World in order to wreak its devastation. He concludes that measles could not have persisted prior to the emergence of civilized population centers.

Some critics of Black's conclusion have proposed that measles and other epidemics might have existed in the prehistoric past if contact between groups was just sufficient to permit the disease to work its way from group to group, meandering across the landscape and never remaining long in any one location. However, although the contemporary studies suggest that measles can on occasion get from one small group to another and can reach relatively isolated groups (see chapter 6), the odds against it continuing to be transmitted from one isolate to another in perpetuity are prohibitively great. Hence, this alternative model seems improbable.

87. Black 1966; Bartlett 1960.

88. Black 1975; Tyrrell 1977.

89. Top 1976; Benenson 1976; Cockburn 1971; Brunell 1976b. Many of these, however, have one or more attributes that make them better candidates for survival in small groups than measles itself. Mims (1980) suggests that rhinoviruses, polioviruses, echo viruses, coxcackie viruses, and rotaviruses are all probably organisms that belong on this list.

90. Black 1975, 1980. Mogabgab 1976; Davenport 1976; Laver 1983; Dowdle 1984. The repeated bouts of colds and flu we experience result from variations in the form of the viruses that "fool" our immune systems. So-called antigenic drift has been observed to produce minor new variations in the influenza virus every one to three years and to produce major shifts in antigen structure every ten to forty years, a pattern that results in the well-known cycle of major and minor flu epidemics witnessed in the last century. The pattern of influenza is also complicated because various animal species—particularly such domestic species as ducks, pigs, and chickens—share the viruses with us, and genetic exchanges between human and animal strains produce new types of virus and new epidemics.

91. Tyrrell (1977). The observation that islands separated from one another by a

sea voyage of more than six weeks are commonly relatively free of such infections, as D.A. Tyrell (1977) has pointed out, provides some indication of the limits of the ability of these organisms to be transmitted between isolated groups.

92. Brunell 1976a; Cockburn 1967; Weller 1976.

93. In a similar manner, the suggestion once offered by MacFarlane Burnet (Burnet and White 1972) that all viral infections of human beings must be of recent origin has been disputed on the grounds that many viruses do seem to persist in human beings and seem capable of persisting in wild animals whose population structure is not unlike that of early human beings. Similarly, too, human tuberculosis was once considered strictly a disease of civilization. But it is now known that tuberculosis is also maintained in a variety of wild animal reservoirs from which human hunter-gatherers could have encountered the disease; and it is known that the disease has a long latency period (a period during which it lies dormant in the human body, producing no symptoms) suggesting that it might well survive even in small human groups. Moreover, as discussed in chapter 7, there is some direct evidence in prehistoric skeletons of its existence in relatively simple early human societies, even though it appears to have been relatively uncommon in such groups.

94. Paul et al. 1951.

95. Black 1975, 1980; see chapter 6.

96. Black 1980. However, another commonly acute fecal-oral disease, typhoid, need not be a disease of recent origin, because it is capable of persisting indefinitely in some individuals who show no symptoms but can nonetheless reinfect others. The famous and historically genuine "Typhoid Mary" of nineteenth-century America is a case in point.

97. Wrigley and Schofield 1981; Braudel 1973, 1981. Joske 1980; Acsadi and Nemeskeri 1970; McAlpin 1983a, 1983b.

98. See chapter 7.

99. Schapera 1930: Kuper 1947; Packard 1984; Prothero 1965.

100. McNeill 1976, 1980; Crosby 1972.

101. Dunn 1965. Cf. de Zulueta (1980), who suggests that falciparum malaria was introduced to the New World at the time of Columbus but that vivax malaria was indigenous. Grove (1980) suggests that schistosomiasis was also absent in the New World before Columbus. However, some scholars argue, based on indirect evidence, that yellow fever may have been present and a major health hazard for some populations in the New World before Columbus (Pavlovsky 1966).

102. Crosby 1972; cf. Hudson 1965; Hackett 1963; Rosebury 1971. The latter calls attention to several possible descriptions of syphilis in the Bible. Some descriptions seem to suggest that Sarah, Abraham's wife, was transmitting some form of venereal disease, although Rosebury suggests that this instance refers to gonorrhea. Paleopathological data (chapter 7) clearly imply that some form of treponemal infection (yaws/syphilis) was present in the New World before Columbus.

103. Benenson 1976a; McNeill 1976, 1980; Fenner 1980.

104. Rausch 1975: Ofosu-Amaah 1980; Burnet and White 1972; Fiennes 1964; Lambrecht 1964; Busvine 1980.

105. Biraben 1968.

106. Wrigley 1966.

107. Civilization may also compound the effects of infectious diseases in other

ways. In addition to encouraging the spread of infections, aspects of civilization may also help lower the resistance of human hosts, helping infections to get established or increasing their severity.

First, poor nutrition generally tends to make infectious disease worse. In approximately three-fourths of existing studies, poor nutrition has been found to exacerbate the effects of infection (Scrimshaw et al. 1968; Taylor 1983; Beisel 1982). If the general trend in human nutrition has been downward (as has probably been the case until very recently, at least for all but the privileged; see chapter 5), people would have become more susceptible to infections. Insufficient iron, zinc, and vitamin A, as well as protein and protein-calorie malnutrition, all hamper the body's defenses against disease. Low iron levels exacerbate gastrointestinal and respiratory infection and increase the risk that wounds will become infected. Malnutrition has been found to contribute to the risk of severity of measles, tuberculosis, diarrhea, most respiratory infections, whooping cough, most intestinal parasites, cholera, leprosy, and even herpes, while exhibiting more marginal effects on typhus, diphtheria, staphylococcal and streptococcal infections, influenza, and syphilis (Rotberg and Rabb 1983; Scrimshaw et al. 1968; Beisel 1982). The co-occurrence and mutual reinforcement of poor nutrition and diarrhea among modern infants in the Third World is widely reported.

Paradoxically, there are some infections against which poor nutrition may actually be beneficial. Deficiencies of protein, iron, vitamins A, C, and E, thiamine, riboflavin, pyridoxine, and pantothenic acid may all help the body to fight malaria; famine has actually been observed to have malaria-suppressing effects (Beisel 1982; Scrimshaw et al. 1968). Similarly, caloric deficiency appears to protect against schistosomiasis, and there is speculation that a diet rich in meat and iron may actually have made wealthy males in the Middle Ages more susceptible to bubonic plague than their poor neighbors (Ell 1984). Moreover, iron in particular is needed by many of the organisms that attack the human body and is actively withheld from invaders by the body through a series of chemical mechanisms. A short-term dietary iron deprivation may actually assist the body in winning this fight, although long-term deprivation eventually acts against the human host (Weinberg 1974).

Second, chemical or physical irritants that abrade the surface of skin (or of internal membranes) may facilitate penetration by parasites. It is clear that some risk of chemical irritation exists even in the simplest societies. Some hunting and gathering populations, such as the San and Eskimo, display lung irritation associated with the smoke of campfires, which facilitates bronchial infection. Members of human groups of all types perversely take irritating smoke into their lungs for recreation. But the range and overall importance of chemical irritations has surely increased as specialized technical and industrial processes have been added to the human repertoire and as larger portions of the human population have been exposed to the effluent of those processes, either through their occupations or their residence in cities. One factor in the upsurge in rates of tuberculosis in recent history is likely to have been such chemical irritation, which would facilitate activitation of the tubercle bacillus. Tuberculosis does, in fact, show an occupation-related distribution.

Third, and more controversial, we can at least speculate about the impact of cultural evolution on the psychological state of individuals, as it effects their resistance to infection via hormonal pathways. Part of the romantic image that we hold of primitive lifestyles is that they are free of the psychological stresses of modern living. But psychological well-being has proved difficult to measure in any objective way; ethnographic descriptions of simple societies do not always conform to the romantic assumptions, even when they are provided by people such as Richard Lee, who otherwise perceive primitive bands to be relatively affluent. Lee (1979) and others have described rather a tight set of emotional regulations—and some tensions —governing interactions among the San (who are described in chapter 6), and it is not clear that their relative freedom of movement from the group can completely offset these tensions. Among some groups of Amazonian Indians (relatively small and mobile groups of hunter-gatherers and farmers alike), warfare and intragroup strife are considerable, and the probability of death by homicide is surprisingly high, suggesting that the lifestyle is hardly stress-free.

Yet, if we compare patterns of psychological stress observable in animal populations and in experimental human groups during aspects of the civilizing process, it is possible to identify some specific patterns of change that may generate psychological stress and contribute to declining resistance to disease. It is clear from work with animals (Christian 1980) and with human beings (Cassell 1976) that enforced change in one's social system—and subordinate status within a social hierarchy—are both likely to generate hormonal changes that depress the immune response. To the extent that both are common functions of civilized organization, they may contribute to an increase in the disease load of civilized groups. Moreover, both animal and human studies demonstrate the importance of peer group support in withstanding the deleterious effects of psychological stress. To the extent that civilization replaces kinship and neighborhood ties by occupational specialization and occupational mobility, it may tend to undermine this support function.

108. Dubos 1965; Neel 1977; McKeown 1976, 1983. Twentieth-century medicine has made enormous inroads against the increasing parasite burden—at least for those individuals who have been protected by it. But, at best, such medicine has only been available in the very recent past. Modern epidemiological models, which facilitated the widespread and rapid scientific development of avoidance strategies, are less than two hundred years old. Effective medicine in the form of chemical therapy is even younger. (Jenner's experiments with vaccination against smallpox make the history of modern disease prevention and theory less than two hundred years old.) Such medical scholars as Theodore McKeown argue that effective Western biomedical intervention in disease (as opposed to the psychotherapy common to most medical systems) is really only a twentieth-century affair.

109. McNeill 1980.

Chapter 5

1. See Boserup 1965; Cohen 1977; Hayden 1981a; Spooner 1972; Bronson 1972, 1977; Bayliss-Smith 1982a, 1982b; Harris 1986; Simon 1983.

2. The efficiency of various hunting and gathering techniques has been the subject of intensive scrutiny in recent years as a result of the emergence of "optimality" theory and "optimal foraging" research in studies of animal and human behavior. Optimal foraging research is designed to test whether animal and human behavior conform to simple economic expectations. The simplest expectation is that foragers will "prefer" activities that give the highest caloric return for their labor. More so-

phisticated models attempt to demonstrate that economic choices represent a balance of competing goals. Many studies do, in fact, demonstrate at least a crude correlation between caloric returns and strategic choices by various human groups, which suggests that caloric efficiency is one major (but not the only) principle guiding foraging strategies (see Winterhalder and Smith 1981; cf. Keene 1981).

3. A large number of studies of different populations in varying environments bear out the argument that when available or encountered, large game are the most efficiently exploited wild prey. See Winterhalder 1981; O'Connell and Hawkes 1981; Hill and Hawkes 1981; Hill 1982; Hurtado and Hill 1987; Hawkes et al. 1982; Jones 1980; Rowly Conwy 1984; Perlman 1980, 1983; Colchester 1984; Lizot 1977, 1978; Hames 1980; Hames and Vickers 1982, 1983; Werner 1979, 1983; Yost and Kelley 1983; Harris 1982; Earle and Christenson 1980; Behrens 1981; Dwyer 1982. Cf. Stocks 1983; Beckerman 1980, 1983.

4. Comparisons of the efficiency of stone and iron tools suggest iron contributes relatively little to the efficiency of hunting, more to the gathering and processing of wild vegetable foods, and most to farming. Colchester (1984) suggests that iron doubles the efficiency of wild vegetable harvesting and triples the efficiency of farming but has little effect on hunting (see also Harris 1988; Bayliss-Smith 1982a, 1982b). The implications are that estimates of primitive hunting efficiency are not significantly inflated by the modern availability of iron tools and that the relative advantage of hunting over gathering or farming would have been even greater in the Stone Age.

Comparisons of the efficiency of spear hunting, bow hunting, net hunting, and blowgun hunting seem to suggest that spear hunting of large animals is more efficient than obtaining small animals by any of the other methods; in addition, the spear may be the weapon of choice when large animals are available. African Mbuti Pygmies hunting large game with spears are, for example, five to six times more efficient than those hunting with a bow and arrow and four times more efficient than those hunting with nets (Harakao 1981; Abruzzi 1979; Webster and Webster 1984; see also Hames and Vickers 1982; Hames 1980; Vickers 1980; Yost and Kelley 1983). Shotguns and modern rifles clearly increase hunting efficiency (Hames 1979; Hill and Hawkes 1983; but cf. Yost and Kelley 1983), but it is not clear that muzzle-loading muskets —the most sophisticated weapons available to many contemporary hunter-gatherers —actually increase efficiency compared to the use of the bow (Marks 1976, 1977, 1979).

Incidentally, observations of the African Hadza and the Paraguayan Ache suggest that technology may not be as essential to meat acquisition as we have thought. O'Connell, Hawkes, and Jones (1988) and Hawkes (personal communication, 1988) describe Hadza scavenging fresh kills by driving off large predators, including lions, without any weapons. The Ache obtain 0.27 kilograms of meat from live game per hour of work using their bare hands (Hill et al. 1984).

The most important prehistoric invention to facilitate hunting, if not the spear, may have been hunting poison. This may have been one of the few inventions that represented actual progress rather than an adjustment to declining prey size. It is interesting to speculate that these inventions might lie at the heart of what many archaeologists now believe to have been the relatively recent and rapid expansion of Homo sapiens at the expense of Homo erectus and Neanderthaloid populations.

5. Very high caloric returns from hunting are reported or estimated by Marks

(1977), Vickers (1988), Jones (1980), Perlman (1983), Rowly Conwy (1984), Hawkes and O'Connell (1985), and Blackburn (1982). Marks' work, which represents one of the few measurements of hunting efficiency in game-rich African savannas (similar to the preferred habitats of early man), is particularly striking. If one omits kills associated with shotguns and rifles but leaves in those resulting from musket fire (which Marks thinks is less productive than bow and arrow), the Bisa of Zambia average 7,500 to 15,000 kilocalories per hour of hunting. Blackburn reports that among Okiek (Dorobo) of Kenya one man with a dog and a spear may obtain 200 pounds of meat in about two hours and that in one to four hours one or more hunting individuals can regularly get 100 to 300 pounds. Behrens (1981) reports that in good seasons the Shipibo of Peru get 6 kilograms of meat per hour of hunting. Rowly-Conway (1984) estimates that hunting may return from 14,000 to 45,000 kilocalories per hour.

The Anbarra of Australia, who obtain more than 10,000 kilocalories per hour from large game when it is (rarely) available, get about 1,000 kilocalories per hour from shellfish (Jones 1980; Meehan 1977a, 1977b). The Alyawara of Australia, who get 3,600 kilocalories per hour from large prey when it is available, obtain about 500 to 800 kilocalories per hour from small game. They obtain 6,000 kilocalories per hour from the choicest vegetable resources when available, but most vegetable resources provide poorer returns. Harvesting and processing small seeds nets only 680 kilocalories per hour, and the Alyawara may not bother with these resources except in times of need. Hawkes and O'Connell estimate that small seeded vegetables may provide only 1,000 to 1,300 kilocalories per hour in other locations. Eder (1978) reports that wild yam harvesting in the Philippines nets about 1,740 kilocalories per hour. Hurtado and Hill (1987) suggest that the Cuiva get about 3,000 kilocalories per hour hunting but about 1,125 kilocalories per hour collecting. Hazelnuts, acorns, and Brazil nuts can sometimes be harvested at rates comparable to rich hunting (Rowly Conwy 1984; Werner 1983) but must still be processed.

Speth (1983, 1988) points out that the apparent efficiency of hunting may be partly misleading, particularly when animals are very lean, because lean meat alone is metabolically inefficient for the body to process. He explains that there is an upper limit to safe meat and protein consumption, especially when other sources of calories are in short supply. He suggests that 1,200 kilocalories per person per day may be the safe upper limit of meat intake and that protein should comprise less than fifty percent of the diet. Speth points out that animal fat may be the scarcer commodity and that hunters may actually abandon a fresh kill if it is found to be too lean. This fact, along with our omnivorous heritage, may explain why, despite the relative efficiency of hunting, human groups outside the Arctic probably never were strict and specialized big game hunters in the manner in which they were once depicted. My own sense is that in rich prehistoric environments people may well have obtained 40 to 50 percent of their diets from meat. The figure of 20 percent that became fashionable among anthropologists in the 1970s based on the San model (see chapter 6) is almost certainly too low to represent prehistory, based as it is on a marginal game-impoverished modern environment with very poor returns from hunting—where heat inhibits hunting and water and calories are scarcer than protein.

6. Clark and Haswell 1970; Boserup 1965, 1983; Bronson 1972; Harris 1986; Bayliss-Smith 1982a, 1982b; Johnson 1983; Grigg 1982. Bronson's figures, for

example, suggest that subsistence farmers without irrigation commonly get 0.2 to 0.9 bushels of grain per day of work, which is roughly equal to 0.5 to 2.25 kilograms of grain for each hour of work (calculations using his figures). This would suggest a range of caloric returns of 1,700 to 8,000 kilocalories per hour, but most values are in the 3,000 to 5,000 kilocalorie per hour range. Eder (1978) reports that rice swiddens in the Phillipines net 1,000 to 2,000 kilocalories per hour. Werner et al. (1979) report one horticultural group in South America that they estimate obtains 17,000 kilocalories per hour.

Direct comparisons of hunting efficiency and farming efficiency by the same group often suggest that farming is the more productive activity (see Johnson 1983; Colchester 1984; Lizot 1977, 1978; Bayliss-Smith 1982a, 1982b). But the hunting being compared is demonstrably poor both because the populations in question inhabit the game-poor Amazon rain forest or New Guinea and because sedentism associated with farming rapidly depletes game in the vicinity of settlements (see note 16).

7. Cohen 1977.

8. Boserup 1965. Boserup did not calculate caloric return per hour but provided estimates suggesting that the number of man-days of labor per planted acre or hectare would go up and the yield per harvest would go down as the same land was cropped more frequently.

9. Bayliss-Smith (1982a, 1982b) estimates that land clearance in agriculture is 500 percent as efficient with iron tools as with stone. Colchester (1984) estimates that iron triples the efficiency of farming. Marvin Harris (1980) suggests that steel tools improve farming efficiency 500 percent. Hames (1979) estimates that the improvement with steel tools is 300–600 percent.

10. Boserup 1983; Simon 1983.

11. Bronson 1972.

12. Simon 1983; Harris 1988. Harris and Simon disagree, however, about who benefits. Harris notes that most or all of the extra production may disappear in taxes. Simon argues that the population as a whole benefits. He argues that the percentage of the human population exposed to the risk of famine has declined over the past fifty years, largely as the result of such investment.

Simon's assessment is controversial, particularly as it applies to the longer span of human history. Comparative data supplied in chapters 6 and 7 suggest that, even if net nutritional benefits have been felt on a world scale in the past fifty years as a function of investment, this trend can hardly be extrapolated back in time or assumed to be the rule of human experience.

13. Harris 1988; Bronson 1972. Bronson's productivity figures for "short fallow" agriculture are generally less than those for "long fallow." But annual cropping and irrigation agriculture seem to be the most efficient systems. For example, in contrast to figures cited in note 6, Bronson estimates that irrigated rice farming may produce 0.5 to 1.5 bushels per man-day of work (equals 1–3 kilograms of rice per hour) or about 3,500 to 10,500 kilocalories per hour of work.

Whether or not modern farming is really more efficient, however, depends on how one counts. If we include the labor costs of the initial land improvements and the labor costs of making the tools, maintaining the necessary animals and machines, obtaining fuel (etc.), as well as the farmer's own yearly labor, the relative efficiency of modern methods is not so certain. If we also include the caloric inputs of animals and of fossil fuels, modern agriculture is manifestly less efficient calorie for calorie than primitive methods. Bayliss-Smith (1982a, 1982b) calculates that primitive farmers get a 10:1 or 14:1 return on calories expended, whereas modern farming averages only about a 2:1 return (counting all sources of calories).

14. Geertz 1963.

15. Boserup (1983) points out, for example, that modern India has as much land per capita as western Europe. The difference in the food economy and in the levels of nutrition enjoyed exist because India, with less investment in fertilizer and special seed, is approximately one hundred years behind Europe in the efficiency with which it uses land. Improved investment in Indian agriculture, she argues, would narrow the gap.

16. J. T. Peterson (1981) and Bailey and Peacock (in press) have both argued that, at least in some environments, domestic fields may increase the local supply of game by providing improved grazing and browsing and by attracting animals to the vicinity of local settlements. Most studies suggest, however, that any such advantage is outweighed by rapid depletion of large game in the vicinity of settlements because of hunting. (See Griffin 1984; Hames 1980; Hames and Vickers 1982; Werner et al. 1979; Abruzzi 1979; Webster and Webster 1984; Hill and Hawkes 1983; Bahuchet and Gillaume 1982; Terashima 1983; Hart 1978; Vickers 1980; Eder 1978; Colchester 1984.)

17. Basic rules of ecology and energy flow, which human behavior has not yet significantly altered, dictate that predatory animals are always scarcer than the herbivorous animals they prey on, and scarcer still than plants. As human beings become more numerous, we are forced to become more herbivorous. Prehistoric decimation of wild herds (human or natural) would have accelerated the process.

The initial domestication of animals would have provided the animals some protection against predators and some help getting food during lean seasons. It helped to maintain the supply of animals within a walking radius of the settlement and may have helped keep the meat supply constant, but it could not have significantly raised the limits of the animals' own food supply without creating disproportionate competition for the human food supply. Animals must still have grazed within walking distance of settlements and/or been fed the produce of human fields. It is arguable whether any net improvement in the availability of animal products was involved (Bronson 1977). There is evidence from human skeletal remains that human populations in some parts of the world enjoyed a temporary reversal of the decline in meat consumption early in the Neolithic period, but the prevailing trend appears to have been downward (see chapter 7).

As the data of the next two chapters make clear, no application of technology has substantially reversed the decline in meat consumption for most of the world population. Despite all of our subsequent improvements in the growth of both plants and animals, we still have not gotten around the fact that raising domestic animals is an inefficient way to use space, unless we confine them to spaces that have no other value—a goal, not fully realized, of modern animal management strategy. Domestic animals convert only a small fraction of their food to human food. Feeding them grain and reserving them grazing room in competition with farming are (calorically) inefficient practices that occur, for the most part, only because of the disproportionate purchasing power of the wealthy.

If domestic animals are kept out of competition with farming, they can contribute significantly to the quantity as well as the quality of human diets. They can convert inedible plant materials into edible meat, increasing the supply of edible calories in environments where edible vegetation is scarce and converting those calories to improved sources of protein and minerals. In addition, by manipulating the spatial movement of animals, human beings can use them to gather and concentrate resources in environments in which resources are too scattered to reward direct human foraging. Some domestic animals, such as pigs, also convert refuse to food, although they may also compete more directly with human beings for food than do grazing such animals as cows and sheep.

18. Alfin-Slater and Kritchevsky 1980; Sever 1973; Winick 1980; Speth 1983. People can live without animal foods, but worldwide few choose to do so; those that do must design an all-vegetable diet with some care in order to avoid malnutrition. Vitamin B_{12} appears to be the hardest nutrient to obtain from vegetable sources. Various green and yellow vegetables provide a substitute for vitamin A, their yellow pigments or carotenoids, which the body can convert to vitamin A, but the uptake of these pigments and their utilization by the body is less efficient than that of vitamin A itself. The absorption of both vitamin A and carotenes is greatly facilitated by the presence of dietary fats and protein. Both the quality and quantity of protein in the body must be adequate for appropriate vitamin A activity to occur. Dietary vitamin D also comes primarily from animal sources, particularly fish oils and other animal fats, although most is manufactured in human skin, such that under normal conditions of exposure to sunlight no dietary source of the vitamin is required.

Animal foods have one other important advantage: because many animals range widely, they tend to provide a good balance of such minerals as iodine, for which availability is affected by soil and water regimes. Domestic animals whose food comes from the same locations as their owners may be less valuable as sources of minerals.

Other nutrients, such as vitamin C, come primarily from vegetable foods, and the diet may have benefited from an increase in their availability as more vegetable foods were consumed. But a look at human diets in small-scale societies (chapter 6) and at those of other primates, as well as the application of modern chemical techniques to the analysis of ancient bones (chapter 7), suggests that vegetables probably always constituted half of the human diet or more among all human populations, except those in arctic and subarctic regions, even in the early stages of our evolution. Relatively, meat has always been the scarcer of the two food classes, except for those human groups living in high latitudes where few edible vegetable foods are to be found; hence, the decline in meat consumption is undoubtedly more important than any associated increase in vegetable foods. Moreover, except for fiber, nutrients usually associated with vegetables, including vitamin C, can be obtained from animal products if one is willing to eat all of the tissues, the bone marrow, and the stomach contents of the animal, and to eat them raw, as many arctic populations do.

Diets rich in meat are popularly associated—in part, erroneously—with several categories of risk to health. Animal products are rich sources of cholesterol, and they are known to promote atherogenesis (the buildup of fatty deposits on blood vessels, which eventually occlude the vessels). Moreover, they are associated, in our common experience, with bowel disorders, including bowel cancers, and with high blood pressure, stroke, and heart disease. But most such risks associated with eating meat are more properly associated with domestic animals than with wild animals, as discussed in the text; or they are problems created by eating large quantities of domesticated meat in combination with other factors that typically do not affect hunter-gatherers or other primitive populations—general obesity, high fat content, high saturated fat intake, lack of exercise, and high salt intake. Hence, these meat-related risks are probably significant only in the modern, civilized world.

High dietary intake of animal protein also tends to cause secondary loss of calcium (Alfin-Slater and Kritchevsky 1980; Winick 1980; Draper 1978), which may be one of the predisposing factors in osteoporosis or the thinning of bone shafts; in this sense, high meat intake may be dangerous, and a decline in meat consumption healthy. The Eskimos and other Arctic hunting populations who are forced by their arctic environment to consume a very high proportion of their diet as meat display osteoporosis, exaggerated by low levels of calcium intake, high phosphate intake, and a lack of sunlight to stimulate vitamin D production—essential to healthy calcium utilization. For most other hunter-gatherer populations, living and dead, osteoporosis does not appear to have been a significant problem, however, presumably because their meat intake was always more moderate than that of the Eskimos and because, in contrast to modern civilized populations, they were and are protected against osteoporosis by exercise. Lack of weight-bearing exercise is one of the factors in the modern, civilized etiology of the disease. In prehistory, high meat intake may have posed other, more important health risks, especially when accompanied by low overall caloric intake. Speth (1983, 1988) has argued that high meat or protein intake in the absence of other sources of calories can be dangerous. See note 5.

19. Meat may be the most threatening source of food-borne infections (as discussed in the last chapter), and there is some risk of poison in animal tissues. Examples include the potentially toxic buildup of vitamin A in the livers of carnivores (Van Veen and Van Veen 1974) and the occasional toxicity of the meat of animals that have consumed poisonous vegetable products. Human beings have occasionally been poisoned by the meat of quail that have fed on hemlock berries or other poisonous plants (NAS-NRC 1973). There is also the possibility of poisoning by toxins associated with spoiled meat or with the intestinal contents of animals (Geist 1978). But animal tissues are usually relatively toxin-free because an animal's tissues are detoxified by the action of its own liver (Hambraeus 1982).

In contrast, toxins and carcinogens are remarkably common in plants (NAS-NRC 1973; Ames 1983). So as vegetable foods, particularly second-choice vegetable foods, became dietary staples, the risk of poison may have increased (Koyama and Thomas 1981). It has been argued that, until human beings learned to process wild plants first with fire and then with a range of grinding, drying, and leaching techniques, they were prevented by the ubiquitous presence of such toxins from ingesting significant portions of the otherwise edible flora (Leopold and Ardrey 1972, 1973; cf. Dornstreich 1973). Certainly, many vegetable species, such as acorns, buckeyes (or horse chestnuts), and wild yams, that became important vegetable resources in prehistory as the proportion of meat in diets declined do require extensive processing to detoxify them.

Focusing on a few chosen staple species tends to reduce or even eliminate one of the risks of broad-spectrum foraging for food: the risk of occasional acute poisoning by such toxins as those associated with some species of mushrooms (NAS-NRC 1973). But acute episodes of toxicity are usually memorable events, and avoidance of such foods is likely rapidly to become part of the cultural teachings of any group. Observed hunter-gatherers, in fact, display fairly sophisticated knowledge of such poisons and avoid them (or use them as hunting weapons). Acute poisoning may be a more common problem among civilized "Sunday" foragers than among hunter-gatherers. Focusing on staple vegetable foods is likely to increase the risks associated with the gradual accumulation of milder toxins.

Hunter-gatherers are undoubtedly exposed to chronic or cumulative toxins—including nutrient antagonists or "antivitamins" and dietary carcinogens from sources not known to us. Both categories of substance are so widespread in known plant foods that it is inconceivable that they are not present in a proportion of the wild foods eaten by these populations (Ames 1983; NAS-NRC 1973). Ripley (1980) has, for example, speculated about whether the low fertility of some hunter-gatherer groups might reflect an as yet unidentified hormone-mimicking substance in vegetable foods that inhibits human fertility. Similar chemicals produced by some grasses appear to inhibit the fertility of the grazing animals that consume them.

On the other hand, both ethnographic studies (chapter 6) and the study of archaeological skeletons (chapter 7) suggest that neither nutrient antagonists nor carcinogenic agents are likely to be or have been a particularly important problem for prehistoric hunter-gatherers compared to more civilized populations; the observable quality of their nutrition is too good, their rates of cancer too low.

20. Lee 1968, 1979; Wehmeyer et al. 1969; Eaton 1988; Eaton and Konner 1985; Eaton et al. 1988; Eder 1978. Speth (1988) has recently characterized the choice of foods in agriculture as a "bizarre" human focus on starch.

21. Winick 1980; Sever 1973; Alfin-Slater and Kritchevsky 1980; NAS-NRC 1973; El-Najjar 1977; Jelliffe and Jelliffe 1982. In addition, all cereals that include maize contain a high ratio of phosphorous to calcium (Eaton 1988). As a rule, plants tend to concentrate phosphorous in their seeds and calcium in their vegetative parts. Cereals, of course, are seeds. Some studies have suggested that this proportion may actually interfere with the utilization of calcium in the body, since a high dietary phosphorous/calcium ratio may induce loss of calcium. A diet rich in phosphorous, like one rich in meat, is associated with osteoporosis. Since low calcium levels are now increasingly thought to be implicated in hypertension, high phosphorous levels may be a factor in that problem as well. Reduced cortical bone maintenance (that is, calcium loss) does, in fact, appear in the archaeological record of several parts of the world fairly shortly after the adoption of agriculture, possibly associated with both high phosphorous intake and with phytate and the related malabsorption of calcium (see chapter 7). High blood pressure or hypertension is unlikely to have become a serious risk until other aspects of civilized diet were added to the equation, as will be discussed in the text.

22. Roe 1973, 1982; Alfin-Slater and Kritchevsky 1980.

23. Reinhold 1972; Young and Pellett 1985; Alfin-Slater and Kritchevsky 1980.

24. Wolf 1980.

25. Jaya Rao 1983; Osman 1981.

26. Oke 1975; NAS-NRC 1973; Jackson and Jackson 1984. Many domestic tubers contain toxins. Chemical precursors of cyanides commonly occur in some modern domesticates, including cassava or manioc, and symptoms of slow, chronic cyanide poisoning can be observed in populations heavily dependent on this crop.

27. Harlan 1967.

28. NAS-NRC 1973; Ames 1983. Selection for palatibility has probably also meant an overall reduction in the presence of toxic substances and carcinogens, which tend to impart a bitter taste to the foods in question.

29. Alfin-Slater and Kritchevsky 1980; Colditz et al. 1985; Wolf 1980. Vitamin C in particular is likely to be lost in storage. Vitamin A is also difficult to obtain from foods stored without refrigeration. Both vitamin A and vitamin C are among the most significant of naturally occurring anticarcinogenic substances. This loss of fresh foods is likely to contribute to increasing rates of carcinogenesis.

Storage and preparation for storage may tend to eliminate labile natural toxins in food. But toxins can be introduced to stored food supplies through bacterial action during storage. I have already referred to ergotism, a toxic condition produced by eating stored rye infected with ergot fungus. Eating sorghum may be associated with a mycotoxin that produces symptoms of pellagra (Jaya Rao 1983). Mold on such stored foods as grains also produces a number of relatively potent natural carcinogens including the aflatoxins that are produced by the mold aspergillis on grain stored in hot, humid conditions and which are associated with high rates of liver cancer in rural populations in Africa and Asia (NAS-NRC 1973; Learmonth 1988).

In the modern world, large-scale storage and transport rely on antibiotics to prevent decay and on various additives to maintain a fresh appearance in products consumed long after they are grown. Many of these chemicals are toxic not only by accident but by design. It is the purpose of antibiotics to be toxic to some life, after all, and it is hardly surprising that many of these chemicals are toxic, at least cumulatively, to human beings (Dwyer 1982). Such food additives may also be carcinogenic. For example, carcinogenic nitrates and nitrites associated with food storage are implicated in increasing modern cancer rates (Hambraeus 1982).

30. Brenton 1987.

31. In the modern world, "storage" of food as money—redeemable on demand—may help a population maintain access to fresh foods. But like other forms of storage, storage in monetary form tends to degrade the quality of the diet in an insidious way. Since all foods are convertible to cash, they tend to become interchangeable with one another and with other nonsubsistence goods. Since calories (which the body craves noticeably) tend to be cheap, whereas protein and other nutrients (which the body does not so obviously miss) are expensive, there is often a tendency on the part of farmers to convert rich and varied nutrients to cheap calories or nonfood items. Hufton (1983) estimates that, in eighteenth century France, purchasing bread alone could easily have required 60 to 80 percent of the budget of a wage-earning family, effectively converting all earning power to energy, at the expense of dietary variety. Wood (1988) and others have pointed out, in addition, that the transition to a cash economy may increase differential distribution of wealth, making it harder for some members of communities or households to obtain adequate nutrition—a situation that has occurred in contemporary New Guinea.

32. Underwood 1971. Dangerously high levels of elements in soil or water are also more likely to produce toxic reactions in groups that are sedentary on such soils than in mobile groups that sample such soils only in passing. Both selenium and fluorine can be dangerous in excess; in addition, chronic natural arsenic poisoning is associated with some soil regimes (Underwood 1971; NAS-NRC 1973).

33. Greenhouse 1981.

34. Katz et al. 1974, 1975.

35. Reinhold 1972.

36. Hodges 1980.

37. Anderson 1952.

38. Newman (1975), for example, describes the negative effects of the intensification of agriculture on the Sandawe of Tanzania.

39. Messer (1977) describes the unfortunate nutritional consequences of the elimination of weeds by recent Mayan farmers. Dennett and Connell (1988) describe the negative consequences of growing population, declining access to protein and wild variety foods, and heavy dependence on sweet potatoes among subsistence farmers in New Guinea, where protein and iodine deficiencies have become common.

40. Pelto and Pelto 1983; Dewey 1979, 1981. Dewey describes the decline in dietary variety and quality among peasants introduced to commercial agriculture in Mexico. Dennett and Connell (1988) conversely suggest that participation in larger markets has tended to improve the diets of populations in highland New Guinea otherwise heavily dependent on (protein-poor) domestic sweet potatoes for their subsistence. They further suggest that a survey of the world literature on the impact of commercial agriculture and cash incomes on subsistence farmers shows that it has mixed results. The impact is not uniformly negative, as some anthropologists have argued; but neither is it uniformly positive.

41. The most obvious example in the modern world is the dissemination of iodized salt across a range of soil zones in which thyroid malfunction related to iodine deficiency and its visible symptom, goiter, would otherwise be a problem. But products homogenized for trade may also be of less nutritional value than what they replace. Kuhnlein (1980) suggests that commercial salt is often poorer in trace minerals than local salts.

42. The recent reintroduction of fresh produce to the diets of the affluent appears to have reduced some cancer rates. The recent decline in stomach cancer in the United States may be related to increased availability of vitamins A and C associated with such fresh foods (Colditz et al. 1985; Wolf 1980; Hodges 1980).

43. Roe 1973, 1982. Specialization also imposes other health risks of course. In the modern world, direct exposure to industrial processes and pollutants is associated with a number of occupation diseases, and such pollution contributes to the development of several cancers, notably those of the skin, bladder, and lung.

Specialization and urbanization are also responsible for some health hazards that we consider natural. Most known rickets or vitamin D deficiency is related to employment and residence in locations that the sun does not reach. It is particularly a problem for dark-skinned people whom civilized transportation has moved to urban locations in northern latitudes and who are employed in indoor activities. Rickets has been more common in nineteenth and early twentieth century black Americans than it was in prehistoric populations, although it is now rare in the United States because of the use of vitamin supplements (see chapter 7).

44. Governmental barriers that have recently prevented available food from reaching starving populations in Ethiopia provide a graphic example.

45. Pelto and Pelto 1983.

46. Van Veen and Van Veen 1974.

47. Alfin-Slater and Kritchevsky 1980.

48. Beisel 1982; Scrimshaw et al. 1968.

49. Binford 1983.

50. In parts of the tropical Third World, storage systems may be so inefficient that they are essentially incapable of preserving food from harvest to harvest, no matter how bountiful the harvests are (Ogbu 1973; see chapter 6).

51. Ames 1983.

52. The best known example historically is probably the introduction of potatoes and maize, American crops, into Europe in the centuries after Columbus, where they substantially improved the food base of European populations (Crosby 1972; Pelto and Pelto 1983). Similarly, maize and sweet potatoes from the New World have had a substantial impact on the food economies of China (Ho 1955). And in the New World, where there were few indigenous domestic food animals, the introduction from the Old World of sheep, cattle, and pigs improved the protein base of farming populations.

But introduction of new species does not always have such salutory effects; pests and blights are also introduced to new regions, and crops are not always as nutritious as those that they displace. Well-balanced packages of nutrients, honed through long histories of trial and error, may be disrupted by the introduction of new crops. The substitution of maize for some indigenous African grains has increased the frequency of nutritional deficiencies for some populations of African farmers.

53. McAlpin argues that the development of railroads in India in the nineteenth century played a major role in alleviating the risk of famine in that subcontinent; examples abound of large-scale relief of famine by transport in the modern world. But transport can also deprive a population.

This pattern of deprivation through trade may be fairly old. In eighteenth-century France bread riots were directed at preventing badly needed grain from leaving rural areas for urban markets, especially during periods of local famine (Hufton 1983). There are also suggestions among archaeological populations (chapter 7) that trade may be negatively correlated with the nutrition of some of the populations involved.

54. Jacobsen and Adams 1958.

55. Dando 1975, 1980; Mellor and Gavian 1987.

56. Rotberg 1983; Mellor and Gavian 1987. Dense concentrations and extended boundaries for modern crops have also tended to mean increased reliance on pesticides, herbicides, biocides, and fertilizers, which are expensive. Perhaps worse, these chemicals then become toxic food additives (Mustafa 1982; Lindsay and Sherlock 1982). In addition, modern hybrid seeds are expensive to buy, and attempts to breed pest-resistant strains of such crops as potatoes or lettuce, capable of surviving intensive cultivation with high pest populations, have introduced or reintroduced mutagenic and carcinogenic properties (Ames 1983).

57. Sen 1981; Tilley 1983.

58. Sen (1981) suggests, for example, that in the Ethiopian famine of the 1970s the risk of starvation was greater for individuals attempting to buy food rather than for those attempting to produce it. Similarly, he argues that in the Bengal famine of 1943 in India much of the burden fell on individuals whose specialized livelihoods were suppressed by wartime conditions and who were unable to command or pur-

chase food. Similarly, in European history during the past 400 years, risk of famine was commonly associated with the failure not just of food supplies but of such other specialized occupations as wine making. These failures rendered particular groups unable to command available food. In Europe, the risk of famine for some segments of the population was further heightened by government policies favoring politically important or dangerous groups (Tilley 1983; Schofield 1984) and concern over exchange relationships became a major factor in social unrest (Hufton 1983; Tilley 1983). As early as the eighteenth century in France, moreover, specialists in food transport, acting as speculators, seem to have introduced a number of "false crises" relating to the food supply (Hufton 1983).

In a world of transport and economic "entitlements," there is an alternative to physical forms of storage, which can assist populations in avoiding short-term scarcity and famine associated with the inadequacy or failure of storage systems. Food can be converted to cash, credit, or other forms of entitlement when abundant and "stored" in that form (Nurse 1975). Cash and credit have the value that they do not deteriorate in quality as stored food does—although money does inflate, which is the equivalent of deterioration—and they have no limited shelf life and little risk of spoilage. Both can be stored in unlimited amounts for periods as long as necessary and thus can be used to ride out not only seasonal shortfalls but also unpredictable crop failure. Cash and credit have, in fact, an important role in protecting some contemporary African farmers against periodic shortages and may contribute substantially to the reliability of their food economies when crops and more traditional means of storage fail.

But the storage of food as cash, credit, or entitlement, which systems of trade and transport encourage, also has its drawbacks. For example, exchanges are often disadvantageous to the farmer at both ends: he sells food at low prices and buys at high prices, resulting in a net loss. Moreover, debt has the tendency to perpetuate shortages and exacerbate future crises. Debts must be paid and often siphon off excess productivity by which the farmer might otherwise protect himself against future shortfalls; debt payment, like taxes, may be demanded, even in the midst of shortfall, deepening a naturally induced crisis. For example, Richards (1982) describes a pattern of debt-influenced food shortages among contemporary rice farmers of Sierra Leone.

59. One of the tensions underlying the French Revolution, as described by Hufton, appears to have been a perception on the part of urban wage earners that peasants, merchants, and the government were conspiring to starve them.

60. Chafkin and Berg 1975.

61. For example, taxation, unremitting even in years of agricultural crisis, is one factor identified by Dando (1976) as contributing to the risk of famine among Russian peasants of the past several centuries.

62. Sen 1981.

63. Pelto and Pelto 1983.

64. Hufton 1983.

65. The boundaries of modern African states were largely determined by European administrations, in European capitols, who looked at nineteenth century maps of Africa with concern for their own political rights and without knowledge or care about the distribution of African social units or ecological regimes. A classic example

of this problem is the contribution of political boundaries to the North African famines. Historical and archaeological evidence suggests that the boundaries of the Sahara desert have been alternately expanding and contracting for millennia. The traditional adjustment of desert-border populations has been to migrate slowly back and forth as particular ecological zones to which each was adjusted gradually moved across the map. Such adjustment was facilitated, in part, by relatively low human population densities but also by a style of social organization and land "ownership" quite distinct from the rigid boundaries that states impose. In the modern world, these traditional patterns of movement find themselves constrained by political frontiers.

66. Cooking in pots is a mixed blessing. More thorough cooking may have helped to eliminate parasites and natural toxins from food and may have eliminated one source of carcinogenesis—burnt or carbonized food, which is a common component of foods roasted or barbecued over an open fire. The new cooking technique, however, is also likely to have increased the loss of heat-labile vitamins, because it results in more thorough heating and because water soluble vitamins are more likely to be lost through moist heat than through roasting.

67. Martin et al. 1984.

68. Brace 1986.

69. Powell 1985; Turner 1979; Rose et al. 1984. Since the bacteria in question, normally lactobacillus or streptococcus mutans, spreads as an infectious disease does, it has been suggested that caries formation, like other infections, would have increased as human population densities increased, provided the necessary carbohydrate substrate was also available in the mouth.

70. Cereals are no more complete weaning foods than they are complete nutrition for adults; indeed, since the protein and mineral demands of rapidly growing infants are disproportionately high in relation to their body size and total food intake, the nutritional limitations of cereals and tubers may be particularly acute for children. The biggest advantage of cereal gruels (or other substitutes for mother's milk) is that they help an infant whose mother cannot nurse it survive.

71. Lee 1980.

72. Colostrum and breast milk are relatively clean; they provide maternal antibodies that help a child fight infection and contains germicidal and antiviral properties that kill such intestinal parasites as the protozoans entamoeba and giardia; it provides a nutrient package that is superior to essentially all known substitutes. Breast milk also appears designed to buffer the infant against some shortages felt by the mother. It is a good source of vitamin A, for example, even when the mother is deprived (there is speculation that the breast itself is capable of making the vitamin). Breast-fed infants are rarely deficient in vitamin B_{12}. A thiamine-deficient mother does not, however, buffer her child from this deficiency. Whether because of the nutritional qualities or antibiotic effects of breast milk or because of dirt associated with misuse of infant formulas, breast-fed children are commonly observed to be less prone to gastroenteric disturbances than are cereal-weaned children, and a fair range of statistics from around the modern and historic world suggest that they have a better chance of surviving infancy.

73. Nursing may benefit the mother if it helps space out pregnancies, however, and it may help prevent breast cancer.

74. Lee 1968, 1979; Wehmeyer, Lee, and Whiting 1969; Eaton and Konner 1985. Wild animals are also fairly lean, as discussed in the text.

75. Food refinement might be particularly important for children, who have caloric and nutritional needs disproportionate to their intestinal capacity.

76. This may explain the human "sweet tooth," a desire for rich sources of energy that may have been one of the scarcest of resources early in our history.

77. One controversial hypothesis suggests that, if levels of female body fat are at or below a critical threshold, maturity may be delayed and cyclic ovulation delayed or interrupted because estrogen and other hormone levels are abnormal. Women who are lean appear to achieve menarche (the onset of menstrual cycles) and fertility (the onset of full ovulatory cycles) relatively late. Such women may also cycle less regularly and have a longer "recovery" phase between one pregnancy and subsequent conception, resulting in longer intervals between successful births (although the degree to which levels of body fat contribute to the latter is a subject of controversy). This mechanism may account for the irregular menstruation and low fertility of modern female athletes in training, as well (Frisch 1978; Frisch and McArthur 1974; Frisch et al. 1980; Howell 1979; cf. Ellison 1982; Hughes and Jones 1985; Trussell 1980; Loucks et al. 1984; Bongaarts and Potter 1983; Prentice and Whitehead n.d.; Graham 1985).

There is evidence (discussed in chapter 6) that some hunter-gatherer groups show not only low fertility but also seasonal fertility linked to changes in dietary intake. In effect, the woman's body may have a failsafe mechanism that monitors body stores and shuts down production when stores are not sufficient to support the physical demands of pregnancy and lactation (Cohen 1980). A pregnancy is estimated to require a woman to provide an extra 250 to 300 kilocalories per day; lactaction, far more expensive, requires an extra 500 kilocalories per day (Prentice and Whitehead n.d.).

It is also possible that the link between lean hunter-gatherers (or athletes) and low fertility has more to do with patterns of exercise and consequent hormonal changes than with leanness. Muscular activity promotes the generation of prolactin, which suppresses ovulation (Malina 1983; Brisson et al. 1980; Graham 1985).

78. Suckling stimulates prolactin production, which in turn tends to delay ovulation. The result can be an important contraceptive effect, providing that nursing is prolonged (that is, weaning is late), is intensive (not supplemented by other foods that reduce the infant's appetite), and is frequent (twenty-four-hour feeding on demand). If the infant controls the nursing pattern, it tends to drink small amounts at very frequent intervals, stimulating constant prolactin flow. Under these conditions, each month of full nursing may delay future conception by more than one month (see Habicht et al. 1985; Masnick 1980; Lee 1980; Konner and Worthman 1980; Wood et al. 1985).

In addition, body fat and nursing may interact in promoting contraception. As the nutritional status of the mother declines, more prolactin is required to evoke equivalent milk synthesis, so equivalent amounts of milk for the baby stimulate more prolactin. And the caloric drain helps keep the mother lean. Although we tend to think of such contraceptive effects as a benefit, it may be a problem for hunter-gatherers (and may be so perceived) in a world in which their competitors are commonly more numerous than they are (Howell 1979).

79. Trowell and Burkitt 1981; Winick 1980; Alfin-Slater and Kritchevsky 1980; Armstrong and McMichael 1980. Eaton (1988) has estimated that Paleolithic diets contained four to ten times as much fiber as modern diets. Cultivated cereals contain less fiber than most wild plants. Cultivated plants other than cereals commonly contain even less fiber.

80. We retain our built-in drive for calories, our appreciation of the sweet, even in a world in which calories are no longer scarce. The availability of sugar on a large scale in the past 150 years, not only as a sweetener but also as a preservative and filler in commercially packaged foods, has contributed significantly to the problem.

81. Neel 1962; Armstrong and McMichael 1980; Kolata 1987a. People whose ancestors have only recently been exposed to such high calorie diets appear commonly to be at great risk, suggesting that populations with a longer history of exposure may have evolved some resistance to diabetes mellitus.

82. Trowell and Burkitt 1981.

83. Lack of fiber also alters the composition of bile acids and the flora of the gut in ways that promote the appearance of carcinogenic substances, and the lack of fiber removes one important substance that absorbs, dilutes, and transports these substances (Trowell and Burkitt 1981; Story and Kritchevsky 1980; Basu et al. 1973; Hughes and Jones 1985).

84. Story and Kritchevsky 1980; Basu et al. 1973; Eaton 1988.

85. Moore and Webb (1986) suggest that a potassium/sodium ratio of 2:1 represents a critical threshold between proper and improper intake.

86. Moore and Webb 1986; see chapter 6.

87. Moore and Webb 1986; Eaton and Konner 1985.

88. Harlan 1967.

89. Winick 1980; Moore and Webb 1986. Low calcium intake may also be related to hypertension (Kolata 1984a).

90. Romsos and Clarke 1980; Basu et al. 1973; Armstrong and McMichael 1980.

91. Wild animals are not only relatively lean, they contain a fatty acid relatively rare in domestic beef (eicosapentaenoic acid), which is now being tested for its anti-atherosclerotic properties (Eaton and Konner 1985; Winick 1980; Alfin-Slater and Kritchevsky 1980). Eaton (1988) suggests that polyunsaturates account for 37 percent of the fat of an array of wild animals but only 7 percent of the fat of domestic animals.

92. It has been estimated that caloric intake in affluent nations averages between 2,500 and 4,000 kilocalories per person per day, in contrast to intakes of 1,600 to 2,100 per person per day in poorer nations (as discussed further in the next chapter). But obesity, once primarily a disease of the affluent (and a status symbol), has become increasingly a disease of the poor as refined foods have become widely available and cheap.

93. The pattern is made worse because affluent people commonly get little physical exercise. Exercise helps to reduce atherosclerosis by stimulating the production of high density lipoproteins, which transport cholesterol from peripheral tissues back to the liver.

Chapter 6

1. I am going to focus only on the smallest of societies—hunting and gathering bands—in order to maximize the contrast to contemporary Western lifestyles. A great deal of data are also available concerning simple farming communities and other societies of intermediate size, but any attempt to outline these data here or summarize them in any simple manner would be impossible. For summary listings of the societies referred to here see Lee and DeVore (1968), Murdock 1968, Bicchieri (1972), Schrire 1984, Leacock and Lee 1982, and Campbell and Wood (in press). The boundaries between hunter-gatherer and farming societies are not always easily drawn. Many societies employ a mixed strategy. I have relied on ethnographers' characterizations of groups as hunter-gatherers.

2. Such extinctions can be demonstrated for Africa and Europe, North and South America, and Australia. See Martin and Wright 1967 for arguments about causes.

3. As described in chapter 3, early human populations in their expansion on each continent seem to have preferred relatively open, game-rich savannas, or temperate woodlands, entering deserts and tropical rain forests only after exploiting choicer locations. Penetration of arctic regions is also quite recent, although groups would have been exposed to more arctic conditions in what are now temperate latitudes during the Pleistocene Ice Age (Cohen 1977; Butzer 1971).

4. Most authorities agree, for example, that Australian aborigine populations were decimated in much the same manner as American Indian groups (Kamien 1980; cf. Denevan 1976; Dobyns 1976). Even the earliest observations of most groups reflect conditions after some population decline.

5. See, for example, descriptions by Schrire (1980), Schrire (1984), Bird (1983), Morris 1982.

6. Fox 1969.

7. Bird 1983.

8. Furer-Haimendorf 1943; Bleek 1928; Morris 1982.

9. For example, about half of the Hadza of Tanzania had been vaccinated by the time the first comprehensive studies of their health were done (Bennett et al. 1970, 1973). And the Tiriyo of Brazil otherwise used as a test case for epidemiological observation had also been vaccinated when studied (Black et al. 1970).

10. Lee 1976.

11. Schrire 1980; Denbow and Wilmsen 1986. Carmel Schrire, one of the most outspoken critics of the research in the Kalahari has argued that the !Kung San described by Lee and his coworkers were, to a large extent, a construct or artifact of the anthropologists, a subset of the larger San population who maintained a hunting and gathering lifestyle at the behest of the research team. She argues on this basis that they have no relevance for the reconstruction of prehistory. I would suggest that, even if she is right, they were, in effect, a controlled experiment in a hunting and gathering/small-group lifestyle involving skilled players. As such, they lose much of the aura that comes with the assumption that they are a pristine remnant of an ancient lifeway. But they still retain much of their value as an experiment, particularly if one recognizes that they provide only one such observation among many. They provide experimental evidence about the efficiency of foraging for wild foods, about the quality and quantity of nutrition obtainable by these methods in this environment,

the effects of that diet on health, the probability of encountering parasites, and so forth.

12. Bleek 1928.

13. Lee 1968, 1969, 1979; Lee and DeVore 1976; Howell 1979, 1986.

14. Tanaka 1980.

15. Silberbauer 1981b.

16. Marshall 1960, 1976.

17. Harpending 1976; Harpending and Wandsnider 1982.

18. Metz et al. 1971; Tobias 1966; Heinz 1961; Bronte-Stewart et al. 1960; Truswell and Hansen 1976.

19. Lee 1968, 1969.

20. Wehmeyer et al. 1969.

21. Tanaka 1980; Metz et al. 1971.

22. Wilmsen 1978.

23. Lee 1980.

24. Howell 1986.

25. Hausman and Wilmsen 1984; Harpending and Wandsnider 1982; Hawkes, personal communication, 1988; Blurton-Jones and Sibley 1978. Blurton-Jones and Sibley suggest that the hot times of the year, which limit foraging effort, may act as a bottleneck in the manner of Leibig's "law of the minimum," limiting population and creating the appearance of abundance and leisure at other times. These observations suggest that the "marginality" of the San environment may have more to do with heat and the scarcity of water to dissipate heat than with the availability of food per se.

26. Hausman and Wilmsen 1984; see also note 78.

27. Esche and Lee 1975.

28. Truswell and Hansen 1976.

29. Bronte-Stewart et al. 1960.

30. Metz, Hart, and Harpending 1971.

31. Hitchcock 1982.

32. Tobias 1966.

33. Metz et al. 1971.

34. Truswell and Hansen 1976; Silberbauer 1981b. Low phosphorous intake may also be beneficial, since a high intake of phosphorous in proportion to calcium may contribute to osteoporosis (see Winick 1980).

35. Nurse and Jenkins 1977.

36. Truswell and Hansen 1976; Nurse and Jenkins 1977; Tobias 1966.

37. Truswell and Hansen 1976; Metz et al. 1971; Nurse and Jenkins 1977.

38. Truswell and Hansen 1976.

39. Heinz 1961; Truswell and Hansen 1976.

40. Truswell and Hansen 1976.

41. The evidence that tuberculosis is likely to be a relatively recent scourge is partly archaeological (see chapter 7).

42. Truswell and Hansen 1976; Tanaka 1980; Bronte-Stewart et al. 1960.

43. Nurse and Jenkins 1977.

44. Truswell and Hansen 1976; Silberbauer 1981b.

45. Truswell and Hansen 1976; Tanaka 1980.

46. Marshall 1960.

47. Lee 1980. Blurton-Jones and Sibley (1978) argue that the heat of the Kala-

hari limits mothers' child carrying and foraging capacities and may induce artificial spacing of children.

48. Howell 1979.

49. Wilmsen 1978; Hausman and Wilmsen 1984.

50. Lager and Ellison (1987) suggest that seasonal weight fluctuations can reduce fertility, even if the basic level of nutrition is not low.

51. Lee 1980; Konner and Worthman 1980.

52. Bentley 1985.

53. Harpending 1976; Harpending and Wandsnider 1982. Harpending and Wandsnider point out that their infant mortality figures probably underestimate true infant mortality because they, unlike Howell, accounted only for named babies (usually those living at least three days). They thus miss the substantial fraction of infant mortality that occurs during this early period. Judging from estimates available elsewhere of the proportion of infant deaths occurring in the first five days, it seems likely that their figures should be raised by an additional one third, suggesting true infant mortality rates of 80 and 160 per 1,000. Elsewhere, Harpending (1976) breaks down the populations discussed into a series of seven populations distinguished more finely by location and economy, and it is worth nothing that the one pure hunting and gathering group in his sample (who are not sharing a water hole with a cattle-keeping group), although suffering infant mortality of about 14 percent, had total prereproductive mortality of only about 24 percent. This figure compares favorably with all but one of the six other groups with varying degrees of interaction with cattle-keeping populations. For the latter, the percentage of individuals dying prior to reproduction are 18, 29, 37, 43, 38, 40, and 39 percent, respectively. In this case, however, the samples available for study are all fairly small.

54. Almost all descriptions of hunter-gatherers report relatively high levels of meat in the diet (higher than those of the San), although they report it in various forms (total meat, protein from meat sources, or total or percentage of calories obtained from meat, etc.).

Population	Source	Meat Intake per Person per Day (unit recorded)
Africa		
San	Lee 1968	34 g meat protein
San	Tanaka 1980	150–200 g meat
San	Wilmsen 1978	15–220 g meat (= 3–40 g meat protein)
San	Silberbauer 1981b	50–500 g meat
Hadza	Woodburn, pers. comm., 1985	100–220 g meat
Hadza	O'Connell et al. 1988	285–1,400 g (carcass weight)
Hadza	Hawkes, pers. comm., 1988	920 g (carcass weight = 650–1,300 kcal)
Mbuti	Hart 1978	300–400 g meat after trading
Mbuti	Harakao 1981	100–500 g meat
Mbuti	Ichikawa 1983	290–580 g meat
Efe	Bailey and Peacock, in press	138% recommended daily allowance (RDA)

(continued)

(*continued*)

Population	Source	Meat Intake per Person per Day (unit recorded)
Asia		
Andaman	Man 1883	⅔ of ample diet
Onge	Sen Gupta 1980	136 g meat protein
Birhor	Williams 1974	59 g meat
Batek (Malay)	Endicott 1980	47 g meat protein (195 g meat)
Agta (Philippine)	Griffin 1984	>100 g meat from largest game alone by my calculations
Agta	J. T. Peterson 1981	6 g animal protein (after loss in trade)
Australia		
Arnhemland	McCarthy and MacArthur 1960	60–300 g animal protein
Anbarra	Meehan 1977a, 1977b; Jones 1980	100–400 g animal foods
Ngatatjara	Gould 1967	1.25 lb game
South America		
Cuiva	Hurtado/Hill 1987	900 g meat
Ache	Hill/Hawkes 1983	1,500 kcal from meat
Siriono	Holmberg 1969	⅓–½ lb
Maku	Milton 1984	33 g faunal protein in poorest season
Arctic		
Eskimo	Draper 1977	200 g meat protein

See also Hill 1982. A number of other sources (Radcliffe-Brown 1948; Man 1883; Morris 1982; Blackburn 1982) make qualitative observations of high protein intake. Moreover, as Morris (1982) notes, meat intake may be underreported because game are often taken in contravention of local laws. In contrast, the Agency for International Development (AID, quoted in J. T. Peterson 1981) suggests that the Third World average animal protein intake is about 7 g.

55. There may actually be an adaptive rationale besides scarcity limiting meat consumption in groups living in deserts. First, heat and dryness may discourage active hunting by a human organism that is designed to cool itself by evaporating body moisture. Second, meat protein acts as a diuretic, producing further "wasteful" elimination of scarce water. Third, consumption of lean meat (which is calorically expensive for the body to process) may be discouraged when energy is in shorter supply than protein (see Speth 1983; Milton 1984).

56. Lee 1968; cf. Hayden 1981b.

57. The San are estimated to obtain only 0.2–0.3 kilograms of meat (equal 200–600 kilocalories) for every hour spent hunting, or about 2.6 kilograms per hunter per day, according to Hawkes and O'Connell (1985). These values are well below average in comparison to other hunters. See Hill 1982; Ichikawa 1983; Hawkes and O'Connell 1985; see also discussion in notes to chapter 5.

The poorest hunting returns, the only ones distinctly below those of the San, are reported by Peter Dwyer (1974, 1983, 1985) among Etolo of New Guinea, who hunt to supplement a farming economy. The only available game is large rodents and marsupials, and the resulting catch ranges from 0.2 kilograms meat (33 grams meat protein) per hour down to 0.024 kilograms meat (3.7 grams meat protein) per hour.

58. Williams 1974.

59. Turnbull 1961, 1965, 1972, 1983; Hart 1978; Ichikawa 1981, 1983; Abruzzi 1979.

60. Griffin 1984; J. T. Peterson 1981; Eder 1978.

61. J. T. Peterson 1981.

62. Several studies suggest that trade acts as a drain on the meat and protein supplies of hunter-gatherers, although it may supplement their caloric intake (see J. T. Peterson 1981; Griffin 1984; Turnbull 1961, 1965, 1972, 1983; Hart 1978; Abruzzi 1979; Williams 1974). Trade rarely, if ever, augments protein supplies.

63. Bunting (1970) suggests that, in contrast to affluent, developed countries where people may average 70 to 100 grams of protein a day, mostly from animal sources, people in poor countries average 40 grams of protein a day, mostly of vegetable origin. Basta (1977) suggests that the urban poor may get only 10 to 12 grams of animal protein a day. AID (1970, quoted by J. T. Peterson 1981) suggests that in the Third World the average animal protein intake is only about 7.2 grams per day.

64. Most descriptions of hunting and gathering populations describe eclectic eating habits producing well-balanced (if lean) diets and well-nourished individuals with well-nourished children (at least by Third World standards). On African populations, see Jelliffe et al. (1962), Woodburn (1968a), Turnbull (1961, 1965, 1983), Bailey and Peacock (in press), Tanno (1981), Ichikawa (1981, 1983), Hiernaux 1974. On Indian populations, see Malhotra (1966), Morris (1982), Radcliffe-Brown (1948), Man (1883), Furer-Haimendorf (1943), Gardner (1972). On Southeast Asian populations, see Endicott (1980), Endicott (1979), Dunn (1975), Griffin (1984). On Australian populations, see Tonkinson (1978), McCarthy and MacArthur (1960), MacArthur (1960), Cook (1970), Irvine (1970), Hart and Pilling (1964), MacPherson (1966), Meehan (1977a, 1977b, 1982), Jones (1980), Davidson (1957), Sullivan (1978), Pierce (1978), MacKay (1938), Packer (1961–62), Spencer and Gillen (1904, 1927), Kamien (1980), Thomson (1975), Davis et al. (1957), Curnow (1957). On Amazon populations, see Neel (1970), Flowers (1983), Hill et al. (1984). Among aborigines in Arnhemland, McCarthy and MacArthur found the iron intake fluctuated in daily samples from 33 to 135 percent of RDA, calcium intake fluctuated from 41 to 490 percent, and vitamin C from 47 to 394 percent. A prominent exception appears to be hunter-gatherers in New Guinea, who have few animal resources available and are heavily reliant on sago palm starch as a dietary staple (Townsend 1971).

65. Several medical sources note levels of total serum protein and serum albumin.

Population	Source	Average Level	
		total protein (g/100 ml)	albumin (g/100 ml)
San	Truswell/Hansen 1976	7.4	3.5–4.0
San	Tobias 1966	7.9–8.2	2.8
Hadza	Barnicot et al. 1972	"healthy"	—
Onge	ARNIN 1969	"healthy"	—

(continued)

(*continued*)

Population	Source	Average Level	
		total protein (g/100 ml)	albumin (g/100 ml)
Australians	Wilkinson et al. 1958	7.7–8.0	4.6–4.7
Australians	Davidson 1957	7.3	3.64
Australians	Elphinstone 1971	6.7–8.0	2.8–4.1
Australians	Curnow 1957	7.56	3.78
Mbuti	Mann et al. 1963	8.2–8.8	3.5–5.5
Central African Republic (CAR) Pygmies	Pennetti et al. 1986	8.8–9.4	3.6–3.8

For individuals, serum albumin at 3.1 g/100 ml has been described as reflecting subclinical malnutrition. An albumin of 1.8 represents moderate deficiency, and 1.5 represents severe deficiency (see McCance and Widdowson 1968).

66. See note 64.

67. For example, ARNIN (1969) reports that the Onge of the Andaman Islands display relatively mild vitamin A and C deficiencies (but no anemia) and that such deficiencies are more common in their more civilized neighbors. Elphinstone (1971) reports two possible cases of scurvy and some anemia in a group of desert-living aborigines but no other clinical evidence of malnutrition: no kwashiorkor or edema. Levels of vitamin B_{12} were high. Silberbauer describes marginal deficiencies indicated by positive response to vitamin pills among San but no frank clinical malnutrition. Polunin (1953) found some iodine deficiency in noncoastal groups of Malay aborigines (hunter-gatherers and farmers) but suggest that the condition gets worse as the frequency of cropping the soil increases. He found marginally low hemoglobin rates among Malay but found no vitamin deficiencies. Pennetti et al. (1986) report some moderate protein malnutrition and occasional kwashiorkor among Pygmies of the CAR, but anemia was rare and they saw no signs of vitamin deficiencies. They reported that goiter was less frequent among the pygmies than among their farming neighbors.

68. Gould (1969), for example, notes bloated stomachs among aborigine children and suggest that malnutrition may be implicated. We are accustomed to seeing pictures of malnourished, listless children with bloated stomachs, lusterless hair, exceedingly thin limbs, and depigmentation of the skin. Among hunter-gatherers, stomach bloating can occur in otherwise active and healthy children (cf. discussion of the San by Truswell and Hansen [1976] described above). It apparently results from the problem of processing extremely high roughage diets. Gould himself was aware of this alternate possibility, although he could not distinguish the etiology in this case.

69. Compare descriptions of Third World populations by May (1970), Weaver (1984), Wenlock (1979), Singh and de Souza (1980), Hassan et al. (1985), Hassan and Ahmad (1984), Basta (1977). For European history, by Hansen (1979), Hufton 1983.

70. See, for example, Pagezy (1978), Paolucci et al. (1969), Cavalli-Sforza (1977, 1986), and Mann et al. (1963) (all concerning the African Pygmy), and Dunn (1972) and Polunin (1953) on Malay. But even in these environments, Mann et al. found

anemia rare among Pygmies; as did Price et al. (1963). Paolucci suggests that protein is generally adequate or marginal, although some kwashiorkor is observed. Mann suggests that overall nutrition is fairly good, despite high parasite rates, and reports that serum vitamin A and carotenoids were at healthy levels. Polunin (1953), who found only marginal nutrition among Malay aboriginals, also argued that they are suffering by crowding and dislocation secondary to civilized contact.

71. Almost all descriptions of Australian aboriginal diets agree that, at least in qualitative terms, they have declined since contact (For example, Davidson 1957; MacKay 1938; Hetzel and Frith 1978. See also Schaeffer 1970; Draper 1977; Esche and Lee 1975 with reference to Eskimo diets; Morris 1982 for India; Milton 1984 for Amazon).

72. Colchester 1985; Flowers 1983; Gross et al. 1979; Harris 1984; Neel 1970.

73. Dennett and Connell 1988.

74. Draper (1977, 1978), for example, argues that the traditional Eskimo diet was well balanced and reports no history of epidemic vitamin deficiencies among Eskimos. He suggests that the quality of diets declined with westernization (see also Schaeffer 1970).

75. The B vitamins and vitamins A and D are all found in meat or fish oils. By eating meat raw or lightly cooked and by eating bone marrow, Eskimos apparently preserved sufficient vitamin C from animal tissues to avoid scurvy (Draper 1977; Speth 1983). Draper suggests that, of all nutrients, only calcium would have been marginal in traditional Eskimo diets and that the problem was not so much low calcium intake as high phosphorous intake, which tended to promote hypocalcemia and bone loss. Low vitamin D production by the body itself, associated with the scarcity of sunlight and the need to keep the body fully covered, may also have been a contributing factor in poor calcium metabolism (see also Foulkes and Katz 1975). Tapeworms, such as the fish tapeworm Diphyllobothrium, may be associated with some reported anemia (Rausch et al. 1967).

76. Heller 1964.

77. Hawkes (personal communication, 1988). Woodburn (1968a, personal communication, 1985) is less explicit but clearly suggests that the Hadza diet is relatively bountiful.

78. A number of teams have provided calculated estimates of caloric intake:

Group	Reporter	Measured Intake (kcal/person/day)
Africa		
San	Lee 1969	2,140 (in average season)
San	Tanaka 1980	2,000
San	Wilmsen 1978	2,200 (in good season)
Pygmy	Ichikawa 1981	1,800–3,000
Pygmy	Ichikawa 1983	2,300
Efe	Bailey and Peacock, in press	126% RDA (even in a lean season)
Hadza	Hawkes, pers. comm., 1988	2,900–3,700 annual average (1,900 during lean season, assuming moderate kcal/kg carcass weight of animals)

(continued)

(*continued*)

Group	Reporter	Measured Intake (kcal/person/day)
India		
Onge	Sen Gupta 1980	2,620
Birhor	Williams 1974	1,518 (in trade for rice)
Southeast Asia		
Philippine Batek	Eder 1978	1,825–2,075 (after losing net calories in trade)
Australia		
Anbarra	Jones 1980 Meehan 1977a, 1977b	1,600–2,500 (above RDA 11 months/ year)
Alyawara	O'Connell and Hawkes 1981	3,000 (average per hour work)
Arnhemland	McCarthy and MacArthur 1960	1,170–2,160*
South America		
Cuiva	Hurtado and Hill 1987	2,000
Ache	Hill et al. 1984	3,800
Maku	Milton 1984	1,600+ (in poorest season from manioc, not including faunal intake)

*See disclaimer (note 80).

The small size of most hunter-gatherers reduces their caloric needs, so that many of these figures are a greater percentage of RDA than we usually assume. Whether hunter-gatherers are small because of their low caloric intake is an unresolved question. And whether small size is a benign adaptation or stunted growth is debated as well (see Dennett and Connell 1988; Garn 1985). The San get larger when fed richer diets, but the small size of the Hadza and the Ache is hard to explain in this manner. Note that the small stature of hunter-gatherer populations is a recent phenomenon. Reduced caloric intake is also offered as an explanation for the extremely small size of eighteenth-century poor in London (R. Fogel 1984; Fogel et al. 1983) and in Germany (Wurm 1984). Hufton (1983) has suggested that, in eighteenth century France, one-third of the adult male population (typically those getting a lion's share of the food) subsisted on fewer than 1,800 kilocalories per day.

79. Even when not explicit about caloric intake, most descriptions of hunter-gatherer diets (except those in very dry or cold environments) suggest that they are adequate and reliable, often more so than those of their neighbors. On Africa, see Barnicot et al. 1972; Turnbull 1961, 1965, 1983; Hiernaux 1974; Hitchcock 1982. On India, see Gardner 1972; Radcliffe-Brown 1948; Malhotra 1966; Man 1883; Morris 1982; Furer-Haimendorf 1943. On southeast Asia, see Dunn 1975; Schebesta 1928; Endicott 1979, Endicott 1980; Griffin 1984. On Australia, see Hart and Pilling 1964; Spencer and Gillen 1904, 1927; Tonkinson 1978; Gould 1967; Thomson 1975; Hodgkinson 1845; Eyre 1845; Bonwick 1870; Goodale 1970; Grey 1841; Lumholtz 1889; Sullivan 1978; Pierce 1978; McBryde 1978.

80. In their study of Arnhemland aborigines returning temporarily to a foraging life, MacArthur (1960) and McCarthy and MacArthur (1960) measured caloric intakes as low as 1,100 kilocalories per person per day. But they note that the aborigines could have obtained more food had they wished on every day they were observed.

81. The San are also inefficient when they obtain and process vegetables, including the famous mongongo nuts, which are estimated to produce only about 1,300 kilocalories per hour of work (Hawkes and O'Connell 1985). Compare figures provided in notes to chapter 5.

82. Gould 1981.

83. Under contemporary conditions, trade often supplements the caloric intake of hunting and gathering groups and in at least some instances hunter-gatherers could not get along without the assistance. Most descriptions of the African Pygmy diet, for example, suggest that it is now heavily dependent on trade with farmers, although there is some disagreement whether the Pygmies would do well in the absence of farmers (compare Turnbull 1961, 1965, 1983; Bailey and Peacock, in press; Hart 1978; Ichikawa 1981, 1983). Turnbull and Ichikawa suggest that the hunting and gathering is quite feasible without farmers; Peacock and Bailey see trade as necessary for the hunting and gathering existence. A similar argument is made by Milton (1984) concerning the Maku of Amazonia.

In India, Sen and Sen (1955) and Sinha (1972) suggest that trade helps Birhor survive but also note that there are restrictions on their hunting. Roy (1925) observed an episode of hunger among Birhor resulting from the expropriation of their goods by a landlord. My own sense (comparing the Onge to the Birhor, for example) is that in India the well-being of hunter-gatherers is inversely proportional to their inclusion in the larger economy. Among Philippine Agta it is suggested that trade helps in lean seasons but that traded food is likely to be withheld precisely at the times most needed (W. Peterson 1981).

84. Bailey and Peacock (in press) base their argument in part on the assertion that hunting itself is richer because of changes in the landscape wrought by farmers. A similar argument has been made by J. T. Peterson (1981) concerning Philippine hunter-gatherers.

85. Eder (1978), for example, argues that Philippine hunter-gatherers lose dietary quality and quantity in market exchange.

86. Comparative studies suggest that as large game is rapidly depleted in the immediate vicinity of settlements, productivity drops off sharply. Hart (1978), Bahuchet and Gillaume (1982), and Terashima (1983) all note that Pygmy hunting efficiency rapidly falls off near settlements. A hunting trip away from a village nets an average of 17 kilograms of meat according to Terashima, whereas a trip near a village nets only 4.5 kilograms of meat (compare Vickers 1988).

87. Williams 1974.

88. Pellet (1983) suggests that about two-thirds of the world population averages fewer than 2,200 kilocalories per person per day. Bunting (1970) estimated the Third World average at 2,000 kilocalories, but that of India at only 1,800. Clark and Haswell (1970) estimate an average intake of 1,950 kilocalories for India and suggest that, in the decade before 1970, the average for China was below 2,000. They also suggest that the average in China fell below 1,800 during 1961 and 1962. Bloom (1988) suggests that one-third of the children in the Third World are malnourished.

89. Basta (1977) has estimated that urban poor in various parts of the world often get only 1,100 to 1,500 kilocalories per person per day.

90. Woodburn (personal communication, 1985). O'Connell and Hawkes affirm that it is hard to imagine complete failure of their resources.

91. See note 64.

92. Seasonal hunger and food anxiety among hunter-gatherers are reported by a number of observers. In Africa: Silberbauer 1981b; Marshall 1976; Wilmsen 1978; Hiernaux 1974; Bahuchet and Guillaume 1982; Pagezy 1984. In Australia: Allen 1974; Spencer and Gillen 1927; Sweeny 1947; Gould 1981; Meggitt 1957–58; Moore 1979; Turner 1979. In South America: Holmberg 1969. In India: Furer-Haimendorf 1943. But few of these reports other than reports from the far north (Balikci 1968; Damas 1972; Watanabe 1969; Osgood 1936) or from very dry deserts (Sweeny 1947; Gould 1969a), document or suggest the occurrence of life-threatening starvation.

93. Compare, for example, descriptions of seasonal hunger among African farmers by Nurse 1975; Ogbu 1973; Annegers 1973. Pagezy 1984 suggests that even 2 kilograms loss by the San would be about half that reported in several other parts of Africa. Hiernaux (1974) argues that Pygmies show less seasonal weight loss than surrounding farmers, as do Bahuchet and Guillaume (1982) and Bailey and Peacock (in press). Pagezy suggests that Pygmies share equally in hunger with their neighbors. It should be noted, however, that weight loss of equal magnitude may be more threatening to people who are already lean.

94. Nurse and Jenkins 1977.

95. Barnicot et al. (1972) suggests Hadza suffer less from seasonal hunger than do their neighbors.

96. Gaulin and Konner 1977.

97. See McAlpin 1983a, 1983b; Alamgir 1980; Dando 1975. Alamgir provides one estimate that there were 22 famines in India during 130 years of British rule. McAlpin suggests that railroads played a major role in reducing famine risk; Alamgir argues that political organization, international war, and profiteering often contributed substantially to the famine.

98. Dando 1975. Dando records 125 famine years and 100 years of hunger in Russia between A.D. 971 and 1970. Moreover, he suggests that the pattern got worse over time, bad years occurring one in three in the nineteenth century and one in five in the first part of the twentieth century.

99. Mallory 1926.

100. Braudel (1973, 1981) estimates that France had an average of 11 general famines per century from the tenth to the eighteenth century; Hufton (1983) suggests that in the eighteenth century, at least, significant mortality was involved. Braudel suggests that people in the vicinity of Florence experienced serious hunger in 111 of 420 years between 1371 and 1791 and notes that in the seventeenth and eighteenth centuries starvation reduced people to cannibalism.

101. Dando 1975.

102. Despite its affluence in the mid-1980s, the United States tolerates surprisingly high rates of hunger and malnutrition within its own borders. The *New York Times* (March 3, 1985) reported an "epidemic" of hunger in the United States,

citing increasing rates of kwashiorkor and marasmas, vitamin deficiency, and stunted growth. It estimated that 20 million Americans (that is, one in every ten to fifteen) went hungry at least two days per month.

103. Hayden (1981b) provides a table comparing rates of hunger and starvation among hunter-gatherers in different environments (see also Balikci 1968; Damas 1972; Steward 1938; Osgood 1936; Gould 1969a).

104. Watanabe (1969) suggests that famine is a major problem for far northern populations, particularly in the arctic tundra, inland without access to coastal resources (see also Heller 1964; Balikci 1968; Damas 1972).

105. Heinz 1961; Dunn 1968.

106. For example, Elphinstone (1971) found no hookworm, no schistosomiasis, essentially no tapeworms, no malaria, no filaria in desert aborigines (see also Davidson 1957). MacKay (1938), Cook (1970), Moodie (1973), and Kamien (1980) all suggest that Australian aborigines were relatively disease-free prior to contact and that isolated groups remained relatively free of such diseases as tuberculosis early in the historic period.

107. Bennett et al. 1973.

108. Very high rates of intestinal parasitization among African Pygmies are reported by Pagezy (1984), Price et al. (1963), Mann et al. (1963), Cavalli-Sforza (1977, 1986). One group of Pygmy were found to have lower malaria rates than their neighbors, but unlike other African hunter-gatherers the Pygmy appear to have high frequencies of the sickle cell trait, suggesting either a long history of exposure to malaria or genetic interchange with their neighbors.

109. McNeill 1976.

110. Rausch et al. 1967.

111. Bennett et al. (1970) and Jelliffe et al. (1962) report that the Hadza have lower rates of many parasites than their neighbors. Hadza children were found to have few parasites and low rates of infection. Human salmonella and shigella were rare or absent and other intestinal parasites less common than in neighboring groups. These authors reported low rates of amoeba, ascaris, hookworm, and tapeworm, and no schistosomiasis, although the latter was found among their neighbors. ARNIN (1969) reports that the Onge of the Andamans had lower rates of many parasitic diseases, including malaria, than their more numerous and more sedentary neighbors.

112. See Gomes 1978; Dunn 1968, 1972; Polunin 1953; Turnbull, 1961, 1965, 1983.

113. Livingstone 1976, 1984.

114. Polunin 1953.

115. Dunn 1968, 1972; Polunin 1953.

116. The Hadza, for example, have had relatively cosmopolitan exposure to tuberculosis, rubella, measles, mumps, influenza, rhinoviruses (the cold), polio virus, whooping cough (see Bennett et al. 1973).

117. Black et al. 1974; Black 1975; Black et al. 1970. As one example, Black reports on the Tiriyo, an agricultural group in Brazil isolated by distance and hostility from their neighbors. He found no history of varicella, no smallpox, no tuberculosis, and virtually no history of influenza, parainfluenza, mumps, or measles. Apparently, rare travelers had been exposed to the latter diseases but were not contagious by the

time they returned home, so that the diseases did not spread. In contrast, everyone over the age of three (but no one younger) had been exposed to rubella, suggesting that an epidemic had burned itself out three years before. But for perspective on how isolated this or any group in the modern world actually can be, the Tiriyo had all been immunized against polio by the time Black studied them!

118. Low blood pressure that does not rise with age has been reported among the San by Truswell and Hansen (1976) and by Tobias (1966); among the Hadza by Barnicot et al. (1972) and Hiernaux (1980); among African Pygmies by Mann et al. (1963), Ghesquiere and Karvoner (1981), and Pennetti et al. (1986); among Malay by Polunin (1953); among Australian aborigines by Scarlett et al. (1982), Casley Smith (1959a, 1959b); Abbie (1971), Abbie and Schroder (1960), Kamien (1980). There are no contradictory data other than one questionable report by Casley Smith (1959a). Low blood pressure has been reported among Eskimos by Draper (1977). This appears to be a blessing also shared by subsistence farmers (see Baker and Neel 1966; Oliver et al. 1975, for the Amazon; Hiernaux and Schweich 1979; Day et al. 1979, for Africa; Armstrong and McMichael 1980; and MacPherson 1966, for New Guinea.

119. Trowell and Burkitt 1981; Burkitt 1982. Baruzzi and Franco (1981) report the absence of gastric or duodenal ulcers, appendicitis, diverticular disease, constipation, varicose veins, and hemorrhoids among Amazonian populations. Australian aborigines also suffered low rates of varicose veins, phlebitis, hemorrhoids, appendicites, and ulcers (Trowell and Burkitt 1981; Kamien 1980).

120. Low rates of diabetes are reported for Malay by Polunin (1953); among aborigines, by Kamien (1980); among Eskimos, by Esche and Lee (1975), citing Quick (1974); Mouratoff et al. (1973).

121. Coronary heart disease is reported to be rare among Malay by Polunin (1953); among Amazonian groups by Baruzzi and Franco (1981); low rates among Australian aborigines are reported by Kamien (1980). Low cancer rates are reported by Baruzzi and Franco among Amazon groups and among Malay by Polunin; among Eskimos, by Schaeffer (1970), Draper (1977, 1978), Esche and Lee (1975). Eskimos, despite our stereotypes, appear to have enjoyed low cholesterol and diets low in saturated fat prior to contact (Draper 1977).

122. Where records have been kept, the overwhelming majority of deaths in tropical hunter-gatherer populations appear to result from infectious diseases, both ancient and recently introduced (see, for example, Van Arsdale 1978 on the Asmat of New Guinea; Gomes 1978 on hunter-gatherers in southeast Asia).

123. Several observers agree that hunting or animal-related risks are minimal (see Woodburn 1968a and personal communication, 1985; Gomes 1978; Turnbull 1965; but cf. Harakao 1981). Death by fire or by infected burns is mentioned as a serious risk to children among the Pygmy (Turnbull 1961, 1965). Among Hadza, major fractures (femur) associated with falls from trees are the only major accidental cause of death (Woodburn 1968a and personal communication, 1985). Gomes (1978) suggests that among Malay groups studied fatality in childbirth was a lesser risk for hunter-gatherers than their neighbors, but trauma-associated fatality a higher risk.

124. Watanabe 1969; Hayden 1981b.

125. Reports of recorded production and loss of children among hunter-gatherers are shown below.

Group	Source	Child Production	Infant Mortality Rate (IMR) (%)	Percent Mortality by Age 15 (includes IMR)
San	Howell 1979	4.6[1]	21	35
San	Tanaka 1980	4	15	28 (by age 10)
San	Harpending and Wandsnider 1982	4.1[3]	6–12[3]	35
San	Harpending 1976	—	14–20	24
San	Hitchcock 1982	4.2	—	—
San	Silberbauer 1981b	—	7	—
Efe	Bailey and Peacock, in press	2.6[1]	14	22
Pygmy (CAR)	Cavalli-Sforza 1986	5[1]	17	45
Pygmy (Ituri)	Cavalli-Sforza 1986	5[1]	—	—
Pygmy (CAR)	Neuwelt-Truntzer (in Cavalli-Sforza 1986)	5[1]	—	—
Pygmy	Turnbull 1972	low[1]	low	low (compared to neighbors)
Hadza	Dyson 1977	6.1	20	—
Chenchu	Furer-Haimendorf 1943	5.5[2]	—	At least 29, not counting perinatal deaths
Chenchu	Sibajuddin 1984	5.75	—	49
Birhor	Williams 1974	5.5[3]	—	—
Andaman	Man 1883	3–4[2]	—	—
Andaman	Radcliffe-Brown 1948	exceptionally low[2]	—	—
Malay	Evans 1937	4.3[2]	—	—
Malay	Gomes 1978	3.7	6	29
Philippines				
Agta	M. Goodman et al. 1985	6.5	30 (age 2)	—
Batek	Eder 1978	—	25	50 (in negative balance with fertility)
New Guinea				
Asmat	Van Arsdale 1978	6.9[4]	30	<50
Hiowe	Townsend 1971	5.3	—	43 by age 5 (of which infanticide claims ¼
Kiunga	Serjeantson 1975	3.5	24	32

(*continued*)

(*continued*)

Group	Source	Child Production	Infant Mortality Rate (IMR) (%)	Percent Mortality by Age 15 (includes IMR)
Australia				
Australians (several groups)	Cowlishaw 1982	3–4.6[2]	—	—
Australians	Grey 1841	4.6[2]	—	—
Australians	Cleland 1930	4.2[2]	28	36
Australians	F. L. Jones 1963	4.45	13	—
Australians	F. L. Jones 1963	5.8[4]	—	—
Australians	Carr-Saunders 1922	4.65–5	—	—
Australians	Eyre 1845	5[2]	—	—
Australians	Rose 1960, 1968	very high[5]	50[5]	—
Australians	Sharp 1940	very low	40[6]	—
Australians	Curr 1886	—	36 (age 2)	50
Australians	Curr, in Early 1985	5	—	—
	Curr, in Early 1985	8	—	—
Australians	Ranke, in Early 1985	5.3	—	—
Australians (missions)	MacArthur 1960	—	11–16	—
Australians	Yengoyan 1972	—	19–29	25 by age 5
Cuiva	Hurtado and Hill 1987	5.1	—	52
Ayoreo	Perez-Diez and Salzano 1978	5.9	—	26 natural plus 25 infanticide totals 51
Xavante	Flowers 1983	5.7[4]	24	31
Ache	Hill et al. 1984	7.8[4]	14 (age 2)	42
Cayapo	Salzano in Early 1985	5.0	—	—
Warao	Heinen, personal communication to Early 1985	8.4[4]	—	—
North American				
Sioux/ Ojibwa	Boas 1894 in Early 1985	5.9	—	—
Old Crow Kutchin (Yukon) pre-1900	Roth 1981	4.4	17	35
Old Crow Kutchin (Yukon) post-1900	Roth 1981	6.6[4]	9	18

Group	Source	Child Production	Infant Mortality Rate (IMR) (%)	Percent Mortality by Age 15 (includes IMR)
James Bay Cree	Romaniuk in Roth 1981	7.2[4]	—	—
Aleut	Laughlin et al. 1979	—	20	—
Eskimo	Laughlin et al. 1979	—	40	—
Eskimo	Binford and Chasko 1976	6.9[4]	—	—
Thule Eskimo	Malaurie et al. 1952 in Early 1985	3.5	—	—

[1] Possibly reduced by recent venereal disease

[2] Many of these reports do not distinguish clearly between the total number of children ever born, the number left after infanticide, and the number surviving immediately after birth or otherwise observed and accounted for. Numbers in this column without a superscript 2 are approximations of completed fertility; those with the superscript are the less formal observations. The latter cannot be used to support a claim of low natural fertility among hunter-gatherers, but they do give an indication of the number of children living and dead ever observed or accounted for.

[3] Harpending and Wandsnider do not count until day 3; Williams does not count until day 6.

[4] Reproductive rates have increased since groups became sedentary.

[5] Rose appears to assume impossibly high rates of fertility outside the known human range, let alone that of hunter-gatherers, and he calculates infant mortality on this basis.

[6] Very small sample size. See note 126.

126. Sharp (1940) reported an infant mortality rate of 40 percent for desert-living aborigines, but he saw only 3 infant deaths. More important, his combined figures for fertility and mortality were consistent with an extremely rapid extinction of the population, suggesting that they could hardly be realistic as a representation of longer experience.

127. Rose (1960, 1968) also reports very high infant and child mortality among Australian aborigines, but he appears to derive the estimate by comparing observed living children to an impossibly high assumption of uncontrolled fertility.

128. Condran and Crimmins-Gardner (1978) found five major United States cities with infant mortality rates of 300 or more per 1,000 in 1890; twenty-four more cities had rates in excess of 200 per 1,000. Flinn (1981) suggested that in seventeenth century Geneva between 289 and 358 per 1,000 died as infants and 63 percent of working-class children died before the age of 10. According to Flinn, 37 to 53 percent of children in London in the first half of the seventeenth century died, only 56 percent surviving to age 10. York in the sixteenth century had an infant mortality rate of 480 per 1,000. Flinn also reports that, in the latter half of the eighteenth century, several German communities had infant mortality rates of 350 or more per 1,000. De Vries (1984) suggests that eighteenth century Amsterdam had an infant mortality rate of about 290 per 1,000 and that 48 percent were dead by the age of five. Hoffer and Hill (1981) report that in London, between 1760 and 1780,

40–50 percent of babies whose births were recorded died as infants. In Berlin and in Schwaben, Bavaria, the infant mortality rate was over 300/1,000 in 1880 (Imhoff 1984).

129. Flinn (1981) suggests that during the eighteenth century in France the infant mortality rate fell from 250 to 200 per 1,000 and that preadult mortality fell from 50 to 36 percent. Goubert (1968, 1984) reports that in Brittany in the eighteenth century three communities had infant mortality rates ranging from 237 to 285 per 1,000 and preadult mortality (by age 10) of 420 to 550 per 1,000. Smith (1977) suggests that in France in the eighteenth century the overall IMR was 210 per 1,000 and that 35 percent were dead by age 5. Rollet (1981) reports an IMR of 130 per 1,000 for France in 1905. Flinn reports that infant mortality in Switzerland fell from 283 to 255 per 1,000 during the eighteenth century and preadult mortality fell from 50 to 30 percent. Lee (1984) estimates infant mortality in Prussia in the nineteenth century as ranging from 130 to 250 per 1,000 and being still at 170 per 1,000 in 1910. Flinn estimates that the IMR in Spain in the eighteenth century fell from 280 to 220 per 1,000. See also Fridlizius (1984), Corsini (1984), Bengtsson (1984), and Turpeinen (1979). Krzywicki (1934) estimated that for Europe as a whole in 1871 an average of 40 percent of children died before age 15. Piontek and Henneberg (1981) provide mortality statistics for a rural polish village where in the 1830s only 39 percent survived to age 15. Hansen (1979) suggests that IMR values for England in the nineteenth century ranged between 148 and 160 per 1,000 (and higher in industrial areas). Harris (1978) has suggested that, for Europe as a whole in the 1770s, fewer than half of the children born survived to age 15.

130. Modern infant mortality rates may be as low as 6 per 1,000 in Japan and Scandinavia. The U.S. rate is about 10 per 1,000. Modern Third World national average rates of infant mortality are still commonly between 100 and 200 per 1,000 (U.N. Demographic Yearbook 1982) with 22 percent dying by age 5 (Bloom 1988). These data may well miss some deaths, just as the ethnographic reports do. For example, in the Demographic Yearbook for 1948 the reported proportion of infant deaths occurring in the first week in many countries is improbably low (see also Singh and de Souza 1980; Wayburne 1968). Wayburne reports that in Johannesburg, South Africa, the black infant death rate fell from about 600 to 400 per 1,000 (registered) births by 1945; it fell from 400 to 250 per 1,000 by 1950. He suggested that the main problem was the mother's need to work and consequent premature weaning and farming out of infants. Singh and de Souza suggest that infant mortality among urban porters in Calcutta is still about 400 per 1,000. Ramalingaswami (1975) suggests that in 1971, in parts of India, 40 percent of infants died before age 4. The *Herald Tribune* reported in 1985 that the contemporary infant mortality rate in Afghanistan under Soviet rule was between 300 and 400 per 1,000.

131. See table, note 125.

132. See notes 128–130.

133. These figures for infant and child survival normally refer to illness or accidental loss of children and often do not include intentional elimination of children by infanticide, abortion, or neglect. (Contemporary Western law, morality, and custom commonly make a sharp distinction between infanticide and abortion. In other cultures some distinction between the illegal murder of children and the legal abortion of fetuses is often made—but the dividing line may occur at some anniversary of

birth rather than at birth itself, so that the distinction between infanticide and abortion is blurred. Even in Europe, infanticide did not become a crime—that is, sharply distinct from abortion—until relatively recent history, when foundling homes were established to accommodate babies that had hitherto simply been abandoned.

From a purely practical point of view, infanticide has several advantages over abortion, particularly when safe sterile means of abortion are not available. Infanticide poses less of a risk to the mother's health than abortion, it permits decisions to be made at the last minute, and it allows eugenic judgments about the quality of the offspring to play a role in the decision.

Almost all observers agree (if they discuss it) that infanticide and/or abortion are at least theoretical possibilities among the hunter-gatherer group they studied, but estimated rates vary widely. Birdsell (1968) estimated that, in prehistory, 15 to 50 percent of all conceived Australian aboriginal children were aborted; Yengoyan has estimated 18 to 20 percent among Pitjandjara aborigines and up to 30 percent elsewhere. Jones (1963) argues that the low observed fertility of aboriginal groups reflects abortion. Among the Amazonian Cuiva, infanticide accounts for only about 4 percent of infants (Hurtado and Hill 1987); among the Ache, 7 percent of infants have been eliminated by age 2. Cavalli-Sforza (1986) and Turnbull (1986) suggest that Pygmies only practice infanticide for eugenic reasons.

But these factors also account for a substantial proportion of children and fetuses in all populations including contemporary urban groups, and they are generally not included in the mortality statistics of any. Almost all populations maintain their success in part by eliminating a large proportion of conceived fetuses at one stage or another. Although it is clear that hunting and gathering groups attain some of their success at childrearing by selective pruning, it is by no means clear that they do so more than their civilized counterparts. In fact, given fertility figures discussed below, the reverse may well be the case.

High reported and unreported rates of infanticide and abortion should also be counted in the health statistics of historic and modern European and American societies. It is well established that infant abandonment was common in fairly recent European history. Also well established but less well known is that foundling homes in European cities were effectively a polite form of infanticide. European foundling homes of the eighteenth century routinely seem to have lost 60 to 90 percent of their inmates. Harris (1978) reports that, of 15,000 infants admitted to the first foundling home in London in the eighteenth century, fewer than one-third survived to adolescence. He also reports that, in France, 330,000 infants were abandoned to foundling homes in the 1820s where 80 to 90 percent died in their first year. It has been estimated that, in Paris in the third quarter of the eighteenth century, one-third of all babies born were delivered to foundling homes, where 30 to 90 percent of them died. In Florence, foundling homes had an IMR of 50 to 80 percent (Corsini 1984; Harris 1978).

In more recent times the health statistics of modern countries do not account for abortion rates, which often represent a very substantial proportion of fetuses conceived. Lafitte has estimated that in England 10 to 30 percent of all pregnancies are ended by abortion. In Japan and some European countries abortion may account for one-third to one-half of all pregnancies. In New York state in 1972 there were 472 legal abortions for every 1,000 live births (Lafitte 1978; Tietze and Murstein

1975; Hoffer and Hill 1981). The real point is that selective elimination of infants or fetuses may be directly related to the health of their siblings. In the United States in the 1970s after abortion was legalized, the rate of accidental infant mortality (excluding mortal vehicle deaths) fell significantly (Robertson 1981).

134. At least two sources, Cavalli-Sforza (1986) and Man (1883) are struck by the scarcity of elderly individuals. In at least one case (an agricultural group, the Yano-mamo, whom I have not otherwise discussed), the absence of older adults appears in large part to reflect interpersonal violence.

135. Several sources, like Lee (1979) and Howell (1979) note the presence of active healthy elderly individuals in hunter-gatherer societies. Woodburn, for example, reports Hadza in their eighties. Gomes (1978), Roy (1925), Morris (1982), Turnbull (1961, 1965), Eyre (1845), Grey (1841), and Laughlin et al. (1979) (referring to aleut) among others all comment on the frequent presence of elderly individuals.

136. Eyre 1845.

137. Weiss (1973) and others provide a collection of figures for life expectancy at age 15, which generally compares unfavorably with the San.

Population	Source	Life expectancy at age 15 (e [15])
San	Howell 1979	35–40
Hadza	Dyson 1977	35–40
Caribou Eskimo	Weiss 1973	28
Greenland Eskimo	Weiss 1973	19
California Indian	Weiss 1973	23.4
Birhor	Weiss 1973	24
Australians, Northern Territory	Jones 1963	49
	Weiss 1973 from Jones	34
Australians, Groote Eylandt	Rose 1960	23
Australians, Tiwi	Weiss 1973	33.1
Pygmy	Cavalli-Sforza 1986	22.5
Asmat	Van Arsdale 1978	27
Aleuts (earliest record)	Laughlin et al. 1979	36*
Eskimo	Laughlin et al. 1979	26*
Eskimo	Laughlin et al. 1979	20*

*Laughlin's figures are for e(10).

Hassan (1981) estimated that average e(15) among known hunter-gatherers was just over 26 years; his figures did not include the higher San, Hadza, Asmat, or Aleut figures. Piontek and Henneberg have provided estimates of life expectancy for a rural Polish village where, between 1830 and 1860, life expectancy at age 15 was 29 to 34 years. Russell (1948) suggests that e(15) was about 33 years in England at the end of the thirteenth century but was generally below 30 years between A.D. 1300 and 1425. For the most part, however, historic European adult life expectancy outside cities seems to have been higher.

138. One puzzling facet of the life expectancy figures for hunter-gatherer groups is that the balance between life expectancy at birth or survivorship for children and

life expectancy for adults (from age 15) does not match modern life tables. The proportion of adult survivorship to child survivorship is too low. It is not clear whether this represents a biological reality outside of contemporary experience or an underestimation of adult ages at death. Howell (1982) has criticized the young adult ages at death reported for almost all archaeological populations (chapter 7) on the grounds that they imply populations with too few parents to care for children. She suggests that we must be underestimating adult ages at death. Similar arguments may apply, although clearly in lesser degree, to the short adult life expectancies reported for some ethnographic hunter-gatherers, given the difficulties of estimating unrecorded adult ages accurately. The more likely explanation in the case of ethnographic populations outside the normal spheres of civilized commerce is that epidemic diseases exert a disproportionate effect on adult mortality because individuals are not routinely immunized (or killed) by childhood exposure.

139. Laughlin's figures for the Aleuts, one of the few hunter-gatherer populations for which there is a significant continuous record of observations, suggests a dramatic decline in life expectancy at age 10 during the last two centuries from ca. 1800 to ca. 1940, associated in large part with bouts of infectious disease. Epidemic disease, which primarily affects and may kill children in a previously exposed population, affects and may kill everyone in a previously unexposed or "virgin soil" population. This may account for the different balance of adult and childhood mortality in small-scale and large-scale societies.

140. Reported life expectancy at birth is shown below.

Group	Source	e(0)
San	Howell 1979	30, 35, 50
San	Tanaka 1980	40*
Andaman	Man 1883	20*
Asmat	Van Arsdale 1978	25
Hadza	Dyson 1977	30
Australians	Jones 1963	50
Pygmy	Cavalli-Sforza 1986	17**
Highland New Guinea tribes	Wood 1988	26–35

*Casual observation.
**This figure combined with observed fertility (see note 125) implies a population in negative balance (one not sustaining itself).

These figures, like those for adult life expectancy, must be evaluated with the knowledge that (presumably recent) epidemic disease accounts for a significant fraction of observed deaths. Access to modern medical care, particularly in the case of the Australians, may aid survival.

141. See life tables in Weiss (1973); cf. Coale and Demeny (1983).

142. An average total fertility rate of 7, the highest reasonable estimate for prehistory based on Third World groups, would require a life expectancy of 20 years at birth simply to be self-maintaining (Coale and Demeny 1983; Oeppen, personal communication, 1985; Wrigley and Schofield 1981).

143. Urban European figures for life expectancy were particularly poor (see Alter 1983; Flinn 1981; Perrenoud 1984; de Vries 1984). Jim Oeppen has made available

some unpublished data suggesting that in Stockholm between 1725 and 1830 life expectancy at birth was consistently below 20. Perrenoud reports that life expectancy at birth in Geneva was less than 30 years until 1725. Alter reports that Amsterdam in the early seventeenth century had life expectancy at birth in the twenties. Ascadi and Nemeskeri (1970) suggest that life expectancy at birth in London in 1604 was about 18 years. De Vries reports that Amsterdam in the late eighteenth century had life expectancy at birth in the mid twenties. Woods and Woodward (1984) report that Sheffield England in the 1860s had a life expectancy at birth of 32 and 35 (male and female, respectively)—ages 47 to 50 for the upper classes but 28 to 30 for lower classes. Woods and Woodward also report that Manchester England in the 1840s had an average age at death for gentlemen of 38 years, for traders of 20 years, and for unskilled laborers of 17 years. Wrigley (1969) reports that lower classes of nineteenth century Manchester and Liverpool had life expectancies at birth of less than 20 years and that Manchester in the middle of the nineteenth century had a life expectancy at birth for men of about 24 years. Connell (1975) reports that the average age of recorded deaths and the estimated life expectancy for Irish cities of the 1830s was about 24 years.

144. McAlpin (1983a, 1983b) reports that life expectancy at birth was 24 years in India in the 1890s. The figure fell to just over 20 years between 1911 and 1921 and did not reach 30 until 1941. Ramalingaswami (1975) reports that life expectancy at birth in India was only 32 years in the late 1940s.

145. The reasonableness of the estimate of a 25 to 30 year life expectancy is based partly on observed values and partly on long-term balance between births and deaths for populations that, for natural or cultural reasons, maintained relatively low fertility at levels described below. For a full discussion see chapter 7.

146. Life expectancy at birth in England as a whole is thought to have been between 20 and 35 years from the thirteenth through the fifteenth centuries (but consistently below 30 during the fourteenth century and ranging as low as 17 years for some cohorts during the plague years). E(o) was in the thirties through the eighteenth century, consistently over 40 only in the mid–nineteenth century (Russell 1948; Wrigley and Schofield 1981). In France, Spain, and Switzerland average life expectancy at birth was below 30 in the eighteenth century. In Italy, Spain, and Hungary, it remained below 30 for most of the nineteenth century (Perrenoud 1984; Livi-Bacci 1968; Acsadi and Nemeskeri 1970). In Russia, life expectancy at birth was only 32 in 1896 (and it was still below 30 for some Soviet nationalities). At the same time e(o) for U.S. blacks was about 34 years (Ladny 1980; Mazur 1969). In one rural Polish community, e(o) was about 30 years between A.D. 1350 and 1650. But in the early nineteenth century it was in the low twenties, reaching 30 again only in the 1860s (Piontek and Henneberg 1981). The average recorded ages at death in Ireland in the 1830s were 30 and 29 (male and female, respectively) in rural areas. Irish life expectancy at birth has been estimated as 29 years (rural) and 24 years (urban) Connell (1975). Life expectancy at birth in much of the contemporary Third World averages about 46 years (Bloom 1988).

147. Most studies suggest values of 6 to 8 for completed fertility in the Third World (see Nag 1968; Bongaarts 1984; Bongaarts and Potter 1983).

148. There are fragmentary bits of evidence to suggest that one or more of the physiological mechanisms thought to limit fertility among the !Kung may be in opera-

tion among other hunter-gatherers. Bailey and Peacock (in press), for example, while noting that recently acquired venereal disease may account in part for very low Efe fertility, also note that the Efe display low levels of fertility-related hormones presumably related to high levels of activity but unaffected by venereal disease. Ellison (1982) has also noted that there are hormonal fertility-reducing effects in operation among Pygmies. One or two observers note that other hunter-gatherers share a late age of menarche with the San (Goodman et al. 1985; Bailey and Peacock, in press). Goodman notes, however, that the Agta differ from the San in having more closely spaced babies and no early cessation of fertility. Krzywici (1934) and Yengoyan (1972) each observe that the fertility of Australian aboriginal women ceases relatively early in life, as does that of the !Kung. Jones (1963) and Thomson (1975) both note the wide birth spacing among aborigines, although Jones attributes it to abortion. Elphinstone (1971) notes that aboriginal women menstruate irregularly, suggesting some suppression of reproductive cycling. Moreover, several behaviors among aborigines have been mentioned by various authors as contributing to physiological limits to fertility. Aboriginal women have been observed to permit nonnutritive suckling by older children; the leanness of women may be enforced by cultural dietary restrictions and priorities; aboriginal partners are often mismatched by age, so that fertile individuals have less fertile partners.

Roth (1985) and Roth and Ray (1985) provide a recent summary of populations with measurable increases in fertility associated with settling down. In addition, see Gomes 1978; Serjeantson 1975; Sharp 1940; Krzywicki 1934; Hill et al. 1984; Jones 1963; Hitchcock 1982; Howell 1979; Binford and Chasko 1976.

149. See table, note 125. Bailey and Peacock (in press) and Campbell and Wood (in press) both point to the possibility that venereal disease is reducing fertility. The problem seems to be particularly acute in the region of central Africa where the Pygmies live.

150. Early 1985.

151. See note 125 above, particularly values for the Hadza, Ache, and Agta.

152. Hill et al. 1984.

153. Goodman et al. 1985.

154. Early 1985; see also Campbell and Wood in press; cf. Handwerker 1983; Roth and Ray 1985; Binford and Chasko 1976; Howell 1986; Harpending 1976; Harpending and Wandsnider 1982; Roth (1981) and Romaniuk (1974, 1981) for discussion of the reality of low hunter-gatherer fertility and the rise of fertility with sedentism. Whether or not fertility increases with the adoption of sedentism or farming, it does appear to increase with the intensification of agriculture, although whether the increase represents altered physiology or altered choices by parents is not clear (Ember 1983).

155. If the low fertility of some contemporary hunter-gatherers reflects their body fat levels, then those of prehistory (who were apparently better nourished) may have been more fertile. But if extensive and intensive nursing or womens' patterns of activity are the key, then prehistoric hunter-gatherers, too, are likely to have been relatively infertile, despite overall good health and nutrition. Moreover, such skeletal indicators of health as Harris lines (see chapter 7) seem to suggest that prehistoric hunter-gatherers did experience seasonal fluctuations in food supply. If the fluctuation (rather than the absolute or average level) of the diet is important, then prehis-

toric hunter-gatherers may also have been infertile. Some demographic profiles of prehistoric groups do seem to suggest an increase in fertility with the adoption of sedentism and/or intensive farming. See chapter 7.

156. See notes 122 and 124. Rose (1960, 1968) presumes extraordinarily high fertility, implying that aboriginal women might have a child a year throughout their reproductive lives and might therefore have eighteen or more children if unchecked by intentional or accidental loss. But these estimates are completely outside the range of other human experience, let alone the values reported for hunter-gatherers.

Chapter 7

1. The size of samples and the degree to which they accurately represent the once-living populations from which they are collected are obvious problems. This is particularly the case in the earliest archaeological samples and in samples from the smallest and most mobile groups, in which total available samples may be no more than a few or a few dozen individuals. Some patterns, such as distribution of ages at death, will be heavily influenced by sampling error; other variables, such as average adult stature or frequency of chronic malnutrition, should be less affected. In later, more sedentary groups, in which each sample compared usually includes one to two hundred individuals or more, the sampling problem is reduced, although not eliminated. Moreover, comparison of mortality profile to contemporay life tables (for example, Goodman et al. 1984b; Buikstra and Mielke 1985; Lovejoy et al. 1977; Mensforth 1985) often enables us to identify the missing segments of the population. The best control on sampling error, however, just as in all sciences, is probably replication—looking for patterns of change that occur in many different archaeological sequences—a practice that should identify and eliminate random (though not systematic) sampling biases.

2. Usable sequences of archaeological skeletons in North America are found in Illinois, Ohio, Alabama, Kentucky, Arkansas, Georgia, Tennessee, California, and the American Southwest. In Latin America useful sequences occur in Oaxaca and other areas of Mexico, Guatemala and Belize, Panama, Ecuador, and Peru. In the Old World, sequences occur in southern Scandinavia, western Europe, central and Mediterranean Europe. In Asia they are found in Israel, Iran, India, and Japan. In Africa only the Nubian region of southern Egypt and the northern Sudan has so far produced a meaningful sequence.

In general, samples are larger and more thoroughly studied in North America than in other parts of the world. Moreover, North American comparative sequences are more tightly controlled in time and in space (the populations compared cover relatively short timespans and come from relatively close proximity to one another), so that direct comparisons are more meaningful than the more eclectic sequences discussed from other parts of the world. For that reason North American comparisons are given disproportionate weight as examples in the discussions that follow.

3. Estimates of disease incidence based on skeletal samples will often appear low in comparison to those for living groups (see discussion of tuberculosis, note 70).

4. More complete descriptions of the techniques in skeletal analysis are provided by Steinbock (1976), Ortner and Putschar (1981), Cohen and Armelagos (1984), Goodman et al. (1984b), Huss-Ashmore, Goodman, and Armelagos (1982), Buikstra

and Cook (1980), Gilbert and Mielke (1985), Ubelaker (1978), Shipman et al. (1985), Krogman (1962), Stewart (1979), Larsen (1987).

5. For tooth wear analysis, see Powell (1985). For caries, see Turner (1979), Rose (1984), Powell (1985).

6. For trace element and isotopic analysis, see Sillen and Kavanaugh (1982), Lambert et al. (1984), Bumstead et al. (1986), Norr (1984), Nelson et al. (1986), Schoeninger et al. (1983), Gilbert (1985).

7. Analysis of age of weaning is attempted by Sillen and Smith (1984). This technique might ultimately be applied to test the hypothesis that differences in nursing patterns underlie changes in human fertility associated with the neolithic revolution. See discussion at the end of this chapter.

8. More precisely, we can assess the net availability of nutrients reflecting not only dietary intake but also secondary nutrient loss to parasites or to such special demands as growth, healing, pregnancy, and lactation.

9. There is now general agreement that porotic hyperostosis reflects anemia. But there is considerable controversy about the age of onset of symptoms of anemia in the skeleton (whether, for example, porotic hyperostosis ever first appears in adults or simply reflects the scars of childhood malnutrition). There is also controversy about whether anemia most commonly results from iron deficiency in the diet, properties of certain foods like maize that inhibit iron absorption, food processing, secondary loss of iron to such parasites as hookworm, or even the body's own withdrawal of iron from circulation as a means of fighting infection (see White 1986; Walker 1985; El Najjar 1977; Weinberg 1974; Cook 1984).

10. Steinbock 1976; Ortner and Putschar 1981.

11. Saul 1972; Ortner and Putschar 1981; Steinbock 1976.

12. Angel 1984; Larsen 1984; cf. Fogel 1984; Steegman 1985; Brodar 1978; Wurm 1984; Stini 1985. In dealing with prehistoric groups we must also consider the possibility that two groups being compared are not genetically related or that they have been affected by long-term genetic evolution related to factors other than nutrition—such as changing climate.

13. Cook 1984; Huss-Ashmore et al. 1982; Martin et al. 1985.

14. Larsen 1983; Garn et al. 1979.

15. Cook 1984; Martin et al. 1984; Goodman et al. 1984a; Ubelaker 1978.

16. Steinbock 1976; Ortner and Putschar 1981; Kelley and Micozzi 1984; Allison et al. 1973.

17. As described in earlier chapters, treponemal infection involves an array of diseases produced by the same or very similar organisms. Yaws is largely a skin surface disease passed by casual touch and is therefore a common childhood disease in many parts of the world. It can affect bone but generally does not affect the nervous system, nor is it transmitted to unborn infants. Syphilis, passed venereally, has far more profound effects on reproduction and the nervous system. The skeletal features of the two are very similar (unless Hutchinson's teeth, characteristic of congenital transmission, are present), so skeletal pathologists do not distinguish between them in most diagnoses, contributing to some of the confusion about where syphilis originated. For descriptions of the pathology, see Steinbock 1976; Ortner and Putschar 1981. For controversies about the history of the disease, see Hudson 1965; Hackett 1963; Crosby 1972; Rosebury 1971.

18. Steinbock 1976; Ortner and Putschar 1981.

19. Jackes 1983.

20. Allison 1984; Allison and Gerszten 1982; Cockburn and Cockburn 1980. In addition, human excrement in archaeological sites often contain eggs or other traces of specific parasites (Reinhard et al. 1987).

21. Steinbock 1976; Ortner and Putschar 1981.

22. Steinbock 1976; Ortner and Putschar 1981; Klepinger 1980.

23. Steinbock 1976; Ortner and Putschar 1981. For an excellent quantitative analysis of a large sample, see Lovejoy and Heiple 1981.

24. Steinbock 1976; Ortner and Putschar 1981; Jurmain 1977; Larsen 1984; Bridges 1983, 1987; Cook 1984.

25. Steinbock 1976; Ortner and Putschar 1981; McHenry 1968; Wells 1975.

26. For discussion of enamel hypoplasia, see Sarnat and Schour 1941; Goodman et al. 1980; Rose et al. 1985. For discussion of Wilson bands, see Rose et al. 1985.

27. Ubelaker 1978; Krogman 1962; Stewart 1979.

28. Ubelaker 1978; Katz and Suchey 1986; Kobayashi 1967; Lovejoy et al. 1985 and accompanying suite of articles in the *American Journal of Physical Anthropology* 68:1; Buikstra and Mielke 1985.

29. For controversies about the interpretation of cemetery age-at-death profiles, see Acsadi and Nemeskeri 1970; Weiss 1973; Goodman et al. 1984a; Van Gerven and Armelagos 1983; Cook 1984; Lovejoy et al. 1977; Buikstra and Konigsberg 1985; Buikstra and Mielke 1985, but cf. Bocquet-Appel and Masset 1982, 1985; Howell 1982; Sattenspiel and Harpending 1983. Howell (1982), Hassan (1981), and Bocquet-Appel and Masset (1982) all note that adult ages at death are very probably underestimated in descriptions of skeletal series.

Other biases are possible. Immigration and emigration can distort a cemetery sample because the people buried are not the same as (all) the people born. If people emigrate when they are old enough to travel, the cemetery will contain a higher proportion of the very young but relatively few adults. The apparent average age at death in the cemetery will go down, even though the actual ages at death of individuals born in the community has not changed. If people immigrate, the reverse will occur. Contemporary Florida presumably has a strikingly high proportion of people dying in old age, but that proportion says nothing about the chances that a Florida-born infant will survive to old age.

A more subtle point about the distribution of ages at death in prehistoric cemeteries is raised by Sattenspiel and Harpending (1983). If a population is growing and each new cohort of infants born is larger than the last, a cemetery will appear to display increasing infant and child mortality (and ultimately even a declining average age at death for adults) because more young people are at risk of dying—even though the percentage of people dying at each age and the life expectancy of any one individual have not changed. For example, if the number of babies being born doubles because fertility has increased, an unchanging 20 percent infant mortality rate will produce twice as many infants in the cemetery, giving the appearance of higher infant mortality. If more babies are born than were born ten years before, the ratio of infant to ten-year-old deaths will appear inflated. Tables by Coale and Demeny (1983) provide estimates of the effects of population growth on the death profile under a variety of conditions.

As a result of these two factors, any attempt to convert a cemetery death profile to a life table or an estimate of life expectancy must assume that no immigration or emigration has taken place and must assume that the population was not growing (or make allowance for the rate of growth—a tricky proposition at best, particularly when we realize that the rate of growth need not be constant). All comparisons of average age at death must bear these often unknown factors in mind, and estimates of life expectancy or the production of life tables should be interpreted with caution (see note 106 below).

30. Although there is reasonably good agreement among paleopathologists about broad categories of pathology, paleopathological indicators have proved hard to quantify and standardize with sufficient precision to permit direct quantitative comparison of the published work of different scholars or teams. The most valuable comparative statements therefore are those that result when a single individual or team has evaluated a series of sequential archaeological populations from the same location. Most of the comparisons discussed in this chapter were generated in this manner. But given the imperfection of the archaeological record, direct genetic and cultural continuity between groups being compared can only rarely be demonstrated.

31. For those not familiar with the terminology, Old World archaeologists usually refer to a sequence of Periods: Paleolithic, Mesolithic, Neolithic, Bronze Age, Iron Age—followed by the periods of recorded history. In a loose sense, *Paleolithic* refers to Stone Age hunter-gatherers of more than 12,000 years ago foraging in a Pleistocene environment still containing large game animals that provided at least a relatively large part of their economies; *Mesolithic* refers to Stone Age hunter-gatherers in game-depleted post-Pleistocene environments beginning 10,000 to 15,000 years ago, usually found to be foraging for a wider range or broad spectrum of smaller animals, plants, fish, and shellfish. *Neolithic* refers to Stone Age farmers who begin to appear at different times in different regions but generally within the past 8,000–10,000 years. *Bronze Age* (beginning in Europe and Asia ca. 5,000–6,000 years ago) and Iron Age (beginning ca. 3,000 years ago) refer to the spread of metal technology but simultaneously to the rise of large urban settlements and large bounded political units or states. The dates of the transitions, of course, vary from region to region, and the labels are only roughly synonymous with lifestyle.

North American archaeologists use a different sequence of terms, which vary from region to region. In the central part of the continent, where most of the archaeological sequences discussed were found, the sequence is as follows: Paleo-Indian, Archaic, Woodland, Mississippian. *Paleo-Indian* is used in a sense roughly synonymous with Paleolithic, although much more recent in years. It refers to prehistoric American populations prior to about 9,000 years ago. Archaic and early Woodland populations (between 9,000 to about 1,000 years ago) tend to be broad spectrum foragers and incipient farmers that used local nuts and seeds, some of which may have been domesticated. The Mississippian period, beginning about A.D. 1000, is the period of fully developed maize-based agriculture. Agriculture appears in Mexico and Peru as early as 7,000 years ago or more but is much more recent in parts of North America that are north of Mexico, where most health studies have been done. Incipient cultivation of indigenous crops begins in some parts of eastern North America by 3,000–4,000 years ago or more, but full-scale agriculture involving maize (derived ultimately from Mexico) did not occur until much later, arriving in late Woodland or Mississippian times, often not much more than 1,000 years ago.

Some aspects of complex civilization appear in North America as early as the

Archaic period among populations that were subsisting primarily by hunting and gathering. Many Woodland period populations have been assumed to be agricultural because they share some features (size, sedentism, and construction) commonly associated with agricultural populations. But archaeological refuse has sometimes suggested a dietary focus on local seed plants that may have been cultivated but not domesticated, and isotopic analysis for the presence of maize in diets has tended to suggest that it was of little importance until relatively late. Mississippian period sites, most often based on intensive maize agriculture, are often the largest and politically most complex of prehistoric North American societies.

Because relatively few sequences are reported from Latin America, Africa, and Asia I will not elaborate standard terminology for these regions but simply use descriptive terminology as necessary in the text or notes. For an overall review of prehistory, see Fagan (1986).

32. Angel 1984; Smith et al. 1984b; Kennedy 1984; Meiklejohn et al. 1984; Frayer 1980, 1981.

CHANGES IN ADULT STATURE (cm)

Area	Source	Sex	Paleolithic	Mesolithic	Neolithic
Europe	Meiklejohn et al. 1984	M	170–74	165–68	164–67
		F	156–57	154–56	153–54
India	Kennedy 1984	M	168–92	declining	declining
		F	162–76	declining	declining
Mediterranean	Angel 1984	M	177	172	169
		F	166	160	156

Meiklejohn et al. (1984) measured 19 Paleolithic males and 46 Mesolithic males. Their female sample sizes were 10 and 36, respectively. Kennedy's estimates of tall-statured early populations are based on a combined Paleolithic sample of about 65 individuals, although it is not clear how many of these were measurable. Angel's estimates are based on measurements of 35 Paleolithic and 61 Mesolithic males. The female samples were 28 and 35, respectively.

33. Angel 1984.
34. Kennedy 1984.
35. See discussion of declining foraging efficiency in chapter 5.
36. Schoeninger 1982.
37. Frayer 1980, 1981.
38. Kennedy 1984; Angel 1984. Angel's figures for average adult age at death in Mediterranean Europe are as follows:

Paleolithic	Neolithic	Bronze	Iron	Medieval	Baroque
(M) 35	33	34–36	39–42	38	34
(F) 31	29	30–31	31–38	31	28

The average age at death of adults reported by Angel gives a good illustration of the problems of relative and absolute adult ages at death. Angel describes Paleolithic men as having an average age at death of about 35 years, implying an extremely low life expectancy at age 15. His relative figures, however, suggest that their average age at death was slightly higher than the average age at death among Mesolithic and Neolithic populations, not substantially below those of the Bronze and Iron Ages, and equal to a sample from the same region dated A.D. 1400–1800. Archaeological skeletal populations from all time periods have a strong tendency to display average adult ages at death in the thirties.

39. Brothwell 1963b.

40. Smith et al. 1984b.

41. One other line of evidence may bear out the argument that the Mesolithic was a time of increasing biological stress. Reconstructing the history of human population growth, Hassan (1981) has suggested that the Mesolithic period in the Old World may have been accompanied by a slowing in the growth of the human species compared even to the slow Paleolithic rate of growth. He estimates Upper Paleolithic population growth at a rate of .01 percent per year, Mesolithic growth at .003 percent per year.

42. Birdsell 1953, 1968.

43. Beaton 1983, 1985; Lourandos 1985a, 1985b; Webb 1984; Flood 1976, 1980. In Australia as elsewhere, large game animals disappeared shortly after the arrival of human beings, and the gradual geographical expansion and economic intensification of foraging populations can be demonstrated.

44. Webb 1984. Webb notes, for example, that 17 percent of 41 scorable individuals in his (earliest) Pleistocene sample had cribra orbitalia (consistent with anemia), whereas 20 to 40 percent of later groups displayed this pathology. He also notes that 29 percent of 24 scorable Pleistocene individuals had enamel hypoplasia of the canine tooth (the tooth usually scored), whereas later groups averaged 40–45 percent. Perhaps more interesting, none of his Pleistocene sample had hypoplasia of the third molar, whereas 5 to 25 percent of individuals in his later samples did. The third molar forms later than the canine, and hypoplasia on that tooth therefore suggests an extension of stress later in childhood. The Pleistocene group did show higher rates of arthritis than later groups.

Most studies of prehistoric Australian aboriginal pathology have suggested generally low rates of porotic hyperostosis. Zaino and Zaino (1975) reported porotic hyperostosis among 26 percent of children but only 2.4 percent of adults. Brothwell (1963a) found only about 5.6 percent of his sample to be afflicted. Sandison (1980) reported no porotic hyperostosis and no severe deficiency diseases. Webb's reported rates of porotic hyperostosis are comparatively high, but his excellent published descriptions of his own grading standards suggests that he uses more sensitive thresholds (that is, includes more marginal cases) than most other scholars.

I have found estimates of age at death for only one prehistoric aboriginal Australian population at Roonka (an assemblage clearly accumulating over a period of time). In this cemetery, 13.3 percent of individuals were under age 3 and a total of 27 percent were under age 15.

45. Mensforth 1985; cf. Lovejoy et al. 1977. The later Libben site displayed an infant mortality rate of 17.5 percent with 47 percent dead before the age of 15. But because of very low apparent adult ages at death, life expectancy at birth was only 20 years, life expectancy at age 15 only an additional 19 years. Similarly, the earlier Carlston-Annis site, despite its low rates of infant and child mortality (22 percent

first year mortality, 38 percent dead by age 15), has a life expectancy at birth of only about 22 years because adult ages at death are described as low. In this population e(15) was described as 19.5 years.

Howell (1982) has argued that this is improbably low infant mortality. Some infants are undoubtedly lost in archaeological preservation, but the reported rates are not markedly out of line with those of ethnographic samples of hunter-gatherers. (see chapter 6). She has also argued that the low adult ages at death are unrealistic, given our experience with living populations, and are a biological impossibility— because there would not be enough parents to go around. The implication is that we are substantially underestimating adult ages at death in skeletal samples.

46. Cook 1984; Cook and Buikstra 1979. Cook reported that 25 percent of individuals in the earliest Archaic sample displayed infections, whereas an average of 50 percent of individuals in all later groups were infected.

Deciduous tooth hypoplasia reflects stress on infants in utero or in very early infancy and implies stress on mothers. Other aspects of the Illinois Archaic population are worth noting. Archaic men are relatively short compared to later populations in the region, but women are relatively tall, suggesting that later economic changes may have affected the relative nutritional status of the sexes as much or more than it affected overall nutrition. Archaic males also had relatively low Harris line counts compared to later populations, but females had comparatively high rates, again possibly suggesting that economic changes affected the sexes in a differential manner.

47. Cook 1984; Blakely 1971. Blakely, comparing Archaic and Woodland populations in Illinois, provided figures suggesting that child survivorship improved in the later population, although differential preservation and recovery may be involved. By his calculations, 23 percent of infants were dead by age 2 in the earlier population, only 14 percent in the later. The proportion dying by age 9 was 49 percent in the earlier group and 26 percent in the later. Blakely also concluded that life expectancy at birth went up in the later group, although in the latest fully agricultural sample in his comparison life expectancy was lower than in either hunter-gatherer group. Working with Blakely's figures but computing only adult life expectancy, Weiss (1973) calculated that life expectancy at age 15 declined slightly from 24 to 23 years between Archaic and Woodland samples, although both displayed higher adult life expectancies than later farmers in the region. Buikstra and Mielke (1985) cite additional life tables from Illinois that tell a slightly different (but not markedly contradictory) story at face value, although the authors suggest caution in their use. An Archaic period sample from Carrier Mills in Southern Illinois (ca. 4800–3700 B.C.) initially reported by Bassett (1982) displayed a life expectancy at birth of about 24 years and a life expectancy of about 20 additional years at age 15. Twenty-eight percent died as infants, 66 percent reached age 15 but only about 4 percent reached age 50. The Middle Woodland Klunk site (ca. A.D. 0–400) originally reported by Asch (1976) had a life expectancy at birth of 28 years and a life expectancy at age 15 of 25 years. Twelve percent of individuals died in their first year, and 66 percent reached age 15. Twenty percent reached age 50. A sample from the agricultural Mississippian period Kane site (thirteenth century) initially reported by Milner (1982), across the river from modern St. Louis, had a life expectancy at birth of 24 years with a further life expectancy at age 15 of about 20 years. Twelve percent died as infants, 64 percent reached age 15, and 10 percent reached age 50. Buikstra and Mielke suggest that the differences between Archaic and Middle Woodland may be an artifact of

poor preservation of and recovery of children's skeletons in the later site and the difficulties of aging older adults. In contrast, they suggest that the contrast between Middle Woodland and Mississippian populations represents a real decline in adult life expectancy associated with increased stress in the later period.

48. McHenry 1968.

49. Dickel et al. 1984.

50. Dickel 1985.

51. Walker 1985; Walker and De Niro 1986.

52. Benfer 1984, 1986. Benfer says that the proportion of children in the Paloma cemetery declines from 48 percent (below age 10) in the earliest phase to 28 percent in the latest. The proportion of people over 40 increases from 6 to 23 percent of the sample.

53. Rates of trauma are reported to increase after the adoption of agriculture in Illinois (Goodman et al. 1984a; Cook 1984). Donisi (1983) suggests that there is little to distinguish Archaic and Mississippian populations in Alabama. Rates are also reported to increase in Ecuador (Ubelaker 1984), India (Kennedy 1984), and Scandinavia (Bennike 1985). Bennike reports that cranial trauma is comparatively frequent in a (very small) Mesolithic sample but that post cranial trauma is infrequent in the Mesolithic sample and increases in frequency through the Bronze Age.

54. Rates of trauma are reported to decrease with the adoption of agriculture in Ohio (Perzigian et al. 1984), and Steinbock (1976) impressionistically reports a general downward trend through time among American Indians. Rates appear to decline also in Iran (Rathbun 1984) and Europe (Meiklejohn et al. 1984).

55. Rathbun 1984.

56. Kennedy 1984.

57. Goodman et al. 1984a. Dickson Mounds site is a single site with three sequential populations dating from the late Woodland and Mississippian periods in Illinois, ca. A.D. 950–1300. The total sample is about 550 individuals. The site spans the adoption and intensification of maize agriculture, as well as increases in size of population and commitment to sedentism and increasing integration into large-scale political networks. A late and relatively marginal site in the adoption of agriculture, it is nonetheless one of the best studied and reported sites and one providing well-controlled samples. In addition, conflicting variables associated with large gaps of time or geographical distance are minimized. Goodman et al. report that trauma afflicted 13 percent of the population of the earlier late Woodland hunting and gathering group at Dickson Mounds but 20 percent of the later Mississippian group.

58. Cook 1984.

59. Compare Cohen 1977; Bronson 1972, 1977; M. Harris 1977. See also discussions of efficiency in chapter 6.

60. Studies in Illinois (by Goodman et al. 1984a; Cook 1984), Kentucky (Cassidy 1984), Georgia (Koerner and Blakely 1985), and Alabama (Bridges 1983) all suggest an increase in workload, as measured by arthritis or muscular robusticity. Rathbun 1984 (Iran) and Rose et al. 1984 (Arkansas) report complex patterns of change.

61. The workload, as measured by arthritis and muscular robusticity, appears to decline in several parts of the world following the adoption of agriculture—Georgia (Larsen 1984), Ohio (Perzigian et al. 1984), India (Kennedy 1984), Israel (Smith et al. 1984), and Europe (Meiklejohn et al. 1984).

62. Larsen 1984.

63. Bridges 1983, 1987.

64. Cook 1984.

65. Infection rates are reported to increase with the adoption of farming—or more accurately with the larger, more sedentary communities associated with farming—in Illinois (Goodman et al. 1984a; Cook 1984), Ohio (Perzigian et al. 1984), Kentucky (Cassidy 1984; Robbins 1978), Arkansas (Rose et al. 1984), Panama (Norr 1984), Ecuador (Ubelaker 1984), and Europe (Meiklejohn et al. 1984), although the trends are not always simple or uniform. Rathbun (1984) surprisingly suggests that, although infections increase in frequency from Paleolithic to Neolithic, they are relatively uncommon in later periods in Iran. In Panama, the apparent infection rate first falls from 26 to 15 percent among incipient agricultural groups and then rises to 42 percent among more established agricultural groups.

Larsen (1984) suggests that 0.5 to 4.5 percent of different bones of the skeleton are infected in his preagricultural sample but 2.7 to 10.5 percent of the same bones are infected in his later, agricultural sample. Perzigian et al. (1984) report that infection rates first rose substantially from 11 to 29 percent of bones surveyed with the adoption of agriculture and then ranged from as low as 13 percent to as high as 70 to 80 percent in later populations in Ohio. Hodges (1987) found no significant change in the frequency of periosteal reactions with the intensification of agriculture in Oaxaco, Mexico.

66. Goodman et al. 1984a indicate that 31 percent of the earlier population and 67 percent of the later population at Dickson Mounds displayed infection.

67. Rose et al. 1984. Rose suggests that in the Caddoan region of the lower Mississippi valley infection affected 11 percent of adults and 12 percent of children in the earliest group observed (ca. 400 B.C.), but infection afflicted 10 to 30 percent of adults and 9 to 33 percent of children in later groups. He also reports that infection increased with nucleation of settlements in the central Mississippi Valley. In the lower Mississippi Valley proper infection rates are surprisingly high (ca. 25 percent in his earliest sample) but rise to 80 to 90 percent of adult individuals in his latest samples.

Most of these reports refer to unspecified infection or to treponemal disease. It is interesting from an epidemiological point of view that the relative freedom of hunter-gatherers from disease appears to extend not only to "crowd" diseases but also to apparently chronic infections like yaws, which are thought to have plagued human beings since earliest times (see Cockburn 1971; Black et al. 1974).

68. Cassidy reports, for example, that disseminated (systemic) periosteal lesions, probably symptomatic of treponemal infection, afflicted 2.4 percent of her earlier Archaic period population at Indian Knoll in Kentucky (ca. 2500 B.C.) but affected 31 percent of individuals at the later Hardin Village site.

69. Allison et al. 1973; Williams 1985.

70. Several scholars have noted that tuberculosis first appears or at least is most common in recent, relatively dense populations in various parts of the world (Cook 1984; Perzigian et al. 1984; Buikstra (ed.) 1981; Pfeiffer 1984; Powell 1987; Robbins 1978; Hartney 1981; Angel 1984; Bennike 1985; Zivanovic 1982). Tuberculosis appears almost exclusively in late Mississippian period urban communities, their satellites in the American Midwest, and relatively late, large and sedentary Iroquois occupations in Canada. In Europe, with rare exceptions, the disease is not observed

until very recent prehistory (see note 111 below). Tuberculosis, however, does not always appear in the skeleton, so the incidence of lesions in bone probably underestimates the true incidence of the disease. Moreover, it may be possible to explain changing rates of skeletal pathology in terms of evolutionary changes in the way the disease attacks human beings, rather than by assuming its recent appearance. Allison and Gerszten (1978) argue that tuberculosis in bone is a sign of resistance, so some increase in the frequency of lesions on bone could reflect acclimatization to the disease rather than its first appearance. However, almost all authorities cited, including Allison and Gerszten, assume that there is a real increase in the importance of tuberculosis as populations become large and sedentary. See Cook 1984; Buikstra 1977; Buikstra and Cook 1979, 1981.

71. Allison 1984.

72. Reinhard et al. 1987; Reinhard, in press.

73. Porotic hyperostosis, suggestive of anemia, almost invariably increases with the adoption of farming: in Illinois (Cook 1984; Goodman et al. 1984a), in Kentucky (Cassidy 1984), in Ohio (Perzigian et al. 1984), in Arkansas (Rose et al. 1984), in the American Southwest (Palkovich 1984; cf. Walker 1985), in Panama (Norr 1984) in Ecuador (Ubelaker 1984), in the Mediterranean (Angel 1984), in Israel (Smith et al. 1984). However, Neves (1987) has reported an abrupt decline in rates of porotic hyperostosis among ceramic period (horticultural?) fishermen in Brazil.

In Panama, for example, Norr reports that porotic hyperostosis affected 12 percent of individuals in the early part of the archaeological sequence but 33 percent of individuals in the later part. Rose reports that in the Caddoan region of the lower Mississippi Valley porotic hyperostosis affected 2 percent of individuals in the earliest population but 5 to 25 percent of individuals in later groups. Hodges (1987) found no significant change in the frequency of cribra orbitalia with the intensification of farming in Oaxaca, Mexico.

In western Europe, porotic hyperostosis is very rare among Paleolithic and Mesolithic populations and apparently does not increase with early farming but clearly increases in later populations (cf. Meiklejohn et al. 1984 and Grauer 1984).

74. Goodman et al. 1984a. At Dickson Mounds, porotic hyperostosis afflicts 14, 32, and 52 percent of children in three successive phases of occupation (a late Woodland phase beginning ca. A.D. 950, a late Late Woodland phase beginning ca. A.D. 1100, and a Mississippian period phase beginning ca. A.D. 1200).

75. El-Najjar 1977.

76. Gilbert 1975.

77. Stuart Macadam 1985; Walker 1986; Cook 1984. Note also Weinberg 1974. See also Walker (1985) with reference to altered cooking styles and White (1986) with reference to cereal processing and tortilla making. See Reinhard (in press) with reference to the role of parasites. Whatever the combination of causes, however, the net result appears to be a common reduction in available iron with the adoption of sedentary farming economies.

78. Several sources report a reduction in cortical bone area and cortical maintenance suggestive of reduced nutritional quality after the adoption of farming: in Illinois (Goodman et al. 1984a; Cook 1984), Kentucky (Cassidy 1984), Ontario (Pfeiffer 1984), Ohio (Stout 1978), Illinois (Nelson 1984). The same trend is reported in Israel (Smith et al. 1984).

79. Cook (1984) reports a temporary decline in childhood bone growth compared to dental development among incipient agriculturalists (late Woodland period) in Illinois.

80. Goodman et al. (1984a) report that childhood growth (measured in the length and circumference of long bones compared to degree of dental development) was retarded in children between the ages of 2 and 5 in later agricultural populations in comparison to earlier hunter-gatherers at Dickson Mounds in Illinois.

81. Larsen (1983) notes a decline in deciduous tooth size and also argues that the timespan represented is too short to imply an evolutionary change. He concludes that the change is a "plastic" one—that is, one representing individual growth response to poor diet. Larsen cites Garn et al. 1979 for clinical studies demonstrating the effects of nutrition on deciduous tooth size.

82. Larsen 1984; and Powell 1987 (Georgia); Rose et al. 1984 (lower Mississippi Valley); Angel 1984 (Mediterranean Europe); Kennedy 1984 (India); Meiklejohn et al. 1984 (western Europe) all report reductions in adult size associated with the transition to agriculture.

83. Angel 1984.

84. Meiklejohn et al. 1984; see also Wurm (1984), who reports a decline in stature in Germany associated with the adoption of cereal agriculture.

85. Smith et al. 1984. Rose (1984) reports an increase in size with the adoption of farming (for the Caddoan region of the lower Mississippi); Bridges (1983) reports an increase in adult robustness in Alabama, which she considers indicative of increased workload. Bennike (1985) reports that in Scandinavia stature went up for men but down for women in the Neolithic. Perzigian et al. (1984) report a temporary increase in stature associated with incipient agriculture but then a decline back to Archaic levels during the Mississippian period in Ohio. Cook (1984) conversely reports a temporary decrease in stature followed by a rebound. Allison (1984) reports no trend in Peruvian stature until the period of Inca administration, when people get smaller. Ubelaker (1984) reports no trend in stature through time in Ecuador.

86. Meiklejohn et al. 1984; cf. Zivanovic 1982; Grauer 1984; Wells 1975. However, y'Edynak (1987) suggests that rickets, osteomalacia, and reduced tooth size may have been common among women and children in a Yugoslavian Mesolithic population practicing incipient cultivation (ca. 6300–5300 B.C.) because men were consuming a disproportionate amount of available animal foods.

87. Several studies report higher rates of Harris line in hunter-gatherers than in subsequent farmers (Goodman et al. 1984a; Cassidy 1984; Rose et al. 1984; Perzigian et al. 1984; Cook 1984; but cf. Rathbun 1984). Benfer 1986 has recently argued that, although Harris lines are less frequent among maize-dependent farmers on the Peruvian coast than in earlier hunting and gathering populations, in the later period they display a severity rarely equaled among the earlier groups. Benfer suggests that later populations experienced fewer lean seasons than their forebears but incurred more episodes of severe stress.

88. Cassidy 1984.

89. Goodman et al. 1984a.

90. Enamel hypoplasias and Wilson bands almost invariably become more frequent and/or severe as farming replaced hunting and gathering as a way of life (Illinois: Goodman et al. 1984; Cook 1984; Georgia: Hutchinson 1987; Kentucky:

Cassidy 1984; Ohio: Perzigian et al. 1984; Sciulli 1977, 1978; Rose and Boyd 1978; Ecuador: Ubelaker 1984; Peru: Allison 1984; Yugoslavia: y'Edynak and Fleisch 1983; England: Brothwell 1963b; Mediterranean Europe: Angel 1984; Israel: Smith et al. 1984; India: Kennedy 1984; Iran: Rathbun 1984). Contrast Molnar and Molnar 1985 and Brothwell 1963b (the latter with reference to the French Neolithic). Kennedy reports that hypoplasia increases during the Neolithic in India but declines again during the Bronze Age.

Hodges (1986) has reported no upward trend in enamel hypoplasia following the adoption of agriculture in Oaxaca, Mexico. She argues that farming may have been less stressful in an area to which agriculture (and the major cultigens) were indigenous than in areas farther north where agriculture arrived later by diffusion.

91. Cassidy (1984) reported that severe hypoplasia afflicted 2 percent of her hunter-gatherer sample from Kentucky but 8 to 13 percent of the later sample. Goodman et al. 1984a report that some hypoplasia affected 45 percent of people in the earlier population in their sample, and 80 percent of people in the later period. The average incidence of hypoplastic areas per person went up from 0.9 to 1.6. Perzigian et al. (1984) report that 20 percent of teeth observed were hypoplastic in the earliest of their samples from Ohio, 60 percent in the later samples.

92. Cassidy 1984.

93. The apparent contradiction between hypoplasia and Harris line trends may also be explained by differences in the formation and durability of the two types of lesions. First, Harris lines mark recovery from stress. The dense line of bone is created by growth acceleration or rebound following a period of retarded growth. In contrast, hypoplasia represents the episode of stress itself. In theory, malnourished individuals would be less likely to record a Harris line than well-nourished individuals because they would display less rapid rebound in growth. In fact, two lines of evidence appear to support this interpretation. First, Harris line formation does appear to correlate with periods of relatively rapid bone growth. Second, tests with intentionally malnourished rhesus monkeys seem to confirm that individuals with better background nutrition are more likely to record stress events in their bones (Murchison et al. 1984; Symes 1984). Given other evidence that prehistoric hunter-gatherers were comparatively well nourished, their high Harris line frequency may reflect superior recovery rather than more frequent stress.

In addition, Harris lines in bone are erased or remodeled during the subsequent growth of the individual. Hypoplasia is not remodeled unless the tooth enamel is worn away entirely—a possibility that can readily be checked. If farming populations are more likely than hunter-gatherers to resorb or remodel Harris lines, the apparent contradiction would be explained. Cereal-based agriculture may, in fact, be associated with increased bone turnover or remodeling, helping to explain the low observed incidence of Harris lines in farming populations (Stout 1978; Cook 1984). Farming populations might therefore display low rates of Harris line formation either because their background nutrition is inferior to hunter-gatherers or because their diets promote erasure of the lines. In fact, at Dickson Mounds, when only juvenile (unremodeled) tibias are evaluated, the frequency of Harris lines increases through time, reversing the trend seen in adult tibias but paralleling the trend in hypoplasia.

One other possible explanation of the contradictory trends in Harris lines and enamel hypoplasia needs to be considered. Hunter-gatherers might display comparatively low rates of enamel hypoplasia (and other types of pathology) because they commonly died before there was time for teeth or other parts of the skeleton to record stress: in short, high mortality might explain the apparent good health of hunter-gatherer skeletons; longer survival encumbered with illness might explain the apparent decline in health among farmers.

I discount this possibility for several reasons. First, the probability of dying from episodic stress depends in part on background levels of infection and malnutrition. Individuals already badly nourished or infected are more likely to succomb (see discussion of synergistic effects of malnutrition and infection in chapter 5). Most evidence suggests that the background health of hunter-gatherers was comparatively good.

Second, the available empirical data, faulty as they are, do not support the impression that hunter-gatherers lost high proportions of their children during childhood. Nor do the data suggest an inverse correlation between the two, as in the case of Dickson Mounds, where rates of hypoplasia and mortality increase together.

The most important argument, however, is based on observed growth rates of prehistoric populations in combination with life table simulations and anticipates data and arguments presented later in this chapter. The point, simply, is that there is no evidence of significant improvement in the survival of children after the adoption of farming and no clear reason to assume this improvement occurred. If the acceleration in population growth commonly observed after the adoption of farming reflects increased fertility and/or relaxed birth control, as many would argue, then the acceleration could easily have been achieved despite higher mortality among later groups, as the skeletal data appear to imply. But even if the acceleration in population growth were due entirely to improved survivorship with no change in the production of children, the slight accleration in average growth (from near zero to 0.1 percent per year) implies only a very small improvement in survivorship. If for the sake of argument we use Howell's data for the San as a basis for analysis, an increase from 44 percent to 45 percent survival of infants to the mean age of maternity (approximately 30) would explain the acceleration in population growth. This increase in the percent surviving is far too small to account for reported increases in rates of pathology. The number of those afflicted (and not just the proportion of the afflicted who survived) must often have increased.

94. Cassidy (1984) reported that 9 to 12 percent of individuals in the later farming population displayed deciduous tooth hypoplasia.

95. Sciulli 1977, 1978.

96. Cook and Buikstra 1979.

97. Goodman et al. 1984a. The two samples are 352 and 221 individuals, respectively. The earlier population had a life expectancy at birth (calculated from the distribution of ages at death in the cemetery) of 26 years. Infant mortality was about 13 percent; sixty-five percent of children born survived to age 15. The expectation of life at age 15 was 23 years, and 14 percent of individuals survived past age 50. The later agricultural group had a life expectancy at birth of 19 years and an infant mortality rate of 22 percent. Fifty percent of infants survived to age 15; expectation of life at age 15 was only 18 more years, and only 5 percent of individuals lived past the age of 50.

98. Cook 1984.

99. Blakely 1971; Weiss 1973; Buikstra and Mielke 1985, citing Asch 1976; Milner 1982; Bassett 1982 (see note 47). These data are obviously not perfectly reliable, since children may be left out of cemeteries, resulting in a false picture of low childhood mortality. In at least one case cited this is clearly the case.

100. Cassidy (1984) reported that the earlier (Indian Knoll) population (Indian Knoll, n = 295) lost 23 percent of infants in the first year and 45 percent of children before the age of 17. Previously, Johnston and Snow (1961) had reported two estimates of mortality in the same hunting and gathering population (n > 1,000 individuals) suggesting an infant mortality of about 20 percent and a preadult mortality of 41 to 54 percent. Cassidy reports that the later population (Hardin Village, n = 296) lost a higher proportion of children (54 percent) before adulthood, despite a lower infant mortality rate (13 percent). As is usual for archaeological populations, life expectancy for adults appears low but was higher for the hunter-gatherers than for the farmers. In the earlier site, e(15) was 20 years for men, 18 for women. In the later site, it was 14 and 16 years, respectively. Cassidy concluded that e(0) was 22 and 18 years for men and women, respectively, in the earlier site, 16 and 17 years in the later site.

101. Ubelaker (1984) for Ecuador; Allison (1984) for Peru. Ubelaker estimates life expectancy at birth of 25 and 28 years in the two earliest populations in his archaeological sequence but of 13, 19, and 23 years in the three latest populations. Allison reports the lowest infant mortality rate in the earliest of his samples, which may not, however, be representative. Magennis (1977) has reported on three other Archaic populations from two sites (Eva and Cherry) in Tennessee. She suggests that the death profiles are probably not realistic representations of living populations. But the data at face value suggests life expectancies at birth ranging from 26 to 33 years, infant mortality rates of 8 to 14 percent, and preadult mortality of 22 to 34 percent. Life expectancies at age 15 are 19 to 26 years; the percentage surviving to age 50 is 8 to 25 percent. Hassan (1981) provides life tables for prehistoric Middle Eastern hunting and gathering populations at Sahaba and Natufian Hayonim with calculated e(0) of 39 and 24 years, respectively, and e(15) of 26 and 14 years. Both show improbably low rates of child mortality (18 and 26 percent). But see also the large populations reported by Lovejoy et al. (1977) and Mensforth (1985) described earlier in note 45. Lovejoy and Mensforth argue that internal checks show no obvious gaps in their large sample of juvenile skeletons.

Despite caveats about sample quality and the likely underrepresentation of infant skeletons, none of these relatively large hunter-gatherer samples displays very high infant or child mortality. In fact, the rates of mortality reported often accord with those reported for contemporary hunting groups (chapter 6). The only exception to this pattern I have been able to find is a small sample of Neanderthals from Krapina who display an extremely low average age at death, suggesting selective burial of subadult individuals, combined with very high rates of enamel hypoplasia (see Wolpoff 1979; Molnar and Molnar 1985). We can point out repeatedly that these data may be misleading because the rates of infant and child mortality seem unrealistically low, given our civilized expectations. But as the data accumulate it becomes harder and harder to argue that prehistoric infant and child mortality were exceptionally high.

102. Where average ages at death for adults or adult life expectancy [e(15) or

e(20)] is reported, that average appears more often than not to decline with the adoption of agriculture, although it often rebounds in later stages of civilization (Illinois: Goodman et al. 1984a; Cook 1984; Blakely 1971; Weiss 1973; Kentucky: Cassidy 1984; Mediterranean Europe: Angel 1984; India: Kennedy 1984; Japan: Kobayashi 1967; Scandinavia: Welinder 1979; see also the more eclectic samples of Acsadi and Nemeskeri 1970 and Weiss 1973, which tell a similar story. Smith et al. 1984 report the opposite trend from Israel). Ubelaker (1984) suggests no trend or a slight increase in e(15) in Ecuador.

Acsadi and Nemeskeri report life expectancies (at age 20) of 9, 24, 27, and 36 years for men and of 6, 17, and 23 for women in pre-Neolithic societies. In Neolithic societies they report values of 16 and 21 years for men and of 14 and 17 for women. The two lowest pre-Neolithic values, (9 and 6) were reported by an earlier source (Vallois 1937) whose methods Acsadi and Nemeskeri believe underestimate adult ages at death in comparison to their own work. Among Old World samples, Weiss reports life expectancies at age 15 of 17 years in a Paleolithic sample, 16 years in a Mesolithic sample, and 12, 14, 15, 17, and 29 in Neolithic samples. Among populations in Illinois, Weiss reports values of 24, 26, and 23 years among hunter-gatherers, 19 among agriculturalists. Hassan (1981), summarizing data from these and other sources, reports e(15) of 17, 27, 30, and 18 years for pre-Neolithic groups and 17, 18, and 26 years for Neolithic. Hassan argues that these values probably underrepresent adult life expectancy but argues that prehistoric life expectancies are not likely to have exceeded those reported ethnographically for contemporary hunter-gatherers. Given arguments developed in earlier chapters about the importance of epidemic disease as a source of adult mortality in contemporary groups, I think he may still be underestimating life expectancy in prehistoric groups.

103. Larsen 1984. Larsen's samples (272 and 344, respectively), which, by his admission, may not be complete, suggest an average age at death for adults of about 31 among the hunter-gatherers (before A.D. 1150), and about 26 for the subsequent farming population.

104. Welinder (1979) suggests that e(15) is 25 to 26 years among preagricultural groups in southern Scandinavia and 13 to 20 years in early farming groups.

105. Kobayashi 1967.

106. Paradoxically, declining average age at death could result either from more severe mortality or increased fertility associated with the adoption of agriculture (see note 29). Higher fertility and accelerating population growth can produce a cemetery with an increased percentage of children or a declining average age at death (because there are proportionally more children and young people in the living population), even though no decrease in individual life expectancy had occurred (Sattenspiel and Harpending 1983; Johansson and Horowitz 1986; Buikstra et al. 1986).

Johansson and Horowitz argue that the apparent decline in life expectancy through three sequential populations at Dickson Mounds reported by Goodman et al. (1984a) may be partly an artifact of accelerating population growth relating to an increase in fertility that they suggest had a profound effect on estimates of life expectancy during the middle or transitional period; even after reevaluating the data they conclude that life expectancy was actually less in the latest population (Mississippian period) than in the earliest population, albeit by a smaller margin than originally calculated.

Moreover, population growth rates can not affect death profiles on any significant scale unless the acceleration of population growth is itself fairly marked and sustained. Such effects cannot have been widespread or long lasting during the Neolithic period, given estimates of average population growth that suggests at best a trivial average acceleration in growth with the adoption of farming. Typical estimates of population growth of 0.1 percent per year for the Neolithic and for early civilizations (Hassan 1981) do not imply a rate of growth sufficient to have a widespread distorting effect on average age at death. Compare Coale and Demeney (1983), who show that, assuming an initial life expectancy at birth of about 30 years (model west), an acceleration of population growth rates of 0.1 percent would raise the proportion of individuals under age 15 only from 47 to 48 percent and would produce a decline in the average age at death in a cemetery of only about one year (and only half a year if only adult deaths are considered).

More rapid population growth at particular sites might distort death profiles on a local basis. For example acceleration from zero to a full 1 percent growth could increase the proportion apparently dying under age 15 from 47 to 58 percent with no increase in mortality and could result in an apparent decrease of 5 years in average adult age at death. But such rapid acceleration cannot have been the case over a wide geographical region unless our estimates of average population growth after the adoption of farming are far too low. The wide geographical distribution of the decline in average age at death after the adoption of farming suggests that we are seeing a real increase in mortality as well as fertility. Similarly, although immigration and emigration might affect the appearance of cemetery profiles, the two effects must balance out when a wide enough geographical region is considered.

Demographers will have noted that the distribution of ages at death among adults in archaeological samples also generates another problem. Although the average age at death of the earliest hunter-gatherers may have been relatively high compared to early farming populations, the absolute levels of average age at death among adults for all archaeological populations discussed appears to be far too low—not just in the sense that they imply an earlier death than we are accustomed to but in the sense that they may represent a biological impossibility and that they are at odds with known demographic patterns (see Howell 1982; compare rates of child and adult mortality in tables in Coale and Demeney 1983). Either prehistoric populations had a different balance of adult and childhood mortality than we are accustomed to or we are substantially underestimating adult ages at death in skeletons. Many demographers with whom I have spoken believe the latter.

107. Angel 1984.

108. Angel 1971, 1984. Angel has reported on one Neolithic site from Khirokitia on Cyprus (n = 123 individuals) in which 28 percent died as infants and life expectancy at birth was 17 to 21 years. Life expectancy at 20 was 16 years. The Greek Bronze Age site of Lerna had an average age at death of about 37 years for adult men and 31 for adult women but displayed an infant mortality rate of 36 percent.

109. Weiss (1973) suggests that e(15) in classical Athens was about 19 years, two years higher than his estimate for a Paleolithic population.

110. Acsadi and Nemeskeri 1970. These authors calculate from *recorded* deaths that the average age at death in Rome was 22.6 years, the average for slaves was 17.5, the average for freed slaves was 25, for tradesmen 31, and for professionals 35. But the recorded averages do not include infant mortality. Acsadi and Nemeskeri

estimated life expectancy at birth by correcting for this omission. They estimate e(o) as 15 to 16 years and e(20) as 15 to 20 years. Brunt (1971, cited by Joske 1980) estimated e(o) for imperial Rome at about 25 years.

111. Wells 1975; Steinbock 1976; Zivanovic 1982; Grauer 1984; Bennike 1985; Brothwell 1972; cf. Meiklejohn et al. 1984.

112. Bennike 1985.

113. Fogel et al. 1983.

114. Wurm 1984.

115. Acsadi and Nemeskeri 1970 provide a sample suggesting that, in comparison to life expectancy (at age 20) of 16 to 20 more years for males and 14 to 17 for females in the Neolithic, Copper Age populations had expectancies of 27 to 29 and 21 to 27, respectively; Bronze Age values were 22 to 26 and 18 to 20, respectively, and Iron Age samples had life expectancies at age 20 of 32 years for both sexes.

116. Weiss (1973) suggests that, in contrast to life expectancy at age 15 of 12, 14, 15, 17, and 29 in the Neolithic, various Copper and Bronze Age populations had life expectancies of 13.2, 21, 18.5, and 23 years. A population from ancient Greece had a life expectancy at age 15 of about 22 years, and a population from Roman Britain had one of about 24 years. Samples from Yugoslavia and Hungary in the tenth to twelfth centuries had life expectancies of 31 and 32 years. But one from medieval Sweden had a life expectancy at age 15 of only 17 years, about equal to Paleolithic levels.

117. Welinder 1979.

118. Bennike 1985.

119. Sellevold et al. 1984 estimated average adult age at death in the Iron Age in Denmark to be in the high thirties.

120. Gejvall 1960. Grauer (1987) has recently provided descriptions of two cemeteries from York, England, dated between A.D. 1100 and 1550. Her analysis suggests that calculated life expectancies at birth are 24 and 28 years, although both cemeteries (particularly the latter) display an unrealistically low proportion of infants, suggesting that actual life expectancy was probably lower.

121. Martin et al. 1984.

122. Rudney (1983). For example, rates of enamel hypoplasia apparently went up in Nubia during periods of administration by the ancient kingdom of Meroe.

123. Smith et al. 1984 report that adult ages at death in Israel, averaging about 30 years among Mesolithic populations, averaged about 39 years during the Hellenistic and Roman periods but fell back to an average of about 32 years early in the period of Arab influence. Enamel hypoplasia afflicted 10 to 30 percent of individuals in pre–Neolithic populations but 40 to 50 percent of most later populations. Premature thinning of cortical bone afflicted about 10 percent of individuals in the preagricultural sample, 15 percent of the Bronze Age sample, 23 percent of the Roman sample, and 53 percent of the early Arab sample. Cribra orbitalia (consistent with anemia) afflicted 60 to 100 percent of individuals in later prehistoric populations.

124. Rathbun (1984) reports average adult ages at death in the low thirties throughout the archaeological sequence in Iran.

125. Lukacs et al. 1983; Kennedy 1984.

126. Powell (1984; 1988) reports that mild infection afflicted 63 percent of adults and 29 percent of children at Moundville.

127. Blakely 1977; Blakely and Brown 1985; Koerner and Blakely 1985; Blakely and Detweiler 1981. Blakely reports that privileged male mound burials at Etowah

had an average age at death of about 40 years; females in the mound averaged about 30 years. Villagers had an average age at death of about 23 years (including 10 percent dead in their first year and 31 percent dead by age 10).

128. Cook 1984; Buikstra 1984; Buikstra et al. 1986.

129. Goodman et al. 1984a.

130. Eisenberg 1985, 1986.

131. Lewis and Kneburg 1946; Storey 1985a, 1985b. At Hiwassee Dallas, e(o) was equal to about 15 years and e(15) equal to 16.5 years (58 percent survived to age 5 and only 38 percent survived to age 15).

132. Palkovich 1984. One population, from the site of Pueblo Bonito, displayed a life expectancy at birth of 26 years, but the population includes only one individual who died as an infant, almost certainly a bias in burial rather than a representation of mortality. The other population, from Arroyo Hondo, displayed a life expectancy at birth of about 16 years. In this population 26 percent of individuals died as infants, 59 percent of individuals died by age 15, and those who reached age 15 had a further life expectancy of 18 years. The famous Pecos Pueblo population originally estimated to have displayed a life expectancy at birth of 43 years (Goldstein 1953) is now estimated to display a life expectancy of less than 25 years (Ruff 1981).

133. Saul 1972; Haviland 1967; Nickens 1976.

134. Storey 1985a, 1985b. Deciduous tooth hypoplasia affected all juvenile skeletons. Overall the infant mortality rate appears to have averaged about 31 percent, with only 46 percent reaching age 15 and only 39 percent reaching age 20. Life expectancy at birth was about 17 years. During the latest period of occupation, life expectancy at birth fell to 14 years; the infant mortality rate rose to 39 percent, and only 38 percent of individuals reached age 15.

135. Allison 1984.

136. Despite gradually improving health around them, excavated slave and free black populations in the United States and in the Caribbean commonly display rates of skeletal pathology similar to or worse than prehistoric groups. For example, Angel and coworkers (Angel and Kelley 1983; Angel et al. 1985) have reported that porotic hyperostosis was found in 67 to 75 percent of individuals from three black American populations (slave and free) in the eighteenth and nineteenth centuries. Rickets was found in 30 percent of the free black group. The incidence of rickets in black Americans reflects poor vitamin D production resulting from high latitude (limited sunlight), urban smog and shade, and dark skin filtering ultraviolet light.

Corrucini et al. (1982, 1985) note extremely high rates of severe hypoplasia among nineteenth century slaves on Barbados, which are rarely if ever matched in prehistoric populations.

Blakey (1987) found rates of enamel defects in eighteenth- and nineteenth-century black Americans in Philadelphia comparable to rates reported in the most stressed prehistoric populations.

Rathbun and Scurry (1985) have reported on the archaeology of a nineteenth-century slave cemetery in South Carolina in which cribra orbitalia occurred in 33 to 36 percent of adults and in 80 percent of children; infection appeared on the skeletons of 60 to 69 percent of adults and 80 percent of children. Hypoplasia (mostly moderate or severe) affected 71 percent of adult women and 100 percent of adult men.

Even more striking, Rose (1985) has reported on rates of pathology in a late nineteenth- and twentieth-century free black American population from Arkansas. The population (eighty skeletons believed to provide a reasonably complete record of deaths in the community between 1890 and 1927) displays a life expectancy at birth of about 14 years, with 55 percent of individuals dying below age 15. The infant mortality rate is about 28 percent, and only 6 to 11 percent reached age 50. Of those dying as children, 41 percent displayed porotic hyperostosis, and 77 percent had active or healed signs of infection. Rickets and scurvy were common. Among those dying as adults, 25 percent displayed porotic hyperostosis, and 80 percent displayed infection. Poor bone mineralization, suggesting low intake of calcium and protein, was common. Fifty percent of adult skeletons displayed arthritis, and 39 percent displayed some trauma. All classes of pathology were substantially above rates reported by a team headed by the same individual (Rose) among almost all prehistoric groups of American Indians in the same region. The cemetery described by Rose, however, may be a good example of the effects of emigration on a death profile, because this is presumably a period of northward emigration by young adults.

137. Lovejoy et al. 1977.

138. Hassan 1981; see also Carneiro and Hilse 1966; Braidwood and Reed 1957. These estimated growth rates are derived from estimates of total population size at the beginning and end of each period of prehistory. The growth rate, similar to a compound interest formula, is the rate needed to generate the observed increase over the period of years in question. Paleolithic and Mesolithic rates are based on estimates of human population at the dawn of agriculture (usually estimated at 5 to 10 million people worldwide), compared to a hypothetical small group of individuals at the moment of human origins thousands of years before. The figure gains some precision from the recent observation based on DNA structures that modern Homo sapiens may all be the descendents of a very small group of individuals in the relatively recent past, rather than evolving out of earlier Homo erectus over a very broad geographical range as once assumed (see Lewin 1988a).

One possible resolution to the paradox is that Hassan's figures are wrong because his estimates of maximum preagricultural population are too low. I have elsewhere estimated 15 million people, a figure higher than Hassan's but still not sufficient to make much difference in the average growth rate. Hassan and I and others were all working from data on the San and other contemporary remnant hunters suggesting that population densities of hunter-gatherers rarely exceeded one person per square mile (Lee and DeVore 1968; Birdsell 1968). Work in Australia and elsewhere (Webb 1984; Lourandos 1985a) now suggests that remaining remnant hunter-gatherers in marginal environments may be well below the average maximum density for prehistoric hunter-gatherers. In contrast to Birdsell, for example, Webb (1984) suggests that, in many parts of Australia, more recent prehistoric hunter-gatherers resembled the dense, historically documented Indian populations of California, rather than the sparsely documented populations of Australian aborigines.

The low average rate of growth could also be a compound of other trends. A likely scenario is to suggest that Paleolithic populations, once they became efficient big game hunters with effective projectiles and arrow poison, in fact grew quite rapidly for a relatively brief period, gradually slowing as their prey disappeared and their hunting returns diminished in the Mesolithic. Some descriptions of the early peopling of the Americas suggest a rapid expansion of game-hunting Paleo-Indians very similar to the scenario just proposed (Lewin 1987a, 1987b; Martin 1973).

139. Goodman et al. (1975). See discussion of zoonoses in chapter 4.

140. See Roth and Ray 1985; Harpending 1976; Harpending and Wandsnider 1982 for a review of cases in which sedentism improves survivorship. These data may be misleading, however. In some cases, at least, the advantages of sedentism are peculiar to the twentieth century. In the case of San populations described by Harpending, for example, improved survivorship in settlements was associated with three factors unique to the twentieth century: slightly better access to modern medicine, the availability of cow's milk as a weaning food, and the availability of reliable water supplies. The milk of other animals is a relatively recent addition to human food economies, much more recent than the beginnings of sedentism and the adoption of less nutritious cereal gruels as weaning foods. The water supplies are more reliable in the settlements partly because the politically more powerful neighboring farmers have commandeered the best waterholes and partly because they have access to modern deep (drilled) wells.

141. Ammerman (1975) and Howell (1979) have also proposed another possible explanation for slow growth. They point out that the small group size of hunter-gatherers poses the risk of stochastic demographic events related to the laws of chance rather than to the stresses of the environment. Small isolated groups might often find themselves with skewed sex ratios and mismatched partners simply by violation of the law of averages. Moreover, even if average death rates were only moderate, random fluctuations in deaths could have disproportionate effects on a small group in much the way that a short string of red or black on an honest roulette wheel might wipe out a gambler with only a few chips to bet (refer to chapter 6 where starvation was described in a small band of aborigines that had lost a few adult males). Howell has demonstrated, using computer simulations based on her San data but allowing for such stochastic events, that the same average values for fertility and mortality can produce various rates of population growth and even, occasionally, extinction, purely by chance. The potential importance of such stochastic events depends in part on just how small and isolated groups actually were. If each band was part of a larger network of groups and communication was reasonably maintained, as commonly observed today, random fluctuations in local demography would be less important than if groups were truly isolated (see work by H. M. Wobst 1974, 1975, 1976).

142. Howell 1979. Cf. Goodman et al. 1985; Neel and Weiss 1975. According to Howell's figures, 4.7 live births per mother combined with a life expectancy at birth of just under 30 years (and a sex ratio and age of menarche like the San) would produce an average rate of population growth very near zero. The key variables in the calculation are that an average San woman who lives to complete her reproduction produces about 2.3 daughters (that is, very slightly less than half of her 4.7 children) and that each daughter has about a 44 percent chance of reaching the average age of maternity (roughly the midpoint of her reproductive career). These figures taken together imply that on the average each mother produces one daughter whose reproductive success equals her own—the definition of zero population growth.

If the average number of babies produced by prehistoric human women was 4 rather than 4.7 (other variables held constant), then it would have been necessary for 51 percent of female children born to reach the average age of reproduction, and the corresponding life expectancy at birth needed to maintain the population would be 34 to 35 years. If total fertility was five, only 41 percent would need to reach this age, and life expectancy would need only to be 26 to 27 years. If total reproduction was 5.5 then only 37 percent need to reach the mean age of reproduction, and life expectancy would need only to be 24 to 25 years.

In contrast, Goodman's figures for the Agta, one of the more fertile of contemporary hunter-gatherer groups (total fertility rate is 6.5; mean age of childbirth is about 26 years) suggest that they would require only 31 percent survival to age 26 (life expectancy at birth of about 20 years) to be self-sustaining. If prehistoric hunter-gatherers were as fertile as the contemporary Yanomamo, a horticultural group with a completed fertility of 8.2, they could have maintained themselves and even expanded as the Yanomamo do with a life expectancy at birth of less than 20 years. But Yanomamo fertility is at least as far above the mean for hunter-gatherers as the !Kung are below it, and their low life expectancy at birth results in large part from an extremely high rate of social mortality (infanticide and warfare).

The possibility that population growth rates increased as life expectancy was falling can be illustrated using the San figures as a model and the tables provided by Coale and Demeny (1983).

If in the process of becoming sedentary, total reproduction had increased from 4.7 to 5.2 (a relatively modest increase), average population growth could have accelerated by the amount estimated for the Neolithic (from zero to 0.1 percent per year) while life expectancy was actually falling. This combination of figures would imply that the probability of a female infant surviving to the mean age of maternity fell from 44 percent to 40 percent, equaling a decline in life expectancy from almost 30 to 25 or 26 years. If in the process of settling down the total number of children born (or kept at birth) had increased to 5.5, the relatively modest observed acceleration in population growth would imply that the probability of survival had dropped to about 38 percent, implying a decline in life expectancy to 24 or 25 years.

Arguments about the balance of reproduction and mortality can also be turned around. Assumptions of extremely high mortality or low life expectancy among primitive groups (see Rose 1968; Acsadi and Nemeskeri 1970) run into problems because they must assume impossibly or improbably high fertility unless the group is known or assumed to be heading for extinction.

143. In addition to the possible physiological mechanisms—body fat, nursing, activity levels—already discussed, Hassan (1981) has provided arguments suggesting why the marginal utility of additional children increases when hunter-gatherers become farmers, an increase that affects birth control choices and leads to the intentional production of more children.

Chapter 8

1. Hobbes 1651.

Bibliography

Abbie, A. A. 1960. Physical changes in Australian aborigines consequent upon European contact. *Oceania* 31:140–44.

———. 1969. *The original Australians*. New York: American Elsevier.

———. 1971. *Blood pressure in Australian aborigines*. Studies in Physical Anthropology, no. 39. Canberra: Australian Institute of Aboriginal Studies.

Abbie, A. A., and J. Schroder. 1960. Blood pressure in Arnhemland Aborigines. *MJA* 11:493–96.

Abruzzi, W. S. 1979. Population pressure and subsistence strategies among the Mbuti. *Hum. Ecol.* 7:183–87.

Ackerknecht, Erwin H. 1965. *History and geography of the most important diseases*. New York: Harper and Row.

Acsadi, Gy, and J. Nemeskeri. 1970. *History of human lifespan and mortality*. Budapest: Akademiai Kiado.

Adels, B. R. et al. 1962. Measles in Australasian Indigenes. *Am. J. Dis. Children* 103:85–91.

Aftergood, Lilian, and R. B. Alfin-Slater. 1982. Adverse effects of some food lipids, 497–510 in Jelliffe and Jelliffe.

Agency for International Development (AID). 1970. *The protein gap*. Washington, D.C.: Bureau of Tech. Assistance.

Akpom, C. A. 1982. Schistosomiasis: Nutritional implications. *RID* 4:776–82.

Alamgir, M. 1980. *Famine in South Asia*. Cambridge: Oelgeschlager Gunn and Hain.

Alcorn, M. L., and A. H. Goodman. 1985. Dental enamel defects among contemporary nomadic and sedentary Jordanians. *AJPA* 66:137.

Alfin-Slater, R. B., and L. Aftergood. 1980. Supplies of energy: Fat, 117–40 in Alfin-Slater and Kritchevsky.

Alfin-Slater, R. B., and D. Kritchevsky, eds. 1980. Human nutrition. New York: Plenum.

Alland, Alexander. 1967. *Evolution and human behavior*. Garden City, New York: American Museum of Natural History.

————. 1970. *Adaptation in cultural evolution: An approach to medical anthropology.* New York: Columbia University Press.

Allen, Harry. 1974. The Bagundji of the Darling Basin: Cereal gatherers in an uncertain environment. *World Arch.* 5:309–22.

Allen, J. et al., eds. 1977. *Sunda and Sahul.* London: Academic Press.

Allison, A. C. 1954. Protection afforded by the sickle cell trait against subtertian malarial infection. *Br. Med. J.* 1:290–94.

————. 1971. Polymorphism and natural selection in human populations, 166–90 in Bajema.

Allison, M. J. 1984. Paleopathology in Peruvian and Chilean populations, 515–30 in Cohen and Armelagos.

Allison, M. J., and E. Gerszten. 1978. Tuberculosis in the Americas. *AJPA* 48:377.

————. 1982. *Paleopathology in South American mummies.* Richmond, Va.: Med. Coll. Va.

Allison, M. J. et al. 1973. Documentation of a case of tuberculosis in pre-Columbian America. *Am. Rev. Resp. Dis.* 107:985–91.

Allison, M. J. et al. 1974. A case of hookworm infestation in a Precolumbian American. *AJPA* 41:115–17.

Allison, M. J. et al. 1974. Infectious diseases in pre-Columbian inhabitants of Peru. *AJPA* 41:468.

Allison, M. J. et al. 1981. Tuberculosis in Precolumbian Andean populations, 49–61 in Buikstra.

Alter, George. 1983. Estimating mortality from annuities, insurance and other life contingent contracts. *Hist. Meth.* 16:45–56.

Ames, Bruce N. 1983. Dietary carcinogens and anticarcinogens. *Science* 221:1256–63.

Amin-Zaki, L. 1982. Mercury in food, 149–63 in Jelliffe and Jelliffe.

Ammerman, A. J. 1975. Late Pleistocene population dynamics: An alternate view. *Hum. Ecol.* 3:310–34.

Andersen, Otto. 1984. The decline of Danish mortality before 1850 and its economic and social background, 115–26 in Bengtsson et al.

Anderson, Athol. 1983. Faunal depletion and subsistence change in the early prehistory of southern New Zealand. *Arch. Ocean.* 18:1–10.

Anderson, Edgar. 1952. *Plants, man and life.* Boston: Little, Brown.

Anderson, J. E. 1965. Human skeletons of Tehuacan. *Science* 148:496–97.

Andrewes, C. H., and J. R. Walton. 1977. *Viral and bacterial zoonoses.* London: Balliere Tindall.

Angel, J. L. 1966. Porotic hyperostosis, anemias, malarias in marshes in the prehistoric eastern Mediterranean. *Science* 153:760–63.

————. 1967. Porotic hyperostosis or osteoporosis symmetrica, 368–89 in Brothwell and Sandison.

————. 1969. Paleodemography and evolution. *AJPA* 31:343–53.

————. 1971. *The people of Lerna.* Washington, D.C.: Smithsonian Institution.

————. 1982. A new measure of growth efficiency: Skull base height. *AJPA* 58:297–305.

————. 1984. Health as a crucial factor in changes from hunting to developed farming in the Eastern Mediterranean, 51–74 in Cohen and Armelagos.

Angel, J. L., and J. O. Kelley. 1983. Health status of colonial iron working slaves. *AJPA* 60:170.

Angel, J. L., and L. M. Olney. 1981. Skull base height and pelvic inlet depth from prehistoric to modern times. *AJPA* 54:197.

Angel, J. L. et al. 1985. Life stresses of the free black community as represented by the First African Baptist Church, 8th and Vine, Philadelphia, 1824–41. Paper presented to the American Association of Physical Anthropologists.

Annegers, J. E. 1973. Seasonal food shortages in West Africa. *EFN* 2:251–58.

Armelagos, George. 1967. Man's changing environment, 66–83 in Cockburn.

––––––. 1969. Disease in ancient man. *Science* 163:255-59.

Armelagos, G. J., A. Goodman, and K. H. Jacobs. 1978. The ecological perspective in disease, 71–84 in Logan and Hunt.

Armelagos, G. J., and C. M. Medina. 1977. The demography of prehistoric populations. *Eug. Soc. Bull.* 9:8–14.

Armstrong, B. K., and A. J. McMichael. 1980. Overnutrition, 491–506 in Stanley and Joske.

Annual Report of the National Institute of Nutrition (ARNIN). 1969. Health survey of the Onge tribe in the Andaman and Nicobar Islands. *Ann. Rep. Nat Inst Nutr. India,* 1969:99–100.

––––––. 1974. Nutrition and diet survey of the Andamans. *Ann. Rep. Nat. Inst. Nutr. India.*

Arnott, M. L. 1975. *Gastronomy: The anthropology of food.* The Hague: Mouton.

Asch, D. L. 1976. *The Middle Woodland population of the lower Illinois valley: A study in paleodemographic methods.* Scientific Papers, no. 1. Evanston, Ill.: Northwestern University Archaeological Program.

Bahuchet, Serge, and Henri Guillaume. 1982. Aka-farmer relations in the northwest Congo Basin, 189–212 in Leacock and Lee.

Bailey, R. C., and N. R. Peacock. In press. Efe Pygmies of northeast Zaire: Subsistence strategies in the Ituri Forest. In *Uncertainty in the food supply,* ed. I. de Garine and G. A. Harrison. Cambridge: Cambridge University Press.

Bajema, Carl. 1971. Natural selection in human populations. New York: John Wiley.

Baker, P. T., and J. S. Weiner. 1966. *The biology of human adaptability.* Oxford: Clarendon.

Balikci, Asen. 1968. The Netsilik Eskimos: Adaptive processes, 78–82 in Lee and DeVore.

Barnes, Frances. 1970. The biology of pre-Neolithic man, 1–26 in Boyden.

Barnicot, N. A. 1969. Human nutrition: Evolutionary perspectives, 525–30 in Ucko and Dimbleby.

Barnicot, N. A. et al. 1972. Blood pressure and serum cholesterol in the Hadza of Tanzania. *Hum. Biol.* 44:87–116.

Barnicot, N. A., and J. Woodburn. 1975. Colour blindness and sensitivity to PTC tasting in Hadza. *AHB* 2:61–68.

Barth, F. 1969. Ecological relations of ethnic groups in Swat, North Pakistan, 363–76 in Vayda.

Bartlett, M. S. 1960. The critical community size for measles in the United States. *JRSSA* 123:37–44.

Barua, D., and A. S. Paguio. 1977. ABO blood groups and cholera. *AHB* 4:489–92.

Baruzzi, Roberto, and L. Franco. 1981. Amerindians of Brazil, 138–53 in Trowell and Burkitt.

Baruzzi, R. G. et al. 1977. The Kren-Akorore: A recently contacted indigenous tribe, 179–211 in CIBA.

Barwick, Diane. 1971. Changes in the aboriginal population of Victoria, 1863–1966, 288–315 in Mulvaney and Golson.

Basedow, Herbert. 1925. *The Australian aboriginal.* Adelaide: F. W. Preece and Sons.

Bassett, E. 1982. Osteological analysis of Carrier Mills burials. In R. Jeffries and B. Butler, *The Carrier Mills archaeological project,* 1029–1114. Carbondale: Southern Illinois University Center for Archaeological Investigations. Research paper 33.

Bassett, E. J. et al. 1980. Tetracycline-labeled human bone from ancient Sudanese Nubia (A.D. 350.). *Science* 209:1532–34.

Basta, S. S. 1977. Nutrition and health in low income urban areas of the third world. *EFN* 6:113–24.

Basu, T. K. et al. 1973. Interrelationships of nutrition and cancer. *EFN* 2:193–99.

Bayliss-Smith, T. 1982a. *The ecology of agricultural systems.* Cambridge: Cambridge University Press.

———. 1982b. Energy use, food production and welfare, 283–317 in Harrison.

Beaton, J. M. 1983. Comment: Does intensification account for changes in Australian Holocene archaeological record? *Arch. Ocean.* 18:94–97.

———. 1985. Evidence for a coastal occupation time-lag at Princess Charlotte Bay, North Queensland, and implications for coastal colonization and population growth theories for aboriginal Australia. *Arch. Ocean.* 20:1–20.

Beckerman, Stephen. 1980. Fishing and hunting by the Bari of Colombia. *Bennington, Vermont, Working Papers on South American Indians* 2:67–109.

———. 1983. Carpe diem: An optimal foraging approach to Bari fishing and hunting, 269–99 in Hames and Vickers.

Behrens, Clifford. 1981. Time allocation and meat procurement among the Shipibo of eastern Brazil. *Hum. Ecol.* 9:189–220.

Beisel, W. R. 1982. Synergisms and antagonisms of parasitic diseases and malnutrition. *RID* 4:746–55.

Belovsky, G. E. 1987. Hunter-gatherer foraging: A linear programming approach. *J. Anthrop. Arch.* 6:29–76.

Benenson, A. S. 1976a. Cholera, 174–83 in Top and Wehrle.

———. 1976b. Smallpox, 623–35 in Top and Wehrle.

Benfer, Robert. 1984. The challenges and rewards of sedentism: The preceramic village of Paloma, Peru, 531–55 in Cohen and Armelagos.

———. 1986. Middle and late archaic adaptation in central coastal Peru. Paper presented to the fifty-first annual meeting of the Society for American Archaeology, New Orleans.

Bengtsson, T. et al. 1984. *Preindustrial population change.* Stockholm: Almquist and Wiksell.

Bennett, F. J. et al. 1970. Helminth and protozoal parasites of the Hadza of Tanzania. *Trans. Roy. Soc. Trop. Med. Hyg.* 64:857–80.

Bennett, F. J. et al. 1973. Studies on viral, bacterial, rickettsial and treponemal disease in the Hadza of Tanzania and a note on injuries. *Hum. Biol.* 45:243–72.

Bennike, Pia. 1985. *Paleopathology of Danish skeletons*. Copenhagen: Almquist and Wiksell.

Bentley, G. 1985. Hunter-gatherer energetics and fertility: A reassessment of the !Kung San. *Hum. Ecol.* 13:79–110.

Berlin, E. A., and E. K. Markell. 1977. An assessment of the nutrition and health status for the Aguaruna Jivaro community, Amazonas, Peru. *EFN* 6:69–81.

Berndt, R. M., and C. H. Berndt. 1964. *The world of the first Australians*. Chicago: University of Chicago Press.

Bicchieri, M. 1969. The differential use of identical features of physical habitat in connection with exploitative, settlement, and community patterns: The BaMbuti case study. In *Ecological Essays*, 65–72. Ottawa: Canadian National Museum Contributions to Anthropology.

———, ed. 1972. *Hunters and gatherers today*. New York: Holt, Reinhart.

Billewicz, W. Z., and I. A. McGregor. 1981. The demography of two West African (Gambian) villages, 1951–1975. *J. Biosoc. Sci.* 13:219–40.

Bina, J. C. et al. 1978. Greater resistance to development of severe schistosomiasis in Brazilian Negroes. *Hum. Biol.* 50:41–49.

Bindon, J. R. 1984. An evaluation of the diet of three groups of Samoan adults: Modernization and dietary inadequacy. *EFN* 14:105–15.

Binford, L. R. 1968. Post-Pleistocene adaptations. In *New perspectives in archaeology*, ed. S. R. Binford and L. R. Binford, 313–36. Chicago: Aldine.

———. 1980. Willow smoke and dogs tails: Hunter-gatherer settlement systems and archaeological site formation. *Amer. Antiq.* 45:4–20.

———. 1983. *In pursuit of the past*. New York: Thames and Hudson.

Binford, L. R., and W. J. Chasko. 1976. Nunamiut Demographic history: A provocative case, 63–144 in Zubrow.

Biraben, Jean-Noel. 1968. Certain demographic characteristics of the plague epidemic in France, 1720–1722. *Daedalus* 97:536–45.

Bird, Nurit. 1983. Wage gathering, socio-economic changes and the case of the food-gathering Naikens of South India. In *Rural South Asia: Linkages and development*, ed. P. Robb, 57–89. London: Curzon.

Birdsell, Joseph. 1953. Some environmental and cultural factors influencing the structure of Australian aboriginal populations. *Amer. Naturalist* 87:171–207.

———. 1968. Some predictions for the Pleistocene based on equilibrium systems among recent hunter-gatherers, 229–40 in Lee and DeVore.

Black, F. L. 1966. Measles endemicity in insular populations: Critical community size and its evolutionary implications. *J. Theoret. Biol.* 11:207–11.

———. 1975. Infectious diseases in primitive societies. *Science* 187:515–18.

———. 1980. Modern isolated pre-agricultural populations as a source of information on prehistoric epidemic patterns, 37–54 in Stanley and Joske.

Black, F. L. et al. 1970. Prevalence of antibody against viruses in the Tiriyo, an isolated Amazonian tribe. *J. Epidem.* 91:430–38.

Black, F. L. et al. 1974. Evidence for persistence of infectious agents in isolated human populations. *Amer. J. Epidem.* 100:230–50.

Black, Francis L. et al. 1977a. Epidemiology of infectious disease: The example of measles, 115–35 in CIBA.

Black, F. L. et al. 1977b. Nutritional status of Brazilian Kayapo Indians. *Hum. Biol.* 49:139–53.

Black, F. L. et al. 1978. Birth and survival patterns in numerically unstable proto-agricultural societies in the Brazilian Amazon. *Med. Anthrop.* 2:95–127.

Black, R. H. 1959. Haptoglobins and hemoglobins in Australian aborigines. *Med. J. Austr.* 1:175–76.

Blackburn, Roderic H. 1982. In the land of milk and honey: Okiek adaptations to their forests and neighbors, 283–306 in Leacock and Lee.

Blakely, R. L. 1971. Comparison of mortality profiles of archaic Middle Woodland and Middle Mississippian skeletal populations. *AJPA* 34:43–54.

———. 1977. Sociocultural implications of demographic data from Etowah, Georgia. *Proc. South. Anth. Soc.* 11:45–66.

———, ed. 1977. *Biocultural adaptation in prehistoric America.* Athens: University of Georgia Press.

Blakely, Robert, and A. B. Brown. 1985. Functionally adaptive biocultural diversity in the Coosa chiefdom of sixteenth century Georgia. *AJPA* 66:146.

Blakely, Robert, and B. Detweiler. 1981. Odontological evidence for differential stress at the King and Etowah sites in sixteenth century Georgia. *AJPA* 69:176.

Blakey, Michael. 1987. Fetal and childhood health in late eighteenth century and early nineteenth century Afro-Americans. *AJPA* 72:179.

Blattner, W. et al. 1988. HIV causes AIDS. *Science* 241:515.

Bleek, D. F. 1928. *The Naron.* Cambridge: Cambridge University Press.

Bloom, B. R. 1988. A new threat to world health. *Science* 239:9.

Blurton-Jones, N., and P. M. Sibley 1978. Testing adaptiveness of culturally determined behavior: Do Bushman women maximize their reproductive success? In *Human behavior and adaptation,* Society for Study of Human Biology, Symposium 18, 135–57. London: Taylor and Francis.

Boas, Franz. 1894. The half-blood Indian: An anthropometric study. *Pop. Sci. Monthly* 45:761–67.

Bocquet-Appel, J-P, and C. Masset. 1982. Farewell to paleodemography. *JHE* 11:321–33.

———. 1985. Paleopathology: Resurrection or ghost. *JHE* 14:107–11.

Bogert, L. J., G. M. Briggs, and D. H. Calloway. 1973. *Nutrition and physical fitness.* Philadelphia: W. B. Saunders.

Bongaarts, J. 1980. Does malnutrition affect fecundity: A summary of evidence. *Science* 208:564–69.

———. 1984. Implications of future fertility trends for contraceptive practice. *Pop. and Dev. Rev.* 10:341–52.

Bongaarts, J., and R. G. Potter. 1983. *Fertility, biology and behavior.* New York: Academic Press.

Bonwick, James. 1870. *Daily life and the origins of the Tasmanians.* London: Samson, Low, Son and Marston.

Borts, I. H., and S. L. Hendricks. 1976. Brucellosis, 143–53 in Top and Wehrle.

Bose, Saradindu. 1964. The economy of the Onge of little Andaman. *Man in India* 44:298–310.

Boserup, E. 1965. *The conditions of agricultural growth.* Chicago: Aldine.

———. 1983. The impact of scarcity and plenty on development, 185–209 in Rotberg and Rabb.

Boyce, A. J. et al. 1976. Association between PTC taster status and goitre in a Papua New Guinea population. *Hum. Biol.* 48:769–73.

Boyden, S. V. 1970. *The impact of civilization on the biology of man*. Canberra: Australian National University.

Brace, C. L. 1986. Egg on the face, *f* in the mouth and the overbite. *Amer. Anthrop.* 88:695–97.

Brachman, P. S. 1976. Anthrax, 137–42 in Top and Wehrle.

Braidwood, R. J., and C. A. Reed. 1957. The achievement and early consequences of food production. *Cold Spring Harbor Symp. Quant. Biol.* 22:19–31.

Brainerd, J. M. 1983. The effects of sedentarization on mortality levels and life expectancy in the Turkana population of Kenya. *AJPA* 60:176.

Braudel, Fernand. 1973. Capitalism and material life, 1400–1800. Translated from the French by Miriam Kochan. London: Weidenfeld and Nicholson.

——— . 1981. *The structures of everyday life*. Translated from the French by Sian Reynolds. New York: Harper and Row.

Brenton, Barry. 1987. Monitoring change in food processing technology by means of skeletal analysis. Paper presented to the twenty-seventh annual meeting of the Northeast Anthropological Association, Amherst, Mass.

Brenton, Barry. 1988. Fermented foods in New World prehistory: North America. In *Diet and subsistence: Current archaeological perspectives*, ed. B. V. Kennedy and G. M. Lemoine. Calgary: Univ. of Calgary, Proceedings of the nineteenth Chacmool Conference.

Bridges, Patricia. 1982. Postcranial dimensions in the Archaic and Mississippian cultures of Northern Alabama: Implications for prehistoric nutrition and behavior. *AJPA* 57:172–73.

——— . 1983. Subsistence activity and biomechanical properties of long bones in two Amerindian populations. *AJPA* 60:177.

——— . 1987. Osteological correlates of prehistoric activities. Paper presented to the annual meeting of the American Anthropological Association, Chicago, Ill.

Brodar, V. 1978. Reduction of body size of the adult as a permanent effect of war-time conditions. *JHE* 7:541–46.

Brody, J. A., and C. J. Gibbs. 1976. Chronic neurological diseases, 519–38 in Evans.

Bronitsky, Gordon, ed. 1983. Ecological models in economic prehistory. *Ariz. St. Univ. Anth. Res. Pap.* 29.

Bronson, Bennet. 1972. Farm labor and the evolution of food production, 190–218 in Spooner.

——— . 1977. The earliest farming: Demography as cause and consequence, 23–48 in Reed.

Bronte-Stewart, B. et al. 1960. The health and nutritional status of the !Kung Bushmen of South West Africa. *S. Afr. J. Lab. Clin. Med.* 6:188–216.

Brothwell, Don R. 1963a. *Digging up bones*. London: British Museum.

——— . 1963b. Macroscopic dental pathology of some earlier human populations, 271–88 in Brothwell.

——— . 1968. *The skeletal biology of earlier human populations*. Oxford: Pergamon.

——— . 1972. Paleodemography of earlier British populations. *World Archaeology* 4: 75–87.

——— , ed., 1963. *Dental anthropology*. Oxford: Pergamon.

Brothwell, Don R., and P. Brothwell. 1969. *Food in antiquity*. New York: Praeger.

Brothwell, Don, and A. T. Sandison. 1967. *Diseases in antiquity*. Springfield, Ill.: C. C. Thomas.

Brunell, P. A. 1976a. Chickenpox, 165–73 in Top and Wehrle.

———. 1976b. Mumps, 461–66 in Top and Wehrle.

Brunt, P. A. 1971. *Italian manpower, 225 B.C.–14 A.D.* Oxford: Clarendon.

Buikstra, Jane E. 1977. Biocultural dimensions of archaeological study: A regional perspective, 67–84 in Blakely.

———. 1984. The lower Illinois river region: A prehistoric context for study of diet and health, 217–36 in Cohen and Armelagos.

———, ed. 1981. *Prehistoric tuberculosis in the Americas.* Evanston, Ill.: Northwestern University Archaeological Program.

Buikstra, Jane, and Della C. Cook. 1980. Paleopathology: An American account. *Ann. Rev. Anthrop.* 9:433–70.

———. 1981. Pre-Columbian tuberculosis in west-central Illinois: Prehistoric disease in biocultural perspective. *Northwestern Univ. Arch. Prog. Sci. Papers* 5:115–39.

Buikstra, Jane, and Lyle Konigsberg. 1985. Paleodemography: Critiques and controversies. *Amer. Anthrop.* 87:316–33.

Buikstra, Jane, and J. Mielke. 1985. Demography, diet and health, 360–423 in Gilbert and Mielke.

Buikstra, Jane, and N. Van der Merwe. 1986. Diet, demography and health: Human adaptations and maize agriculture in the Eastern Woodlands. Paper presented to the nineteenth Chacmool Conference, Calgary.

Buikstra, Jane et al. 1985. Diet sedentism and demographic change: The identification of key variables. *AJPA* 66:151.

Buikstra, Jane et al. 1986. Fertility and the development of agriculture in the prehistoric Midwest. *Amer. Antiq.* 51:528–46.

Bumstead, Pam et al. 1986. Multi-element enhancement of 13c/12c dietary interpretation: Pilot study. Paper presented to the nineteenth Chacmool Conference, Calgary.

Bunney, S. 1985. The older we were the faster we grew. *New Sci.* 1481:26.

Bunting, A. H. 1970. Food, agriculture, population and poverty, 717–22 in Bunting.

Bunting, A. H., ed. 1970. *Change in agriculture.* London: Duckworth.

Burgdorfer, Willy. 1975. Introduction to the Rickettsioses [and following essays], 382–429 in Hubbert et al.

Burkitt, Denis P. 1973. Some diseases characteristic of modern Western civilization. *Brit. Med. J.* 1:274–78.

———. 1982. Dietary fiber as a protection against disease, 483–96 in Jelliffe and Jelliffe.

Burks, John et al. 1976. Iron deficiency in an Eskimo village. *J. Pediatrics* 88:224–28.

Burnet, Sir MacFarlane, and D. White. 1972. Natural history of infectious diseases. Cambridge: Cambridge University Press.

Buskirk E. R., and J. Mendez. 1980. Energy and caloric requirements, 49–95 in Alfin-Slater and Kritchevsky.

Busvine, J. R. 1980. The evolution and mutual adaptation of insects, microorganisms, and man, 55–68 in Stanley and Joske.

Butzer, Karl. 1971. *Environment and archaeology.* 2d ed. Chicago: Aldine.

Calloway, D. H. 1982. Functional consequences of malnutrition. *RID* 4:736–45.

Campbell, K. L, and J. W. Wood. In press. Fertility in traditional societies. In *Natural human fertility: Social and biological mechanisms*, ed. P. Diggory, M. Potts, and S. Teper. London: Macmillan.

Campbell, V. 1978. Ethnohistorical evidence on the diet and economy of the aborigines of the Macleay River Valley, 82–100 in McBryde.

Carneiro, Robert. 1967. On the relationship between size of population and complexity of social organization. *SWJA* 22:234–43.

———. 1970. A theory of the origin of the state. *Science* 169:733–38.

———. 1978. Political expansion as an expression of the principle of competitive exclusion, 205–44 in Cohen and Service.

———. 1981. The chiefdom: Precursor of the state, 37–79 in Jones and Kautz.

Carneiro, Robert, and Daisy Hilse. 1966. On determining the probable rate of population growth during the Neolithic. *Amer. Anthrop.* 68:179–81.

Carr-Saunders, A. M. 1922. *The population problem.* Oxford: Clarendon.

Casley Smith, J. R. 1959a. Blood pressure, serum cholesterol and atherosclerosis in Australian aborigines. *MJA 1959* 2:695.

———. 1959b. Blood pressure in Australian aborigines. *MJA 1959* 1:627–37.

Cassell, John. 1976. The contribution of social environment to host resistance. *Am. J. Epidem.* 104:107–23.

Cassidy, Claire M. 1984. Skeletal evidence for prehistoric subsistence adaptation in the Central Ohio River Valley, 307–46 in Cohen and Armelagos.

Cavalli-Sforza, L. L. 1977. Biological research on African Pygmies, 273–84 in Harrison.

———. 1986. *African Pygmies.* New York: Academic Press.

Chafkin, S. H., and A. D. Berg. 1975. The innocent bystander: Some observations on the impact of international financial forces on nutrition. *EFN* 4:1–4.

Childe, V. G. 1950. *Man makes himself.* New York: Mentor.

———. 1964. *What happened in history.* Rev. ed. Baltimore: Penguin.

Christian, John. 1980. Endocrine factors in population regulation, 55–116 in Cohen et al.

CIBA. 1977. *Health and disease in tribal societies.* New York: Elsevier.

———. 1978. *Health and industrial growth.* Amsterdam: Elsevier.

Cilento, R. W., and A. H. Baldwin. 1930. Malaria in Australia. *Med. J. Aust.* 1:274.

Claessen, H. J. M., and P. Skalnik, eds. 1978. *The early state.* The Hague: Mouton.

Clark, C. 1970. Health, population and agricultural growth, 11–24 in Bunting.

Clark, C., and M. Haswell. 1970. *The economics of subsistence agriculture.* 4th ed. London: MacMillan.

Clark, G. A. 1981. The paleoepidemiology of Harris lines in Dickson Mounds infant and child populations and tibial growth. *AJPA* 54:209.

Cleland, J. Burton. 1928. Disease amongst Australian aborigines. *J. Trop. Med. Hyg.* 31:53–59, 65–70, 125–30, 141–45, 157–60, 173–77.

———. 1929. A short history of scurvy in Australia. *MJA* 2:867. Adelaide University Collected Papers 198.

———. 1930. Notes on pathological lesions and vital statistics of Australian natives in central Australia. *MJA* Adelaide University Collected Papers 196.

Coale, A., and P. Demeny. 1983. *Regional model life tables and stable populations.* 2d ed. New York: Academic Press.

Cockburn, Aiden, and Eve Cockburn. 1980. *Mummies, disease and ancient cultures.* Cambridge: Cambridge University Press.

Cockburn, T. A. 1967. *Infectious diseases: Their evolution and eradication.* Springfield, Ill.: C. C. Thomas.

———. 1971. Infectious diseases in ancient population. *CA* 12 (1):45–62.

Cohen, M. N. 1977. *The food crisis in prehistory.* New Haven and London: Yale University Press.

———. 1980. Speculations on the evolution of density measurement and population regulation in Homo sapiens, 275–304 in Cohen et al.

———. 1981. The ecological basis for New World state formation: General and local model building, 105–22 in Jones and Kautz.

———. 1985. Prehistoric hunter-gatherers: The meaning of social complexity, 99–122 in Price and Brown.

Cohen, M. N., and G. J. Armelagos. 1984. *Paleopathology at the origins of agriculture.* New York: Academic Press.

Cohen, M. N. et al., eds. 1980. *Biosocial mechanisms of population regulation.* New Haven and London: Yale.

Cohen, Mitchell, and R. V. Tauxe. 1986. Drug-resistant Salmonella in the United States: An epidemiological perspective. *Science* 234:964–69.

Cohen, R., and E. Service, eds. 1978. *Origins of the state.* Philadelphia: Institute for the Study of Human Issues.

Colchester, Marcus. 1984. Rethinking stone age economics: Some speculations concerning the pre-Columbia Yanoama economy. *Hum. Ecol.* 12:291–314.

———, ed. 1985. *The health and survival of the Venezuelan Yanoama.* Copenhagen: ARC/SI/IWGIA Doc 53.

Colditz, G. A. et al. 1985. Increased green and yellow vegetable intake and lowered cancer deaths in an elderly population. *AJCN* 41:32–36.

Condran, G. A., and E. Crimmins-Gardner. 1978. Public health measures and mortality in U.S. cities in the late nineteenth century. *Hum. Ecol.* 6:27–54.

Connell, K. H. 1975. *The population of Ireland.* Westport, Conn.: Greenwood.

Cook, C. E. 1966. Medicine and the Australian aboriginal: A century of contact in the Northwest Territory. *MJA* 1:559–65.

———. 1970. Notable changes in the incidence of diseases in northern territory aboriginals, 116–30 in Pilling and Waterman.

Cook, D. C. 1984. Subsistence and health in the lower Illinois Valley: Osteological evidence, 237–70 in Cohen and Armelagos.

Cook, D. C., and J. E. Buikstra. 1979. Health and differential survival in prehistoric populations: Prenatal dental defects. *AJPA* 51:649–64.

Corruccini, R. S. et al. 1982. Osteology of a slave burial population from Barbados, West Indies. *AJPA* 59:443–59.

Corruccini, R. S. et al. 1985. Distribution of enamel hypoplasia in an early Caribbean slave population. *AJPA* 667:158.

Corsini, C. A. 1984. Structural changes in infant mortality in Tuscany from the eighteenth to the nineteenth century, 127–50 in Bengtsson et al.

Cowlishaw, G. 1982. Family planning: A post-contact problem, 31–48 in Reid.

Crawford, M. H. et al. 1981. A comparison of mortality patterns of human populations residing under diverse ecological conditions. *AJPA* 54:212.

Crosby, A. W. 1972. *The Columbian exchange: Biological and cultural consequences of 1492.* Westport, Conn.: Greenwood.

Culbert, T. P. 1973. *The classic Maya collapse.* Albuquerque: University of New Mexico Press.

Cumpston, J. H. L. 1931. Public health in Australia. *MJA* 1:491–99.

Curnow, D. H. 1957. The serum protein of Abos in the Warburton range area. *MJA* 2:608–9.

Curr, E. M. 1886. *The Australian race.* Melbourne: J. Ferres.

Curtin, Philip. 1968. Epidemiology of the slave trade. *Pol. Sci. Quart.* 83:190–216.

Czarnecki, S. K., and D. Kritchevsky. 1980. Trace elements, 319–50 in Alfin-Slater and Kritchevsky.

Czarnetski, A. 1980. Pathological changes in the morphology of the young paleolithic skeletal remains from Stetten (s.w. Germany). *JHE* 9:15–17.

Dalton, H. P. et al. 1976. The documentation of communicable diseases in Peruvian mummies. *MCV Quart.* 123:43–48.

Damas, David. 1972. The copper Eskimo, 3–50 in Bicchieri.

Damon, Albert, ed. 1975. *Physiological anthropology.* New York: Oxford.

Dando, W. A. 1975. Manmade famines: Russia's past and the developing world's future. *Proceedings of the Association of American Geographers* 7:60–63.

————. 1980. *The geography of famine.* London: Arnold.

————. 1983. Biblical famines 1850 B.C. to A.D. 46. *EFN* 13:231–49.

Danforth, Marie. 1988. A comparison of Lake Classic and colonial Mayan health patterns using enamel microdefects. Ph.D. diss., Department of Anthropology, Indiana Univ., Bloomington.

Davenport, F. M. 1976. Influenza viruses, 273–96 in Evans.

Davidson, S. R. et al. 1975. *Human nutrition and dietetics.* 6th ed. Edinburgh: Churchill, Livingstone.

Davidson, W. S. 1957. Health and nutrition of Warburton range natives of central Australia. *MJA* 2:601–5.

Davis, D. H. S. et al. 1975. Plague, 147–73 in Hubbert et al.

Davis, R. E. et al. 1957. Some hematological observations on aborigines in the Warburton range area. *MJA* 2:605–10.

Day, Jose et al. 1979. Biological variety associated with change in lifestyle among the pastoral and nomadic tribes of East Africa. *AHB* 6:29–39.

Deisch, L., and H. C. Ellinghausen. 1975. Leptospiroses, 436–64 in Hubbert et al.

Delgado, H. L. 1985. Physical growth, age at menarche and age at first union in rural Guatemala. *EFN* 16:127–33.

de Luca, H. F. 1980. Vitamin D, 205–44 in Alfin-Slater and Kritchevsky.

Denbow, J. R., and E. M. Wilmsen. 1986. Advent and course of pastoralism in the Kalahari. *Science* 234:1509–15.

Denevan, William, ed. 1976. *The native population of the Americas in 1492.* Madison: University of Wisconsin Press.

Dennett, Glenn, and John Connell. 1988. Acculturation and health in the highlands of New Guinea. *CA* 29:273–99.

Derban, L. K. 1978. Some environmental health problems associated with industrial growth in Ghana, 49–71 in CIBA.

Desowitz, Robert S. 1980. Epidemiological-ecological interactions in savanna environments, 457–77 in D. Harris.

————. 1981. *New Guinea tapeworms and Jewish grandmothers.* New York: Norton.

de Vries, Jan. 1984. *European urbanization, 1500–1800.* London: Methuen.

Dewey, Kathryn, 1979. Commentary: Agricultural development, diet and nutrition. *EFN* 8:265–74.

———. 1981. Nutritional consequences of the transformation from subsistence to commercial agriculture in Tabasco, Mexico. *Hum. Ecol.* 151–87.

de Zulueta, Julian. 1956. Malaria in Sarawak and Brunei. *Bull. WHO* 15:651–71.

———. 1980. Man and malaria, 175–86 in Stanley and Joske.

Dickel, David. 1985. Growth stress and central California pre-historic subsistence shifts. *AJPA* 63:152.

Dickel, David et al. 1984. Central California: Prehistoric subsistence changes and health, 439–62 in Cohen and Armelagos.

Dickeman, Mildred. 1975. Demographic consequences of infanticide. *Ann. Rev. Ecol. Syst.* 11:107–38.

Divale, William T. 1972. Systematic population control in the Middle and Upper Paleolithic. *World Arch.* 4:22–43.

Divale, William, and M. Harris. 1978. The male supremacist complex: Discovery of a cultural invention. *Amer. Anthrop.* 80:668–71.

Dobyns, Henry C. 1976. *Native American historical demography.* Bloomington: Indiana University Press.

———. 1983. *Their numbers become thinned: Native population dynamics in eastern North America.* Knoxville: University of Tennessee Press.

Donisi, M. P. 1983. The incidence and pattern of long bone fractures in selected prehistoric human skeletal series from the central Tennessee River Valley of Alabama. *AJPA* 60:189.

Dornstreich, Mark. 1973. Food habits of early man: Balance between hunting and gathering. *Science* 179:306–7.

Dowdle, W. D. 1984. Influenza viruses. *Science* 223:1402–3.

Downs, W. G. 1976. Arboviruses, 71–102 in Evans.

Draper, H. H. 1977. The aboriginal Eskimo diet. *AA* 79:309–16.

———. 1978. Nutrition studies: The aboriginal Eskimo diet—a modern perspective. In *Eskimos of Northwestern Alaska,* ed. P. L. Jamison et al., 139–61. Stroudsberg P.A. USIBP Series 8.

Dubos, Rene. 1965. *Man adapting.* New Haven and London: Yale University Press.

———. 1968. *Man, medicine and environment.* New York: Mentor.

Duesberg, Peter. 1988. HIV is not the cause of AIDS. *Science* 241:514–17.

Dunn, F. L. 1965. On the antiquity of malaria in the western hemisphere. *Hum. Biol.* 37:385–93.

———. 1966. Patterns of parasitism in primates: Phylogenetic and ecological interpretations with particular reference to the Hominoidea. *Folia Primatologica* 4:329–45.

———. 1968. Epidemiological factors: Health and disease in hunter-gatherers, 221–28 in Lee and DeVore.

———. 1972. Intestinal parasitism in Malay aborigines (Orang Asli). *Bull. WHO* 46:99–113.

———. 1975. *Rainforest collectors and traders.* Kuala Lampur: Royal Asiatic Society of Malaysia.

Durham, William. 1976. The adaptive significance of cultural behavior. *Hum. Ecol.* 4:89–121.

————. 1982. Toward a coevolutionary theory of human biology and culture. In *Biology and the social sciences*, ed. T. C. Weigele, 77–94. Boulder: Westview.

Dutta, P. C. 1978. *The great Andamanese*. Calcutta: Anthropological Survey of India.

Dwyer, Johanna. 1982. Commercial additives, 163–94 in Jelliffe and Jelliffe.

Dwyer, Peter. 1974. The price of protein: Five hundred hours of hunting in the New Guinea Highlands. *Oceania* 44:278–93.

————. 1983. Etolo hunting performance and energetics. *Hum. Ecol.* 11:145–74.

————. 1985. The contribution of nondomestic animals to the diet of the Etolo, Southern Highlands Province, Papua New Guinea. *EFN* 17:101–15.

Dyson, Tim. 1977. The demography of the Hadza—in historical perspective, 139–54 in *African Historical Demography*, proceedings of a seminar held in the Centre of African Studies, University of Edinburgh.

Earle, Tim, and Andrew Christenson, eds. 1980. *Modeling change in prehistoric subsistence economies*. New York: Academic Press.

Early, John D. 1985. Low forager fertility: Demographic characteristic or methodological artifact. *Hum. Biol.* 57:387–99.

Eaton, S. B. 1988. Nutritional changes at the origin of agriculture. Paper presented at symposium on population growth, disease, and the origins of agriculture, Rutgers Univ., New Brunswick, N.J.

Eaton, S. B., and M. Konner. 1985. Paleolithic nutrition: A consideration of its nature and current implications. *NEJM* 312:283–89.

Eaton, S. B. et al. 1988. *The Paleolithic prescription*. New York: Harper and Row.

Eder, James F. 1978. The caloric returns to food collecting: Disruption and change among the Batek, of the Philippine tropical forests. *Hum. Ecol.* 6:55–69.

Eisenberg, L. E. 1985. Bioarchaeological perspectives on disease in a "marginal" Mississippian population. *AJPA* 66:166–67.

————. 1986. The patterning of trauma at Averbuch: Activity levels and conflict during the late Mississippian period. Paper presented to the annual meeting of the American Association of Physical Anthropologists.

Eklund, C. M., and W. J. Hadlow. 1975. Slow viral and related diseases, 1018–30 in Hubbert et al.

Ell, S. R. 1984. Immunity as a factor in the epidemiology of medieval plague. *RID* 6:866–77.

Ellinghausen, W. C., and F. W. Top. 1976. Lepstospirosis, 395–409 in Top and Wehrle.

Ellison, P. T. 1982. Skeletal growth, fatness and menarchaeal age: A comparison of two hypotheses. *Hum. Biol.* 54:269–81.

El-Najjar, M. Y. 1977. Maize, malarias and the anemias in the pre-Columbian New World. *Yrbk. Phys. Anth* 28:329–37.

————. 1979. Human treponematosis: Evidence from the New World. *AJPA* 51:599–618.

El-Najjar, M. Y. et al. 1976. The etiology of porotic hyperostosis among the prehistoric and historia Anasazi Indians of the southwestern United States. *AJPA* 44:477–87.

El-Najjar, M. Y. et al. 1978. Prevalence and possible etiology of enamel hypoplasia. *AJPA* 185–92.

Elphinstone, J. J. 1971. The health of aborigines with no previous association with Europeans. *Med. J. Aust.* 2:293–303.

Ember, Carol. 1983. The relative decline in womens' contribution to agriculture with intensification. *Amer. Anthrop.* 85:285–304.

Endicott, Karen L. 1980. *Batek Negrito sex roles: Behavior and ideology.* Lavalle: Second International Congress on Hunter-gatherers, 625–70.

Endicott, Kirk. 1979. *Batek Negrito religion.* Oxford: Clarendon.

Esche, Helga, and Richard Lee. 1975. Is maximal optimal? Paper presented to the annual meetings of the American Anthropological Association.

Evans, Alfred S., ed. 1976. *Viral infections of humans.* New York: Plenum.

Evans, I. 1937. *The Negritos of Malaya.* Cambridge: Cambridge University Press.

Eyre, E. J. 1845. *Journals of expeditions of discovery into central Australia and overland from Adelaide to King George's Sound.* London: T. and W. Boone.

Fagan, Brian. 1986. *People of the earth.* Boston: Little, Brown.

Fannin, S. L. 1982. Food infections, 261–80 in Jelliffe and Jelliffe.

FAO. 1967. Joint FAO-WHO expert committee on zoonoses. *FAO Agric. Stud.* 74.

———. 1969. *Production Yearbook,* vol. 232. Rome: United Nations.

Feldman, H. A. 1976. Toxoplasmosis, 702–8 in Top and Wehrle.

Fenner, Frank. 1970. The effects of changing social organization on the infectious diseases of man, 48–76 in Boyden.

———. 1980. Sociocultural change and environmental diseases, 7–26 in Stanley and Joske.

Ferro-Luzzi, A. et al. 1978. The nutritional status of some New Guinea children as assessed by anthropometric, biomedical and other indices. *EFN* 7:115–28.

Fiennes, Richard. 1964. *Men, nature, disease.* New York: Signet.

———. 1967. *Zoonoses of the primates.* Ithaca, N.Y.: Cornell University Press.

———. 1978. *Zoonoses and the origins and ecology of human disease.* New York: Academic Press.

Fildes, V. 1980. Neonatal feeding practices and infant mortality during the eighteenth century. *J. Biosoc. Sci.* 12:313–24.

Finkelstein, R. R. et al. 1983. The role of iron in microbe-host interactions. *RID* 5(S):759–77.

Fix, Alan G. 1975. Fission-fusion and lineal effect: Aspects of the population structure of the Samei Senoi of Malaysia. *AJPA* 43:295–302.

Flannery, K. V. 1965. The ecology of early food production in Mesopotamia. *Science* 147:1247–56.

———. 1969. Origins and ecological effects of early domestication in Iran and the Near East, 73–100 in Ucko and Dimbleby.

———. 1973. The origins of agriculture. *Ann. Rev. Anthrop.* 2:271–310.

Flinn, Michael. 1981. *The European demographic system.* Baltimore: Johns Hopkins.

Flood, Josephine. 1976. Man and ecology in the highlands of south Australia, 30–44 in Peterson.

———. 1980. *The moth hunters.* Canberra: Australian Institute for Aboriginal Studies.

Flowers, Nancy M. 1979. Child growth and nutrition in relation to subsistence in a central Brazilian Indian community. Paper presented to the American Anthropological Association, Cincinnati, Ohio.

———. 1983. Seasonal factors in subsistence, nutrition and child growth in a central Brazilian Indian community, 357–90 in Hames and Vickers.

Fogel, R. W. 1984. Nutrition and the decline in mortality since 1700: Some preliminary findings. Working Paper 1402. Cambridge, Mass.: National Bureau of Economic Research.

Fogel, R. W. et al. 1983. Secular changes in American and British stature and nutrition, 247–83 in Rotberg and Rabb.

Foley, Robert. 1982. A reconsideration of the role of predation on large mammals in tropical hunter-gatherer adaptation. *Man* (N.S.) 17:393–402.

Ford, E. 1942. Medical conditions on Bathurst and Melville Islands. *MJA* 2:235–40.

Fornaciari, Gino et al. 1981. Cribra orbitalia and elemental bone iron in the Punics of Carthage. *OSSA* 8:63–78.

Foulkes, Edward, and S. H. Katz. 1975. Biobehavioral adaptations in the Arctic, 183–93 in Watts, Johnston, and Lasker.

Fox, R. G. 1969. Professional primitives: Hunter-gatherers of nuclear South Asia. *Man in India.* 49:139–60.

Frankel, J. K. et al. 1970. Toxoplasma gondii in cats: Fecal stages as coccidian oocysts. *Science* 167:893–96.

Fraser, Antonia. 1984. *The weaker vessel.* New York: Knopf.

Frayer, David. 1980. Sexual dimorphism and cultural evolution in the late Pleistocene and Holocene of Europe. *J. Hum. Evol.* 9:399–415.

——. 1981. Body size, weapon use and natural selection in the European Upper Paleolithic and Mesolithic. *AA* 83:57–73.

Fridlizius, Gunnar. 1984. The mortality decline in the first phase of the demographic transition: Swedish experiences, 77–114 in Bengtsson et al.

Fried, M. 1967. *The evolution of political society.* New York: Random House.

Friedl, John. 1981. Lactase deficiency: Distribution, associated problems and implications for nutritional policy. *EFN* 11:37–48.

Frisancho, A. R., and V. R. Leonard. 1985. The influence of dietary sodium and potassium on blood pressure of American blacks and whites. *AJPA* 66:170.

Frisch, Rose E. 1978. Population, food intake and fertility. *Science* 199:22–30.

Frisch, Rose E., and Janet W. McArthur. 1974. Menstrual cycles: Fatness as a determinant of minimum weight for height necessary for their maintenance and onset. *Science* 185:949–51.

Frisch, Rose E. et al. 1980. Delayed menarche and amenorrhea in ballet dancers. *NEJM* 303:17–19.

Furer-Haimendorf, C. von. 1943. *The Chenchus.* London: Macmillan.

Gaisie, S. K. 1969. Estimating vital rates for Ghana. *Pop. Stud.* 23:21–42.

Gajdusek, D. C. 1977. Urgent opportunistic observations: The study of changing transient and disappearing phenomena of medical interest in disrupted primitive communities, 69–71 in CIBA.

Gajdusek, D. C., and R. M. Garruto. 1975. The focus of hyperendemic goiter, cretinism and associated deaf mutism in western New Guinea, 267–86 in Watts, Johnston, and Lasker.

Gall, Patricia, and Arthur Saxe. 1977. The ecological evolution of culture: The state as predator in succession theory. In *Exchange systems in prehistory*, ed. T. Earle and J. Erickson, 255–68. New York: Academic Press.

Gangarosa, E. J. 1976. Food poisoning, bacterial, 287–98 in Top and Wehrle.

Gardner, P. M. 1972. The Paliyans, 404–47 in Bicchieri.

Garn, S. M. 1985. On undernutrition among the unacculturated. *CA* 26:665.

Garn, S. M. et al. 1979. The effects of prenatal factors on crown dimensions. *AJPA* 51:665–78.

Gaulin, S., and M. Konner. 1977. On the natural diet of primates including humans. In *Nutrition and the brain*, Vol. 1, ed. R. J. Wurtman and J. J. Wurtman. New York: Raven.

Geertz, Clifford. 1963. *Agricultural involution*. Berkeley: University of California Press.

Geist, Valerius. 1978. *Life strategies, human evolution, environmental design*. New York: Springer-Verlag.

Gejvall, N-G. 1960. *Westerhus: Medieval population and church in the light of skeletal remains*. Lund: Hakan Ohlssons Boktryckeri.

Ghesquiere, J. L., and M. J. Karvonen. 1981. Some anthropometric and functional dimensions of the Pygmy (Kivu Twa). *AHB* 8:119–34.

Giblett, E. R. 1977. Genetic polymorphisms in human blood. *Ann. Rev. Genet.* 11: 13–28.

Gilbert, R. I. 1975. Trace element analysis of three skeletal Amerindian populations at Dickson Mounds. Ph.D. diss., University of Massachusetts.

———. 1985. Stress, paleonutrition and trace elements, 339–59 in Gilbert and Mielke.

Gilbert, R. I., and J. H. Mielke. 1985. *The analysis of prehistoric diets*. New York: Academic Press.

Gillen, F. D., D. S. Reiner, and C. S. Wang. 1983. Human milk kills parasitic intestinal protozoa. *Science* 221:1290–92.

Godber, M. et al. 1976. The blood groups, serum groups, red cell enzymes and haemoglobins of the Sandawe and Nyaturu of Tanzania. *AHB* 3:463–73.

Goldstein, M. S. 1953. Some vital statistics based on skeletal material. *Hum. Biol.* 25:3–12.

Goldstein, M. S. 1969. Human paleopathology and some diseases in living primitive societies: A review of the recent literature. *AJPA* 31:285–94.

Gomes, Albert. 1978. *Demographic and environmental adaptation: A comparative study of two aboriginal populations in west Malaysia*. Kuala Lampur: Seaprap Research Report 35.

Goodale, Jane C. 1970. An example of ritual change among the Tiwi of Melville Island, 350–66 in Pilling and Waterman.

Goodman, A. et al. 1975. The role of infectious and nutritional diseases in population growth. Paper presented to the annual meeting of the American Anthropological Association, San Francisco.

Goodman, A. et al. 1980. Enamel hypoplasias as indicators of stress in three prehistoric populations from Illinois. *Hum. Biol.* 52:515–28.

Goodman, A. et al. 1984a. Health changes at Dickson Mounds, Illinois (A.D. 950–1300), 271–306 in Cohen and Armelagos.

———. 1984b. Indications of stress from bone and teeth, 13–50 in Cohen and Armelagos.

Goodman, M. et al. 1985. Menarche, pregnancy, birth spacing and menopause among Agta women foragers of Cagayan Province, Luzon, the Philippines. *AHB* 12:169–78.

Gopaldas, T. 1983. The impact of Sanskritization in a forest dwelling tribe of Gujarat, India. *EFN* 12:217–27.

Goubert, P. 1968. Legitimate fecundity and infant mortality in France during the eighteenth century: A comparison. *Daedalus* 47:2:593–603.

———. 1984. Public hygiene and mortality decline in France in the nineteenth century, 151–60 in Bengtsson et al.

———. 1967. Notes on hunting, butchering and sharing of game among Ngatatjara and their neighbors in the West Australian desert. *Kroeber Anthrop. Society Reports* 36:41–63.

———. 1969a. Subsistence behavior among the western desert aborigines of Australia. *Oceania* 39:253–74.

———. 1969b. Yiwara: *Foragers of the Australian desert.* New York: Charles Scribner's Sons.

———. 1981. Comparative ecology of food sharing in Australia and northwest California, 422–54 in Harding and Teleki.

Gracey, Michael. 1980. Malnutrition, 415–34 in Stanley and Joske.

Graham, Susan. 1985. Running and menstrual disturbance: Recent discoveries provide new insights into the division of labor by sex. *AA* 87:878–82.

Grauer, A. L. 1984. Health and disease in an Anglo-Saxon cemetery population from Raunds, Northamptonshire, England. *AJPA* 63:166.

———. 1987. The demography of Jewbury and St. Helen-on-the-Walls Cemeteries, York, England. *AJPA* 72:204–5.

Greenhouse, R. 1981. Preparation effects on iron and calcium in traditional Pima foods. *EFN* 10:221–25.

Gregg, David. 1982. *The dynamics of agricultural growth.* London: Hutchinson.

Grey, Sir George. 1841. *Journals of two expeditions of discovery in Northwest and western Australia during the years 1837, 1838, and 1839.* London: Boone.

Griffin, P. Bion. 1984. Forager resource and land use in the humid tropics: The Agta of Northeastern Luzon, the Philippines, 99–122 in Schrire.

Grigg, David B. 1982. *The dynamics of agricultural growth.* London: Hutchinson.

Gross, B. A., and C. J. Eastman. 1985. Prolactin and the return of ovulation in breast-feeding women. *J. Biosoc. Sci. Supp.* 9:25–42.

Gross, Daniel et al. 1979. Ecology and acculturation among native peoples of central Brazil. *Science* 206:1043–49.

Grove, David. 1980. Schistosomiasis, snails and man, 187–204 in Stanley and Joske.

Gugliardo, Mark. 1982. Tooth crown size differences between age groups as a possible new indicator of stress in skeletal samples. *AJPA* 58:388–89.

Gust, Ian. 1980. Acute viral hepatitis, 85–114 in Stanley and Joske.

Habicht, J-P. et al. 1985. The contraceptive role of breast feeding. *Pop. Stud.* 39: 213–32.

Hackett, C. J. 1936. A critical survey of some references to syphilis and yaws among Australian aborigines. *MJA* 1:733–45.

———. 1963. On the origin of the human treponematoses. *Bull. WHO* 29:7–41.

Hahn, C. H. L., H. Vedder, and L. Fourie. 1966. *The native tribes of southwest Africa.* New York: Barnes and Noble.

Haldane, J. B. S. 1932. *The inequality of man.* London: Chatto and Windus.

Hambraeus, Leif. 1982. Naturally occurring toxicants in food, 13–36 in Jelliffe and Jelliffe.

Hames, R. B. 1979. A comparison of the efficiency of the shotgun and the bow in neotropical forest hunting. *Hum. Ecol.* 7:219–52.

———. 1980. Game depletion and hunting zone rotation among the Ye'kwana and Yanomamo of Amazonas, Venezuela. *WPSAI* 2:31–60.

Hames, R. B., and W. T. Vickers. 1982. Optimal diet breadth theory as a model to explain variability in Amazonian hunting. *Amer. Ethnol.* 90:358–78.

———, eds. 1983. *The adaptive responses of native Amazonians.* New York: Academic Press.

Hancock, Beverly. 1985. Food preparation and consumption practices among southeast United States aboriginals as a possible contribution to porotic hyperostosis. *AJPA* 66:178.

Handwerker, W. P. 1983. The first demographic transition: Analysis of subsistence changes and reproductive consequences. *AA* 85:5–27.

Hansen, Elizabeth. 1979. Overlaying in nineteenth century England: Infant mortality or infanticide. *Hum. Ecol.* 7:333–52.

Harakao, Reizo. 1981. The cultural ecology of hunting behavior among Mbuti pygmies in the Ituri Forest, Zaire, 499–555 in Harding and Teleki.

Hardesty, Donald L. 1978. Human evolutionary ecology. In *Human Evolution*, ed. N. Korn, 234–44. New York: Holt, Rinehart and Winston.

Harding, R. S. O., and G. Teleki. 1981. *Omnivorous primates.* New York: Columbia University Press.

Hare, Ronald. 1967. The antiquity of diseases caused by bacteria and viruses: A review of the problem from a bacteriologist's point of view, 115–31 in Brothwell and Sandison.

Harlan, Jack. 1967. A wild wheat harvest in Turkey. *Archaeol.* 20:197–201.

———. 1971. Agricultural origins: Centers and noncenters. *Science* 174:468–74.

———. 1977. The origins of cereal agriculture in the Old World, 357–384 in Reed.

Harner, Michael. 1970. Population pressure and the social evolution of agriculturalists. *SWJA* 26:67–86.

Harpending, H. C. 1976. Regional variation in !Kung populations, 152–65 in Lee and DeVore.

Harpending, H. C., and L. Wandsnider. 1982. Population structures of Ghanzi and Ngamiland !Kung. In *Current developments in anthropological genetics*, Vol. 2, ed. M. H. Crawford and J. H. Mielke, 29–50. New York: Plenum.

Harrell, Barbara. 1981. Lactation and menstruation in cultural perspective. *AA* 83:796–823.

Harris, David. 1977. Subsistence strategies across the Torres Strait, 421–63 in Allen et al.

———. 1982. Resource distribution and foraging effort in hunter-gatherer subsistence, 189–208 in Harrison.

———, ed. 1980. *Human ecology in savanna environments.* New York: Academic Press.

Harris, Marvin. 1974. *Cows, pigs, wars and witches.* New York: Random House.

———. 1978. *Cannibals and kings.* New York: Random House.

———. 1980. *Culture, people, nature.* 3d ed. New York: Harper and Row.

———. 1984. Animal capture and Yanomamo warfare: retrospective and new evidence. *JAR* 40:183–201.

———. 1985. *Culture, people, nature.* 4th ed. New York: Harper and Row.

————. 1988. *Culture, people, nature*. 5th ed. New York: Harper and Row.

Harrison, G. 1975. Primary lactase deficiency: A problem in anthropological genetics. *AA* 77:812–35.

————. 1977. *Population structures and human variation*. Cambridge: Cambridge University Press.

————. 1982. *Energy and effort*. London: Taylor and Francis.

Harrison, G. A., and A. J. Boyce. 1972. *The structure of human populations*. Oxford: Clarendon.

Hart, John. 1978. From subsistence to market: A case study of the Mbuti net hunters. *Hum. Ecol.* 6:325–54.

Hart, C. W. M., and A. R. Pilling. 1964. *The Tiwi of northern Australia*. New York: Holt, Rinehart and Winston.

Hartney, P. C. 1981. Tuberculosis in a prehistoric population sample from southern Ontario, 141–60 in Buikstra.

Hartwig, G. W., and K. D. Patterson. 1978. *Disease in African history*. Durham, North Carolina: Duke University Press.

Harvey, P. W., and P. F. Heywood. 1983. Twenty-five years of dietary change in Simbu province, Papua, New Guinea. *EFN* 13:27–35.

Hassan, F. 1981. *Demographic archaeology*. New York: Academic Press.

Hassan, N. et al. 1985. Seasonal patterns of food intake in rural Bangladesh: Its impact on nutritional status. *EFN* 17:175–86.

Hassan, N., and K. Ahmad. 1984. Studies in food and nutrient intake by rural populations of Bangladesh and comparison between intakes of 1962–64, 1975–76, and 1981–82. *EFN* 15:143–58.

Hattwick, M. A. W. 1976. Rabies, 555–66 in Top and Wehrle.

Hausman, A. J., and E. N. Wilmsen. 1984. Impact of seasonality of foods on growth and fertility. *AJPA* 63:169.

Haviland, William. 1967. Stature at Tikal. *Amer. Antiq.* 35:316–25.

Hawkes, Kristen, and J. F. O'Connell. 1985. Optimal foraging models and the case of the Kung. *AA* 87:401–5.

Hawkes, Kristen et al. 1982. Why hunters forage: The Ache of eastern Paraguay. *Am. Ethnol.* 9:379–98.

Hayden, Brian. 1981a. Research and development in the Stone Age. *Cur. Anthrop.* 22:519–48.

————. 1981b. Subsistence and ecological adaptation of modern hunter-gatherers, 344–422 in Harding and Teleki.

Heinz, H. J. 1961. Factors governing the survival of Bushman worm parasites in the Kalahari. *S. Afr. J. Sci.* 8:207–13.

Heiser, Charles. 1973. *Seed to civilization*. San Francisco: Freeman.

Heithersay, G. 1959. A dental survey of the aborigines of Haasts Bluff, Central Australia. *MJA* 1:721–29.

Helbaek, H. 1969. Plant collecting, dry farming and irrigation agriculture in prehistoric Deh Luran. In *Prehistory and human ecology of the Deh Luran Plain*, ed. F. Hole et al., 383–428. Ann Arbor: Memoir, Museum of Anthropology, University of Michigan.

Heller, C. A. 1964. The diet of some Alaskan Eskimos and Indians. *J. Amer. Diet. Assoc.* 45:425–28.

Herald Tribune. 1985. Genocide in Afghanistan. Editorial, October 12.

Hetzel, B. S., and H. J. Frith. 1978. The nutrition of aborigines in relation to the ecosystem of central Australia. Melbourne: Commonwealth Scientific and Industrial Research Organization.

Hiatt, Betty. 1967–68. The food quest and the economy of the Tasmanian aborigines. *Oceania* 38:99–133, 190–219.

Hiernaux, J. 1974. *The people of Africa.* London: Weidenfeld.

Hiernaux, J., and D. Boedhi Hartono. 1980. Physical measurements of the adult Hadza of Tanzania. *AHB* 7:339–46.

Hiernaux, J., and A. Schweich. 1979. Variation of blood pressure and heart rate in and between ethnic groups of Rwanda, Burundi, and Zaire. *JHE* 8:767–77.

Higginson, John. 1980. Cancer and the environment, 447–66 in Stanley and Joske.

Higgs, Robert, and D. Booth. 1979. Mortality differentials within large American cities in 1890. *Hum. Ecol.* 7:353–83.

Hildes, J., and O. Schaefer. 1973. Health of Igloolik Eskimos and changes with urbanization. *JHE* 2:241–46.

Hill, K. 1982. Hunting and human evolution. *JHE* 11:521–44.

Hill, K., and K. Hawkes. 1983. Neotropical hunting among the Ache of eastern Paraguay, 139–188 in Hames and Vickers.

Hill, K., and H. Kaplan. 1988. Tradeoffs in male and female reproductive strategy among the Ache. In *Human reproductive behavior*, ed. L. Betzig et al. Cambridge: Cambridge University Press.

Hill, K. et al. 1984. Seasonal variance in the diet of Ache hunter-gatherers in eastern Paraguay. *Hum. Ecol.* 12:101–37.

Hillson, S. W. 1981. Human biological variation in the early Nile valley in relation to environmental factors. Ph.D. diss., University of London.

Hitchcock, Robert K. 1982. Patterns of sedentism among the Besarwa of eastern Botswana, 223–68 in Leacock and Lee.

Ho, P. T. 1955. The introduction of American food plants into China. *Amer. Anthrop.* 57:191–201.

Hobbes, Thomas. 1950 [1651]. *Leviathan.* New York: Dutton.

Hodges, Denise. 1986. Chronological distribution of childhood stress episodes in pre-Classic and Classic period samples from the valley of Oaxaco, Mexico. *AJPA* 69:215.

———. 1987. Health and agricultural intensification in the prehistoric valley of Oaxaca, Mexico. *AJPA* 73:323–32.

Hodges, R. 1980. Vitamin C, 73–96 in Alfin-Slater and Kritchevsky.

Hodgkinson, Clement. 1845. *Australia from Port Macquarie to Moreton Bay, with description of the natives.* London: Boone.

Hoffer, Peter C., and N. E. Hill. 1981. *Murdering mothers: Infanticide in England and New England, 1558–1803.* New York: New York University Press.

Holmberg, Alan. 1969. *Nomads of the long bow.* Garden City, N.Y.: American Museum.

Horne, G., and G. Aiston. 1924. *Savage life in central Australia.* London: Macmillan.

House, J. S. et al. 1988. Social relationships and health. *Science* 241:540–45.

Howell, Nancy. 1976. Toward a uniformitarian theory of human paleodemography. *J. Hum. Evol.* 5:25–40.

———. 1979. *Demography of the Dobe !Kung.* New York: Academic Press.

———. 1982. Village composition implied by a paleodemographic life table: The Libben site, Ohio. *AJPA* 59:263–70.

———. 1986. Feedback and buffers in relation to scarcity and abundance: Studies of hunter-gatherer populations. In *State of population theory*, ed. Coleman and Schofield. London: Blackwell.

Hubbert, William T. et al., eds. 1975. Diseases transmitted from animals to man. 6th ed. Springfield, Mass.: C. C. Thomas.

Hudson, E. H. 1965. Treponematosis and man's social evolution. *AA* 67:885–901.

Hufton, O. 1983. Social conflict and the grain supply in eighteenth-century France, 105–31 in Rotberg and Rabb.

Hughes, R. E., and E. Jones. 1985. Intake of dietary fibre and age of menarche. *AHB* 12:325–32.

Hugh-Jones, P. et al. 1977. Medical studies among the Indians of the Upper Xingu. *Brit. J. Hosp. Med.* 7:317–34.

Hummert, J. R., and D. P. Van Gerven. 1983. Skeletal growth in a medieval population from Sudanese Nubia. *AJPA* 60:471–78.

———. 1985. Observations on the formation and persistence of radio-opaque transverse lines. *AJPA* 66:297–306.

Hurtado, A., and K. Hill. 1987. Early dry season subsistence ecology of the Cuiva (Hiwi) foragers of Venezuela. *Hum. Ecol.* 15:163–87.

Hussain, M. A., and K. Ahmad. 1977. Protein problems in Bangladesh. *EFN* 6: 31–38.

Huss-Ashmore, R. 1984. Seasonal cycles of nutrition and resource procurement in Lesotho. *AJPA* 68:177.

Huss-Ashmore, Rebecca, A. H. Goodman, and G. J. Armelagos. 1982. Nutritional inference from paleopathology. *Adv. Arch. Meth. Theor.* 5:395–474.

Hutchinson, D. L. 1987. Stress and lifeway change on the Georgia coast: The evidence from enamel hypoplasia. *AJPA* 72:214.

Ichikawa, M. 1981. Ecological and sociological importance of honey to the Mbuti net hunters, Eastern Zaire. *KUASM* 1:55–68.

———. 1983. An examination of the hunting-dependent life of the Mbuti Pygmies of eastern Zaire. *KUASM* 4:55–76.

Imhoff, A. E. 1984. The amazing simultaneousness of the big differences and the boom in the nineteenth century, 191–222 in Bengtsson et al.

Ingold, Tim. 1983. The significance of storage in hunting societies. *Man* 18:553–71.

Irvine, F. R. 1957–58. Wild and emergency foods of Australian and Tasmanian aborigines. *Oceania* 28:113–42.

———. 1970. Evidence of change in the vegetable diet of Australian aborigines, 278–84 in Pilling and Waterman.

Isaac, E. 1970. *The geography of domestication*. Englewood Cliffs, N.J.: Prentice-Hall.

Isaac, Glyn. 1972. Early phases of human behavior: Models in lower Paleolithic archaeology. In *Models in archaeology*, ed. D. Clarke, 167–99. London: Methuen.

Jackes, M. 1983. Osteological evidence for smallpox: A possible case from seventeenth century Ontario. *AJPA* 60:75–81.

Jackson, L. L., and R. T. Jackson. 1984. Health implications of chronic dietary cyanide ingestion. *AJPA* 63:174.

Jacobs, Wilbur R. 1978. The fatal confrontation: Early native-white relations on the frontiers of Australia, New Guinea and America (a comparative study). *Pacific Hist. Rev.* 47:283–309.

Jacobsen, Thorkild, and R. M. Adams. 1958. Salt and silt in ancient Mesopotamian agriculture. *Science* 128:1251–58.

Jaiswal, H. K. 1979. *Demographic structure of tribal society.* New Delhi: Meenakshi Prakashan.

Janowitz, B. et al. 1981. Breast feeding and child survival in Egypt. *J. Biosoc. Sci.* 13: 287–97.

Janssens, Paul A. 1970. *Paleopathology.* London: John Baker.

Jarcho, Saul. 1964. Some observations on diseases in prehistoric America. *Bull. Hist. Med.* 38:1–19.

——. 1966. *Human paleopathology.* New Haven and London: Yale University Press.

Jaya Rao, K. S. 1983. Pellagra in sorghum eating: A mycotoxicosis? *EFN* 13:59–64.

Jelliffe, D. B., and E. F. Patrice Jelliffe. 1982. Major food-borne parasitic infections, 281–88 in Jelliffe and Jelliffe.

Jelliffe, E. F., and D. B. Jelliffe, eds. 1982. *Adverse effects of foods.* New York: Plenum.

Jelliffe, D. B. et al. 1962. The children of the Hadza hunters. *Trop. Paed.* 60:907–13.

Jenkins, Trefor et al. 1975. Sero Genetic Studies on the G/wi and G//ana San of Botswana. *Hum. Hered.* 25:318–28.

Johansson, S. R., and S. Horwitz. 1986. Estimating mortality in skeletal populations: Influence of the growth rate on the interpretation of levels and trends during the transition to agriculture. *AJPA* 71:233–50.

Johnson, Allen. 1982. Reductionism in cultural ecology: The Amazon case. *CA* 23: 413–28.

——. 1983. Machiguenga gardens, 29–64 in Hames and Vickers.

Johnson, Allen, and T. Earle. 1987. *The evolution of human societies.* Stanford: Stanford University Press.

Johnson, K. M. 1975. Yellow fever, 929–38 in Hubbert et al.

Johnson, K. M., and P. A. Webb. 1975. Rodent transmitted hemorrhagic fevers, 911–16 in Hubbert et al.

Johnston, F. E., and C. E. Snow. 1961. The reassessment of the age and sex of the Indian Knoll skeletal population: Demographic and methodological aspects. *AJPA* 19:237–44.

Jones, F. L. 1963. *A demographic survey of the aboriginal populations of the Northern Territory with special reference to Bathurst Island Mission.* Canberra: AIAS.

Jones, Grant, and Robert Kautz. 1981. *The transition to statehood in the New World.* Cambridge: Cambridge University Press.

Jones, Rhys. 1971. The demography of hunters and farmers in Tasmania, 271–87 in Mulvaney and Golson.

——. 1980. Hunters in the Australian coastal savanna, 107–47 in D. Harris.

Joraleman, Donald. 1982. New world depopulation and the case of disease. *JAR* 38: 108–28.

Joske, E. A. 1980. The physician and human disease and death, 551–66 in Stanley and Joske.

Jukes, T. H., and J. L. King. 1975. Evolutionary loss of ascorbic acid synthesizing ability. *J. Hum. Evol.* 4:85–88.

Jurmain, Robert D. 1977. Stress and the etiology of osteoarthritis. *AJPA* 46:353–365.

———. 1980. The pattern of involvement of appendicular degenerative joint disease. *AJPA* 53:143–50.

Kamien, Max. 1980. The aboriginal Australian experience, 253–70 in Stanley and Joske.

Katz, Darryl, and J. M. Suchey. 1986. Age determination of the male os pubis. *AJPA* 69:427–36.

Katz, S. H. 1986. Fava bean consumption: A case for the coevolution of genes and culture. Paper presented to the Chacmool Conference, Calgary.

Katz, S. H. et al. 1974. Traditional maize processing techniques in the New World. *Science* 184:765–73.

Katz, S. H. et al. 1975. The anthropological and nutritional significance of maize processing techniques in the New World, 195–232 in Watts, Johnston, and Lasker.

Keene, A. 1981. Optimal foraging in a nonmarginal environment: A model of prehistoric subsistence strategy in Michigan, 171–93 in Winterhalder and Smith.

Keith, M. S., and G. J. Armelagos. 1983. Naturally occurring dietary antibiotics and human health. In *The anthropology of medicine,* ed. L. Romanucci Ross et al., 221–30. New York: Praeger.

Kelley, J. O., and J. L. Angel. 1985. Stresses of slavery. Paper presented to the American Association of Physical Anthropologists, Knoxville, Tenn.

Kelley, Marc, and Marc Micozzi. 1984. Rib lesions in chronic pulmonary tuberculosis. *AJPA* 65:381–86.

Kelley, Marc, and M. R. Zimmerman. 1982. *Atlas of human paleopathology.* New York: Praeger.

Kennedy, K. A. R. 1982. Recently discovered late Pleistocene hominid remains from India: Morphological evolution and technological change. *AJPA* 57:201–2.

———. 1984. Growth nutrition and pathology in changing paleodemographic settings in South Asia, 169–92 in Cohen and Armelagos.

Kies, Constance, and H. M. Fox. 1972. Interrelationships of leucine with lysine, tryptophan and niacin as they influence protein value of cereal grains for humans. *Cereal Chemistry* 49:223–31.

King, J. et al. 1985. Household consumption profile of cowpea (Vigna unguiculata) among low income farmers in Nigeria. *EFN* 16:209–21.

Kirk, R. L. 1966. Population genetic studies in Australia and New Guinea, 395–430 in Baker and Weiner.

———. 1971. Genetic evidence and its implications for aboriginal prehistory, 326–43 in Mulvaney and Golson.

———. 1981. *Aboriginal man adapting.* Oxford: Clarendon.

———, ed. 1973. *The human biology of aborigines in Cape York.* Canberra: Australian National University.

Kirk, R. L., and A. G. Thorne. 1977. The biology of aboriginal man in Australia. *J. Hum. Evol.* 6:i–ii.

Kleeburg, H. H. 1975. Tuberculosis and other mycobacterioses, 303–60 in Hubbert et al.

Klepinger, Linda L. 1979. Paleopathologic evidence for the evolution of rheumatoid arthritis. *AJPA* 50:119–22.

————. 1980. The evolution of human disease: New findings and problems. *J. Biosoc. Sci.* 12:481–86.

————. 1982. Tuberculosis in the New World: More probabilities, possibilities and predictions. *AJPA* 57:202.

Knodel, John. 1977. Breast feeding and population growth. *Science* 198:1111–15.

Knowler, W. C. et al. 1983. Diabetes mellitus in the Pima Indians: Genetic and evolutionary considerations. *AJPA* 62:107–14.

Kobayashi, K. 1967. Trend in the length of life based on human skeletons from prehistoric to modern times in Japan. *Univ. Tokyo J. Fac. Sci.* 3:2.

Koerner, B. D., and R. L. Blakely. 1985. DJD, subsistence and sex roles in the protohistoric King Site in Georgia. *AJPA* 66:190.

Koike, H., and N. Ohtaishi. 1985. Prehistoric hunting pressure estimated by the age composition of excavated sika deer (Cervus Nippon) using the annual layer of tooth cement. *J. Arch. Sci.* 12:443–56.

Kolata, Gina Bari. 1974. !Kung hunter-gatherers: Feminism, diet, and birth control. *Science* 185:932–34.

————. 1984a. Does a lack of calcium cause hypertension? *Science* 225:705–6.

————. 1984b. Lowered cholesterol decreases heart disease. *Science* 223:381–82.

————. 1985. A disease in many guises. *Science* 230:1019.

————. 1987a. Diabetics should lose weight and avoid fad diets. *Science* 235:163–64.

————. 1987b. Dietary fat–breast cancer link questioned. *Science* 235:436.

Konner, Melvin, and Carol Worthman. 1980. Nursing frequency, gonad function and birth spacing among !Kung hunter-gatherers. *Science* 207:788–91.

Koyama, S., and D. H. Thomas, eds. 1981. *Affluent foragers.* Kyoto: Senri Ethnol. Series 9.

Kretchmer, Norman. 1972. Lactose and lactase. *Sci. Amer.* 227:70–78.

Kritchevsky D., and S. K. Czarnecki. 1980. Nutrients with special functions: Cholesterol, 239–58 in Alfin-Slater and Kritchevsky.

Kroeger, A., and F. Barbira-Freedman. 1982. *Culture change and health: The case of the Southamerican rainforest Indians.* Frankfurt: Verlag Peter Lang.

Krogman, Wilton. 1962. *The human skeleton in forensic medicine.* Springfield, Mass.: C. C. Thomas.

Kromhout, D. et al. 1985. Potassium, calcium, alcohol, and blood pressure, the Zutphen Study. *AJCN* 41:1299–304.

Krzywicki, Ludwig. 1934. *Primitive society and its vital statistics.* London: Macmillan.

Kuhnlein, H. V. 1980. The trace element content of indigenous salts compared with commercially refined substitutes. *EFN* 10:113–21.

Kunitz, S. J. 1984. Mortality change in America, 1620–1920. *HB* 56:559–82.

Kuntz, Robert E. 1982. Significant infections in primate parasitology. *JHE* 11:185–94.

Kuper, Hilda. 1947. *The uniform of color.* Johannesburg: Witwatersrand University Press.

Kurtz, T. W., and R. C. Morris, Jr. 1983. Dietary chloride as a determinant of "sodium-dependent" hypertension. *Science* 222:1139–41.

Ladny, I. D. 1980. Health care in the USSR, 345–70 in Stanley and Joske.

Lafitte, Francois. 1978. Recent and possible future trends in abortion. *J. Med. Ethics* 1:25–29.

Lager, C., and P. T. Ellison. 1987. Effects of moderate weight loss on ovulatory frequency and luteal function in adult women. *AJPA* 72:221–22.

Lallo, John W. et al. 1977. The role of diet, disease and physiology in the origin of porotic hyperostosis. *Hum. Biol.* 49:471–83.

Lallo, John, G. J. Armelagos, and J. C. Rose. 1978. Paleoepidemiology of infectious disease in the Dickson Mounds populations. *MCV Quart.* 14:17–23.

Lambert, Joseph et al. 1984. Copper and barium as dietary discriminants: The effects of diagenesis. *Archaeometry* 26:131–38.

Lambert, S. M. 1921. Intestinal parasites in N. Queensland. *MJA* 1:332–35.

Lambrecht, F. L. 1964. Aspects of evolution and ecology of tsetse flies and trypanosomiasis in prehistoric African environments. *J. Afr. Hist.* 5:1–22.

———. 1967. Trypanosomiasis in prehistoric and later human populations: A tentative reconstruction, 132–51 in Brothwell and Sandison.

Lampl, Michelle, and Baruch S. Blumberg. 1979. Blood polymorphism and the origins of New World populations. In *The first Americans*, ed. W. S. Laughlin and A. B. Harper, 107–23. New York: Gustav Fischer.

Larsen, Clark. 1983. Deciduous tooth size and subsistence change in prehistoric Georgia coast populations. *CA* 24:225–26.

———. 1984. Health and disease in prehistoric Georgia: The transition to agriculture, 367–92 in Cohen and Armelagos.

———. 1987. Bioarchaeological interpretations of subsistence economy and behavior from human skeletal remains. *Adv. Arch. Meth. Theor.* 10:339–445.

Laslett, Peter. 1965. *The world we have lost*. New York: Charles Scribner's Sons.

———. 1977. *Family life and illicit love in earlier generations*. Cambridge: Cambridge University Press.

———. 1984. *The world we have lost further explored*. New York: Charles Scribner's Sons.

———, ed. 1972. *Household and family in past time*. Cambridge: Cambridge University Press.

Laughlin, William S. 1968. The demography of hunters: An Eskimo example, 241–43 in Lee and DeVore.

Laughlin, William S., and A. B. Harper. 1979. *The first Americans: Origins, affinities, adaptations*. New York: Gustav Fischer.

Laughlin, William S. et al. 1979. New approaches to the pre- and post-contact history of arctic peoples. *AJPA* 51:579–87.

Laver, W. G., ed. 1983. *The origin of pandemic influenza viruses*. New York: Elsevier.

Lawrence, Roger. 1969. *Aboriginal habitat and economy*. Canberra: Australian National University.

Leacock, Eleanor, and R. B. Lee, eds. 1982. *Politics and history in band societies*. Cambridge: Cambridge University Press.

Learmonth, Andrew. 1988. *Disease ecology*. New York: Basil Blackwell.

Ledger, W. J. 1976. Anaerobic infections, 125–36 in Top and Wehrle.

Lee, R. B. 1968. What hunters do for a living or how to make out on scarce resources, 30–48 in Lee and DeVore.

———. 1969. !Kung Bushman subsistence: An input-output analysis. In *Ecological studies in cultural anthropology*, ed. A. P. Vayda, 47–79. New York: Natural History Press.

———. 1972a. The intensification of social life among the !Kung Bushmen, 343–50 in Spooner.

———. 1972b. Population growth and the beginning of sedentary life among the !Kung bushmen, 329–42 in Spooner.

———. 1973. Mongongo: The ethnography of a major wild food source. *Ecol. Food. Nutr.* 2:307–21.

———. 1976. !Kung spatial organization, 73–97 in Lee and DeVore.

———. 1979. *The !Kung San.* London: Cambridge University Press.

———. 1980. Lactation, ovulation, infanticide and women's work: A study of hunter-gatherer population regulation, 321–48 in Cohen et al.

Lee, R. B., and I. DeVore, eds. 1968. *Man the hunter.* Chicago: Aldine.

———. 1976. *Kalahari hunter-gatherers.* Cambridge: Harvard University Press.

Lee, R. D. 1977. *Population patterns in the past.* New York: Academic Press.

Lee, W. R. 1984. Mortality levels and agrarian reform in early nineteenth century Prussia: Some regional evidence, 161–90 in Bengtsson et al.

Leeds, A., and A. P. Vayda, eds. 1965. *Man, culture, and animals.* Washington, D.C.: AAAS.

Leibowitz, Uri et al. 1971. Multiple sclerosis in Israel. *Isr. Med. J.* 7:1562–67.

Leopold, A. C., and R. Ardrey. 1972. Toxic substances in plants and the food habits of early man. *Science* 176:512–13.

———. 1973. Reply to Dornstreich. *Science* 179:306–7.

Lepowsky, M. 1985. Food taboos, malaria and dietary change: Infant feeding and cultural adaptation on a Papua New Guinea Island. *EFN* 16:105–26.

Levine, M. M. et al. 1979. Genetic susceptibility to cholera. *AHB* 6:369–74.

Levine, Norman. 1973. *Protozoan parasites of domestic animals and man.* Minneapolis: Burgess.

Levy, R. I., and Jay Moskowitz. 1982. Cardiovascular research: Decades of progress, a decade of promise. *Science* 217:121–29.

Lewin, Roger. 1987a. Domino effect involved in ice age extinctions. *Science* 238:1509–10.

———. 1987b. The first Americans are getting younger. *Science* 238:1230–32.

———. 1988a. Modern human origins under close scrutiny. *Science* 239:1240–41.

———. 1988b. New views emerge on hunters and gatherers. *Science* 240:1146–48.

Lewis, T. M. and M. Kneburg. 1946. *Hiwassee Island: An archaeological account of four Tennessee Indian populations.* Knoxville: University of Tennessee Press.

Lieberman, L. S. 1976. Diet, natural selection and adaptation in human populations. Paper presented to the seventy-fifth annual meeting of the American Anthropological Association.

———. 1985. Dietary changes and disease consequences among Afro-Americans. *AJPA* 66:196.

Lindsay, D. G. and J. C. Sherlock. 1982. Environmental contaminants, 85–110 in Jelliffe and Jelliffe.

Livi-Bacci, M. 1983. The nutrition-mortality link, 95–104 in Rotberg and Rabb.

Livingstone, F. B. 1958. Anthropological implications of sickle cell gene distribution in West Africa. *AA* 60:533–62.

———. 1964. Human populations. In *Horizons of anthropology,* ed. S. Tax, 60–70. Chicago: Aldine.

———. 1976. Hemoglobin history in West Africa. *Hum. Biol.* 48:487–500.

———. 1984. The Duffy blood groups, vivax malaria, and malarial selection in human populations: A review. *Hum. Biol.* 56:413–25.

Livi-Bacci, Massimo. 1968. Fertility and population growth in Spain in the eighteenth and nineteenth centuries. *Daedalus* 97:523–35.

Lizot, J. 1977. Population resources and warfare among the Yanomami. *Man* 12: 497–517.

———. 1978. Economie primitive et subsistance. *Libre* 4:69–113.

Logan, Michael, and E. E. Hunt, eds. 1978. *Health and the human condition.* North Scituate, Mass.: Duxbury.

Loomis, W. F. 1967. Skin pigment regulation of vitamin D biosynthesis in man. *Science* 157:501–6.

———. 1970. Rickets. *Sci. Amer.* 223:77–91.

Loucks, A. B. et al. 1984. Menstrual status and validation of body fat prediction in athletes. *Hum. Biol.* 56:383–92.

Lourandos, H. 1983. Intensification: A late Pleistocene-Holocene archaeological sequence from southwestern Victoria. *Arch. Ocean.* 18:81–94.

———. 1985a. Intensification in Australian prehistory, 385–423 in Price and Brown.

———. 1985b. Comment: Problems with the interpretation of late Holocene changes in Australian prehistory. *Arch. Ocean.* 20:37–39.

Lovejoy, C. O., and K. G. Heiple. 1981. The analysis of fractures in skeletal populations with an example from the Libben site, Ottowa Co., Ohio. *AJPA* 55:529–42.

Lovejoy, C. O. et al. 1977. Paleobiology at the Libben site, Ottawa Co., Ohio. *Science* 198:291–3.

Lovejoy, C. O. et al. 1985. Multifactorial determination of skeletal age at death: A method and blind tests of its accuracy (and following essays). *AJPA* 68:1–106.

Lozoff, B., and G. M. Brittenham. 1977. Field methods for the assessment of health and disease in pre-agricultural societies, 49–68 in CIBA.

Lukacs, J. R. et al. 1983. Crown dimensions of deciduous teeth of prehistoric and living populations of western India. *AJPA* 61:383–87.

Lumholtz, Carol. 1889. *Among cannibals.* London: John Murray.

McAlpin, M. B. 1983a. Famines, epidemics and population growth: The case of India, 153–68 in Rotberg and Rabb.

———. 1983b. *Subject to famine.* Princeton: Princeton University Press.

MacArthur, Margaret. 1960. Report of the nutrition unit, 1–13 in Mountford.

McBean, L. D., and E. W. Speckmann. 1982. Diet, nutrition, and cancer, 511–28 in Jelliffe and Jelliffe.

McBryde, Isabel, ed. 1978. *Records of times past.* Canberra: Australian Institute for Aboriginal Studies.

McCall, M. G. 1980. Cardiovascular disease, 507–26 in Stanley and Joske.

McCance, R. A., and Elsie M. Widdowson, eds. 1968. *Caloric deficiency and protein deficiencies.* Boston: Little, Brown.

McCarthy, F. D. 1963. Ecology, equipment, economy and trade. In *Australian aboriginal studies,* ed. W. E. Stanner and H. Sheils, 171–91. Melbourne: Oxford University Press.

McCarthy, F. D., and M. MacArthur. 1960. The food quest and the time factor in aboriginal economic life, 145–94 in Mountford.

McCollum, Robert. 1976. Viral hepatitis, 235–52 in Evans.

MacDonald, Ian. 1980. Supplies of energy: Carbohydrates, 97–116 in Alfin-Slater and Kritchevsky.

MacDonald, Kenneth. 1976. Hookworm, 359–61 in Top and Wehrle.

McGregor, J. A. 1982. Malaria: Nutritional implications. *RID* 4:798–804.

McHenry, Henry. 1968. Transverse lines in the long bones of prehistoric California Indians. *AJPA* 29:1–18.

Machlin, L. J., and M. Brin. 1980. Vitamin E, 245–66 in Alfin-Slater and Kritchevsky.

McInnes, Mary E. 1975. *Essentials of communicable disease*. St. Louis: C. V. Moseby.

McIntosh, B. M., and J. H. S. Gear. 1975. Mosquito borne arboviruses, primarily in the Eastern hemisphere, 939–67 in Hubbert et al.

MacKay, C. V. 1938. Some pathological changes in Australian aboriginal bones. *MJA* 2:537–55.

McKenzie, D. 1985. The simple solution for vitamin deficiencies. *New Sci.* 1478:24.

McKenzie, John. 1980. Possible future changes in the epidemiology and pathogenesis of human influenza A viral infections, 129–50 in Stanley and Joske.

McKeown, T. 1976. *The modern rise of population*. New York: Academic Press.

———. 1983. Food, infection and population, 29–50 in Rotberg and Rabb.

McLaren, Donald S. 1982. Excessive nutrient intakes, 367–88 in Jelliffe and Jelliffe.

McLean, D. M. 1975. Group A mosquito-borne arboviruses primarily in the Western hemisphere, 968–83 in Hubbert et al.

McNeill, William. 1976. *Plagues and peoples*. Garden City, N.Y.: Anchor.

———. 1979. *The human condition*. Princeton: Princeton University Press.

———. 1980. Migration patterns and infection in traditional societies, 28–36 in Stanley and Joske.

MacPherson, R. K. 1966. Physiological adaptation, fitness, and nutrition in the peoples of Australia and New Guinea, 431–68 in Baker and Weiner.

McSheehy, T. W. 1974. Nutrition and breast cancer. *EFN* 3:41–46.

Magennis, Ann. 1977. Middle and late Archaic mortuary patterns. Master's thesis, Department of Anthropology, University of Tennessee.

Malaurie, J. et al. 1952. L'isolat equimau de Thule (Groenland). *Population* 7:675–712.

Malhotra, M. S. 1966. Peoples of India including primitive tribes: A survey on physiological adaptation, physical fitness, and nutrition, 329–56 in Baker and Weiner.

Malina, R. M. 1983. Menarche in athletes: A synthesis and hypothesis. *AHB* 10:1–24.

Mallory, W. H. 1926. *China, land of famine*. New York: American Geographical Society.

Malthus, Thomas. 1960 [1830]. *A summary view of the principle of population in three essays on population*. New York: Mentor.

Man, E. H. 1883. On the aboriginal inhabitants of the Andaman Islands. *JAI* 12:69ff.

Manchester, Keith. 1983. The archaeology of disease. Bradford, England: University of Bradford.

Mann, G. V. et al. 1963. Cardiovascular disease in African Pygmies. *J. Chron. Dis.* 14:341–71.

Marks, M. K. 1984. Congenital treponematosis in an early twentieth century rural black American cemetery. *AJPA* 63:90.

Marks, Stuart. 1976. *Large mammals and a brave people*. Seattle: University of Washington Press.

———. 1977. Hunting behavior and strategies of the valley Bisa of Zambia. *Hum. Ecol.* 5:1–30.

———. 1979. Profile and process: Subsistence hunters in a Zambian community. *Africa* 49:53–67.

Marshall, Lorna. 1960. !Kung Bushman bands. *Africa* 30:325–56.

———. 1976. *The !Kung of Nyae Nyae*. Cambridge: Cambridge University Press.

Martin, D. et al. 1984. The effects of socioeconomic change in prehistoric Africa: Sudanese Nubia as a case study, 193–216 in Cohen and Armelagos.

Martin, D. et al. 1985. Skeletal pathologies as indicators of quality and quantity of diet, 227–80 in Gilbert and Mielke.

Martin, Paul. 1973. The discovery of America. *Science* 179:969–74.

Martin, Paul, and H. E. Wright, eds. 1967. *Pleistocene extinctions: The search for a cause*. New Haven and London: Yale University Press.

Marx, Jean. 1986. Viruses and cancers briefing. *Science* 231:919–20.

———. 1988. The AIDS virus can take on many guises. *Science* 241:1039–40.

Masali, M., and B. Chiarelli. 1969. Demographic data on the remains of ancient Egyptians. *JHE* 1:161–69.

Masnick, G. S. 1980. The demographic impact of breast feeding: A critical review. *Hum. Biol.* 51:109–25.

Mathies, J. R., Jr., and K. MacDonald. 1976. Trichinosis, 719–23 in Top and Wehrle.

May, J. 1958. *Ecology of human disease*. New York: M.D. Publishers.

———. 1970. *The ecology of malnutrition in eastern Africa and four countries in western Africa*. New York: Hafner.

Mazur, D. P. 1969. Expectancy of life at birth in thirty-six nationalities of the Soviet Union, 1958–1960. *Pop. Stud.* 23:225–46.

Means, M. R., and D. M. Austin. 1979. Nutrition and growth of migrant and sedentary Tzeltal children in Chiapas, Mexico. *AJPA* 50:463.

Meehan, Betty. 1977a. Hunters by the seashore. *JHE* 6:363–70.

———. 1977b. Man does not live by calories alone: The role of shellfish in a coastal cuisine, 493–532 in Allen et al.

———. 1982. Ten fish for one man: Some Anbarra attitudes toward food and health, 96–120 in Reid.

Megaw, J. V. S. 1977. *Hunters, gatherers, and first farmers beyond Europe*. Leicester: Leicester University Press.

Meggitt, M. J. 1957–58. Notes on the vegetable foods of the Walbiri of Central Australia. *Oceania* 28:143–45.

———. 1962. *Desert people*. Chicago: University of Chicago.

Meiklejohn, C. et al. 1984. Socioeconomic change and patterns of pathology and variation in the Mesolithic and Neolithic of western Europe: Some suggestions, 75–100 in Cohen and Armelagos.

Mellor, J. W., and S. Gavian. 1987. Famines: Causes, prevention, and relief. *Science* 235:539–59.

Mensforth, R. 1985. Relative long bone growth in the Libben and Bt-5 prehistoric skeletal populations. *AJPA* 68:247–62.

Messer, Ellen. 1977. The ecology of vegetarian diet in a modernizing Mexican community. 117–24. In *Nutrition and anthropology in action*, ed. T. K. Fitzgerald, Amsterdam: Elsevier.

——. 1984. Anthropological perspective on diet. *Ann. Rev. Anthrop.* 15:205–49.

Metz, J., D. Hart, and H. C. Harpending. 1971. Iron, folate, and vitamin B_{12} nutrition in a hunter-gatherer people: A study of !Kung bushmen. *Amer. J. Clin. Nutr.* 24:229–42.

Micozzi, M. S., and A. Shatzkin. 1985. International correlation of anthropometric variables and adolescent growth patterns with breast cancer incidence. *AJPA* 66: 206.

Middleton, Margaret, and Sarah H. Francis. 1976. *Yuendumu and its children*. Canberra: Australian Government Publishing Service.

Mielke, J. H., and P. G. Trapp. 1981. Infant mortality patterns in Aland, Finland. *AJPA* 54:254.

Miles, J. A. R. 1953. Observations on serum iron in aborigines in the northern territory of Australia. *MJA* 2:773–75.

Miles, J. A. R., and D. W. Howes. 1953. Observations on virus encephalitis in South Australia. *MJA* 1:7–12.

Miller, George. 1976. Epidemiology of Burkitt's lymphoma, 481–500 in Evans.

Milner, G. 1982. Measuring prehistoric levels of health: A study of Mississippian period skeletal remains from the American Bottom, Illinois. Ph.D. Diss., Northwestern University.

Milton, Katharine. 1984. Protein and Carbohydrate resources of the Maku Indians of Northwestern Amazonia. *Amer. Anthrop.* 86:7–27.

Mims, Cedric. 1980. The emergence of new infectious diseases, 231–50 in Stanley and Joske.

Mogabgab, W. J. 1976. Influenza, 369–78 in Top and Wehrle.

Molnar, S., and I. Molnar. 1985. The incidence of enamel hypoplasia among the Krapina Neanderthals. *AA* 87:536–49.

——. 1985. Observations of dental diseases among prehistoric populations of Hungary. *AJPA* 67:51–63.

Moodie, Peter. 1973. *Aboriginal health*. Canberra: Australian National University.

——. 1981. Australian aborigines, 154–67 in Trowell and Burkitt.

Moodie, Peter, and E. P. Pedersen. 1971. *The health of aborigines: An annotated bibliography*. Canberra: Australian Government Publishing Service.

Moore, David R. 1979. *Islanders and aborigines at Cape York*. Canberra: Australian Institute Behavioral Studies.

Moore, Richard D., and G. D. Webb. 1986. *The K factor*. New York: Macmillan.

Morgan, L. H. 1877. *Ancient society*. New York: Holt, Rinehart.

Morley, David. 1980. Severe measles, 115–28 in Stanley and Joske.

Morris, B. 1982. *Forest traders: A socioeconomic study of the Hill Pandaram*. London: Athlone.

Morse, Dan. 1961. Prehistoric tuberculosis in America. *Amer. Rev. Resp. Dis.* 83: 489–504.

Mosley, J. W. 1976a. Hepatitis A, 316–25 in Top and Wehrle.

——. 1976b. Hepatitis B, 326–38 in Top and Wehrle.

Mountford, C. P., ed. 1960. *Records of the American-Australian scientific expedition to Arnhemland*. Melbourne: Melbourne University Press.

Mouratoff, G. J. et al. 1973. Diabetes mellitus in Eskimos after a decade. *JAMA* 226: 1345–46.

Mulvaney, D. J., and J. Golson, eds. 1971. *Aboriginal man and environment in Australia*. Canberra: Australian National Univ.

Murchison, M. A. et al. 1984. Transverse line formation in protein-deprived rhesus monkeys. *Hum. Biol.* 56:173–82.

Murdock, G. P. 1968. The current status of the world's hunting and gathering peoples, 13–22 in Lee and DeVore.

Murray, M. J. et al. 1982. Adverse effects of normal nutrients and foods on host resistance to disease, 313–24 in Jelliffe and Jelliffe.

Mustafa, M. G. 1982. Agricultural chemicals, 111–28 in Jelliffe and Jelliffe.

Muul, Illar. 1970. Mammalian ecology and the epidemiology of zoonoses. *Science* 170:1275–79.

Myers, F. R. 1988. Critical trends in the study of hunter-gatherers. *Ann. Rev. of Anthrop.* 17:261–82.

Nag, Moni. 1968. *Factors affecting human fertility in nonindustrial societies: A cross cultural study*. New Haven: Human Relations Area Files Press.

National Academy of Science-National Research Council (NAS-NRC). 1973. *Toxicants occurring naturally in foods*. Washington, D.C.: NAS-NRC.

Neel, James, V. 1962. Diabetes mellitus: A "thrifty" genotype rendered detrimental by "progress"? *Amer. J. Hum. Genet.* 14:353–62.

———. 1970. Lessons from a primitive people. *Science* 170:815–22.

———. 1977. Health and disease in unacculturated Amerindian populations, 155–68 in CIBA.

Neel, James V., and N. A. Chagnon. 1968. The demography of two tribes of primitive relatively unacculturated American Indians. *Proc. N.A.S.* 59:680–89.

Neel, J. V., and K. Weiss. 1975. The genetic structure of a tribal population of Yanomamo Indians. *AJPA* 42:25–52.

Neel, J. V. et al. 1964. Studies on the Xavante Indians of the Brazilian Mato Grosso. *Am J. Hum. Genet.* 16:52–140.

Neel, J. V. et al. 1968. Further studies of the Xavante. *Amer. J. Trop. Med. Hyg.* 17: 486–98.

Neel, J. V. et al. 1970. Notes on the effect of measles and measles vaccine on a virgin-soil population of South American Indians. *Amer. J. Epidem.* 91:418–29.

Neel, J. V. et al. 1977. Man in the tropics: The Yanomamo Indians, 108–42, in Harrison.

Neer, Robert M. 1975. The evolutionary significance of Vitamin D, skin pigment, and ultraviolet light. *AJPA* 43:409–16.

Nelson, A. J. 1985. A study of stature, sex, and age ratios and average age at death from Romano-British to late Anglo-Saxon period. Master's thesis, Sheffield University.

Nelson, B. K. et al. 1986. Effects of diagenesis on strontium, carbon, nitrogen, and oxygen concentrations and isotopic composition of bone. *Geo., et Cosmo. Acta.* 50: 1941–49.

Nelson, D. A. 1984. Bone density in three archaeological populations. *AJPA* 63:198.

Nelson, J. S. 1975. Schistosomiasis, 620–40 in Hubbert et al.

Neumann, H. W. 1967. *The paleopathology of the archaic Modoc Rock Shelter inhabitants*. Springfield: Illinois State Museum Report #11.

Neuwelt-Truntzer, S. 1986. Ecological influences on the physical, behavioral and cognitive development of Pygmy children. Ph.D. diss., Dept. of Behavioral Sciences, University of Chicago, cited in Cavalli-Sforza.

Neva, F. A. 1975. American trypanosomiasis, 765–72 in Hubbert et al.

Neves, W. A. 1987. Nutritional inferences from paleopathologies in a tropical marine environment. *AJPA* 72:235–36.

Newman, J. L. 1975. Dimensions of Sandawe diet. *EFN* 4:33–39.

Newman, M. T. 1962. Ecological and medical anthropology. *AJPA* 22:351–54.

———. 1975. Nutritional adaptation in man, 210–59 in Damon.

———. 1976. Aboriginal New World epidemiology and medical care and the impact of Old World disease imports. *AJPA* 45:667–72.

Newman, Russell. 1970. Why man is such a sweaty and thirsty naked animal: A speculative review. *Hum. Biol.* 4:12–27.

Nickens, Paul R. 1976. Stature reduction as an adaptive response to food production in Mesoamerica. *J. Arc. Sci.* 3:31–41.

Nielsen, O. V. 1970. *Human remains.* Scand. Joint Exped. to Sudanese Nubia, Vol. 9. Copenhagen: Scandinavian University.

Nietschmann, Bernard. 1972. Hunting and fishing focus among the Miskito Indians of eastern Nicaragua. *Hum. Ecol.* 1:41–68.

Norden, C. W., and F. L. Ruben. 1976. Staphylococcal infection, 636–54 in Top and Wehrle.

Norman, C. 1985. Politics and science clash on African AIDS. *Science* 230:1140–42.

Norr, L. 1984. Prehistoric subsistence and health status of coastal peoples from the Panamanian isthmus of lower Central America, 463–90 in Cohen and Armelagos.

Nurse, George T. 1975. Seasonal hunger among the Ngoni and Ntumba of central Malawi. *Africa* 45:1–11.

Nurse, George T., and Trefor Jenkins. 1977. *Health and the hunter-gatherer.* Basel, Switzerland: Karger.

O'Connell, J. F., and K. Hawkes. 1981. Alyawara plant use and optimal foraging theory, 99–125 in Winterhalder and Smith.

———. 1984. Food choice and foraging sites among the Alyawara. *J. Anthrop. Res.* 40:504–35.

O'Connell, J. F. K. Hawkes, and N. Blurton Jones. 1988. Hadza scavenging: Implications for Plio/Pleistocene hominid subsistence. *CA* 29:356–63.

Ofosu-Amaah, S. 1980. The African experience, 299–322 in Stanley and Joske.

Ogbu, John. 1973. Seasonal hunger in tropical Africa as a cultural phenomenon. *Africa* 43:317–32.

Oke, O. L. 1975. Hydrocianic acid and the incidence of ataxic neuropathy in Nigeria. *Proc. Ninth Inter. Cong. Nutrition*, 267–71.

Olivier, G. 1980. The increase of stature in France. *JHE* 9:645–49.

Olsen, P. F. 1975. Tularemia, 191–223 in Hubbert et al.

Ortner, Donald. 1972. Ecological factors in disease among North American archaeological skeletal samples. *AJPA* 37:447.

Ortner, Donald, and W. Putschar. 1981. Identification of pathological conditions in human skeletal remains. Washington, D.C.: Smithsonian Contributions to Anthropology 28.

Osgood, C. B. 1936. *Contributions to the ethnography of the Kutchin.* New Haven: Yale University Publications in Anthropology 14.

Osman, A. K. 1981. Bulrush millett (Pennisetum typhoides): A contributing factor in the endemicity of goiter in Western Sudan. *EFN* 11:121–28.

Overfield, T., and M. R. Klauber. 1980. Prevalence of tuberculosis in Eskimos having blood group B gene. *Hum. Biol.* 52:87–92.

Overturf, G. D., and A. W. Mathies. 1976. Salmonellosis, 598–611 in Top and Wehrle.

Owen-Smith, N. 1987. Pleistocene extinctions: The pivotal role of megaherbivores. *Paleobiology* 13.

Owsley, D., and B. Bradtmiller. 1983. Mortality of pregnant females in Arikara villages: Osteological evidence. *AJPA* 61:331–36.

Packard, R. M. 1984. Maize, cattle and mosquitos: The political economy of malaria epidemics in colonial Swaziland. *JAH* 25:189–212.

Packer, A. D. 1961–62. The health of the Australian native. *Oceania* 32:60–70.

Pagezy, H. 1978. Morphological, physical and ethoecological adaptations of Oto and Twa women living in the equatorial forest, Tumba Lake, Zaire. *JHE* 6:83–94.

——. 1983. Attitude of Ntumba society toward the primiparous woman and its biological effects. *J. Biosoc. Sci.* 15:421–31.

——. 1984. Seasonal hunger as experienced by the Oto and Twa women of Ntumba in the equatorial forest (Lake Tumba), Zaire. *EFN* 15:13–27.

Palkovich, Ann. 1984. Agriculture, marginal environments and nutritional stress in the prehistoric Southwest, 425–38 in Cohen and Armelagos.

Paolucci, A. M. et al. 1969. Serum free amino acid patterns in a Babinga pygmy adult population. *AJCN* 22:1652–59.

Pappagainis, D. 1976. Coccidioidomycosis, 184–94 in Top and Wehrle.

Parkin, W. E. 1975. Mosquito borne arboviruses other than group A primarily in the Western hemisphere, 984–93 in Hubbert et al.

Passarello, P. 1977. Paleodemographic aspects of the iron age in Italy: The Veio's Villanovians. *JHE* 6:175–79.

Patrucco, Raul et al. 1983. Parasitological studies of coprolites of pre-hispanic Peruvian populations. *CA* 24:393–94.

Paul, J. R. 1955. *The epidemiology of poliomyelitis*. WHO monograph 26. Geneva: WHO.

Paul, J. R. et al. 1951. Antibodies to three different antigenic types of poliomyelitis virus in serum from North Alaskan Eskimos. *Amer. J. Hyg.* 54:275–85.

Pavlovsky, E. U. 1966. Natural nidality of transmissible diseases. Urbana: Univ. of Illinois Press.

Pecotte, J. 1985. Nutritional stress and health during the first intermediate period in Ancient Egypt. *AJPA* 66:213.

Pellett, P. 1983. Commentary: Changing concepts of world malnutrition. *EFN* 13: 115–25.

Pelto, G. H., and P. J. Pelto. 1983. Diet and delocalization: Dietary change since 1750, 309–30 in Rotberg and Rabb.

Pennetti, V. et al. 1986. General health of African Pygmies of the Central African Republic, 128–38 in Cavalli-Sforza.

Perez-Diez, A. A., and F. M. Salzano. 1978. Evolutionary implications of the ethnography and demography of Ayoreo Indians. *JHE* 7:253–68.

Perlman, Stephen. 1980. An optimum diet model coastal variability and hunter-gatherer behavior. *Adv. Arch Meth, Theor.* 3:257–310.

———. 1983. Optimum diet models and return rate curves: A test on Martha's Vineyard, 115–67 in Bronitsky.

Perrenoud, Alfred. 1984. Mortality decline in its secular setting, 41–69 in Bengtsson et al.

Perzigian, A. et al. 1984. Prehistoric health in the Ohio River Valley, 347–66 in Cohen and Armelagos.

Petersen, William. 1975. *Population.* New York: Macmillan.

Peterson, J. T. 1978. Hunter-gatherer—farmer exchange. *AA* 80:335–51.

———. 1981. Game, farming and interethnic relations in northeastern Luzon, Philippines. *Hum. Ecol.* 9:1–22.

Peterson, Nicolas, ed. 1976. *Tribes and boundaries in Australia.* Canberra: Australian Institute of Aboriginal Studies.

Peterson, Warren. 1981. Recent adaptive shifts among Palanan hunters of the Philipines. *Man* 6:43–61.

Pfeiffer, Susan. 1984. Paleopathology in an Iroquoian ossuary with special reference to tuberculosis. *AJPA* 65:181–89.

Pfeiffer, Susan, and P. King. 1983. Cortical bone formation and diet among protohistoric Iroquois. *AJPA* 60:23–28.

Picot, H., and J. Benoist. 1975. Interaction of social and ecological factors in the epidemiology of helminth parasites, 223–48 in Watts et al.

Pierce, Russel. 1978. The evidence of J. Ainsworth on the diet and economy of the Ballina horde, 116–21 in McBryde.

Pilling, A., and R. Waterman. 1970. *Diptrodon to detribalization.* East Lansing: Michigan State University Press.

Piontek, J., and M. Henneberg. 1981. Mortality changes in a Polish rural community, 1350 to 1972, and estimation of their evolutionary significance. *AJPA* 54:129–36.

Piot, Peter et al. 1988. AIDS: An international perspective. *Science* 239:573–79.

Poland, J. 1976. Tularemia, 754–60 in Top and Wehrle.

Polanyi, Karl. 1953. *Semantics of general economic history.* New York: Columbia University Council for Research in the Social Sciences.

Polgar, S. 1964. Evolution and the ills of mankind. In *Horizons of anthropology,* ed. S. Tax, 200–211. Chicago: Aldine.

———. 1972. Population history and population policies. *CA* 13:203–15.

Polunin, Ivan. 1953. The medical natural history of Malayan aborigines. *Med. J. Malaysia* 8:55–174.

———. 1977. Some characteristics of tribal peoples, 5–20 in CIBA.

Post, P. W. et al. 1975. Cold injury and the evolution of white skin. *Hum. Biol.* 47:65–80.

Potts, M. et al. 1985. Breast feeding and fertility. *J. Biosoc. Sci.,* supp. 9.

Powell, M. L. 1984. Health, disease and social stratification in the complex Mississippian chiefdom at Moundville. *AJPA* 63:205.

———. 1985. The analysis of dental wear and caries for dietary reconstruction, 307–38 in Gilbert and Mielke.

———. 1987. On the eve of the conquest: Life and death at Irene Mound, Georgia. *AJPA* 72:243–44.

———. 1988. *Status and health in prehistory.* Washington, D.C.: Smithsonian Institution Press.

Prentice, A. M., and R. G. Whitehead. N.d. The energetics of human reproduction. Manuscript, Cambridge, England, MRC Dunn Nutrition Unit.

Price, D. L. et al. 1963. Parasitism in Congo Pygmies. *Am. J. Trop. Med. Hyg.* 12(3): 83–87.

Price, T. D., and J. A. Brown. 1985. *Prehistoric hunter-gatherers: The emergence of cultural complexity*. New York: Academic Press.

Prokopec, Miroslav. 1979. Demographic and morphological aspects of the Roonka population. *Arch. and Phys. Anth. Ocean.* 14:11–26.

Prothero, R. M. 1965. *Migrants and malaria*. London: Longmans.

Quevado, W. C., Jr., et al. 1975. The role of light in human skin color variation. *AJPA* 43:393–408.

Quick, W. W. 1974. Diabetes in Eskimos. *JAMA* 227:1392.

Quinn, T. C. et al. 1986. AIDS in Africa: An epidemiological paradigm. *Science* 234: 955–63.

Radcliffe-Brown, A. R. 1948. The Andaman Islanders. Glencoe, Ill.: Free Press.

Ramalingaswami, V. 1978. Health and industrial growth, the current Indian scene, 89–106 in CIBA.

Rappaport, R. A. 1968. *Pigs for the ancestors*. New Haven and London: Yale University Press.

Rathbun, T. A. 1981. Harris lines and dentition as indirect evidence of nutritional states in early Iron-Age Iran. *AJPA* 54:266.

———. 1984. Skeletal pathology from the paleolithic through the metal ages in Iran and Iraq, 137–68 in Cohen and Armelagos.

Rathbun, T. A., and J. D. Scurry. 1985. Status and health in colonial South Carolina: Belleview Plantation, 1738–1756. In *Skeletal analysis of the effects of socioeconomic status on health*, ed. D. Martin. Research Report 25, Department of Anthropology, University of Massachusetts, Amherst.

Rausch, R. L. 1975. Taenidae, 678–707 in Hubbert et al.

Rausch, R. et al. 1967. Helminths in Eskimos in western Alaska with particular reference to diphillobothrium infection and anemia. *Trans. Roy Soc. Trop Med. Hyg.* 61:351–57.

Read, M. 1966. *Culture, health and disease*. Philadelphia: Lippencott.

Redman, Charles et al., ed. 1978. *Social archaeology: Beyond subsistence and dating*. New York: Academic Press.

Reed, Charles, ed. 1977. *Origins of agriculture*. The Hague: Mouton.

Reid, Janice, ed. 1982. Body, land and spirit: Health and healing in aboriginal society. St. Lucia: University of Queensland Press.

Reinhard, Karl J. In press. Cultural ecology of prehistoric parasites on the Colorado plateau as evidenced by coprology. *Amer. J. Phys. Anthrop.*

Reinhard, Karl J. et al. 1987. Helminth remains from prehistoric Indian coprolites on the Colorado Plateau. *Journal of Parasitology* 73, no. 3:630–39.

Reinhold, J. G. 1972. Phytate concentrations of leavened and unleavened Iranian breads. *EFN* 1:187–92.

Richard, J. L. 1975. Introduction to the mycoses and mycotoxicoses, 465–68 in Hubbert et al.

Richards, Paul. 1982. Quality and quantity in agricultural work: Sierra Leone rice farming, 209–28 in Harrison.

Rindos, David. 1984. *The origins of agriculture*. Orlando: Academic Press.

Ripley, Suzanne. 1980. Infanticide in langurs and man: Adaptive advantage or social pathology, 349–90 in M. Cohen et al.

Robbins, L. M. 1978. The antiquity of tuberculosis in prehistoric peoples of Kentucky. *AJPA* 48:429.

Robbins, Richard H. 1973. Identity and the interpersonal theory of disease. Paper presented to the annual meeting of the Southern Anthropological Association.

Robertson, L. S. 1981. Abortion and infant mortality before and after the U.S. Supreme Court decision on abortion. *J. Biosoc. Sci.* 13:275–80.

Roe, Daphne. 1973. *A plague of corn: The social history of pellagra*. Ithaca, N.Y.: Cornell University Press.

———. 1982. Nutrient deficiencies in naturally occurring foods, 407–26 in Jelliffe and Jelliffe.

Rollet, Catherine. 1981. Infant feeding, fosterage and infant mortality in France at the end of the nineteenth century. *Population*, Select papers 2.

Romaniuk, A. 1974. Modernization and fertility: The case of the James Bay Indians. *Can. Rev. Sociol. and Anthrop.* 11:344–59.

———. 1981. Increases in natural fertility during the early stages of modernization: Canadian Indian Studies. *Demography*: 18:157–72.

Romaniuk, A., and V. Piché. 1972. Natality estimates for the Canadian Indians of James Bay by stable population models. *Can. Rev. Sociol. Anthrop.* 9:1–20.

Romsos, D. R., and S. D. Clarke. 1980. Supplies of energy: Carbohydrate-fat inter-relationships, 141–58 in Alfin-Slater and Kritchevsky.

Rose, F. G. 1960. *Classification of kin, age structure, and marriage among the Groote Eylandt aborigines*. Oxford: Pergamon.

———. 1968. Australian marriage, land-owning groups and initiations, 200-208 in Lee and DeVore.

Rose, J. C. 1984. Black American history and paleopathology in Arkansas. *AJPA* 63: 210.

———, ed. 1985. *Gone to a better land*. Little Rock: Arkansas Archaeological Survey Research Series 2.

Rose, J. C., G. J. Armelagos, and J. W. Lallo. 1978. Histological enamel indicators of childhood stress in prehistoric skeletal samples. *AJPA* 49: 511–16.

Rose, J. C., and L. F. Boyd. 1978. Dietary reconstruction utilizing histological observations of enamel and dentin. *AJPA* 48: 431.

Rose, J. C. et al. 1984. Paleopathology and the origins of maize agriculture in the lower Mississippi valley and Caddoan culture areas, 393–424 in Cohen and Armelagos.

Rose, J. C. et al. 1985. Diet and dentition: Developmental disturbances, 281–306 in Gilbert and Mielke.

Rosebury, T. 1971. *Microbes and morals*. New York: Ballantine.

Rosen, M. N. 1975. Colstridial infections and intoxications, 251–62 in Hubbert et al.

Rosenberg, J. H., and B. B. Bowman. 1982. Intestinal physiology and parasitic diseases. *RID* 4:763–67.

Rosenberg, J. H. et al. 1976. Interaction of infection and nutrition: Some practical concepts. *EFN* 4:203–6.

Ross, A. 1981. Holocene environments and prehistoric site patterns in the Victorian Mallee. *Arch. Ocean.* 16:45–154.

Rotberg, R. I. 1983. *Imperialism, colonialism and hunger.* Lexington, Mass.: Heath.

Rotberg, R. I., and T. K. Rabb. 1983. *Hunger and history.* Cambridge: Cambridge University Press.

Roth, E. A. 1980. Sedentism and changing patterns of fertility in a northern Athapascan isolate. *AJPA* 52:272.

———. 1981. Sedentism and changing fertility patterns in a northern Athapascan isolate. *J. Hum. Evol.* 10:413–25.

———. 1985. A note on the demographic concomitants of sedentism. *AA* 87:380–82.

Roth, E. A., and A. K. Ray. 1985. Demographic patterns of sedentary and nomadic Juang of Orissa. *Hum. Biol.* 57:319–25.

Roth, H. L. 1899. *The aborigines of Tasmania.* 2d ed. Halifax: L. F. King and Sons.

Rothschild, Henry R. 1981. *Biocultural aspects of disease.* New York: Academic Press.

Rowley-Conwy, P. 1984. The laziness of the short-distance hunter: The origins of agriculture in western Denmark. *J. Anth. Arch.* 38: 300–24.

Roy, S. C. 1925. *The Birhors.* Ranchi, India: G.E.L. Mission Press.

Rudney, Joel. 1981. Early childhood stress in ancient Nubia. *AJPA* 54:270.

———. 1983. Dental indicators of growth disturbance in a series of ancient lower nubian populations: Changes over time. *AJPA* 60:463–70.

Rudolf, A. H. 1976. Syphilis, 672–97 in Top and Wehrle.

Ruff, C. B. 1981. New demographic estimates for Pecos Pueblo. *AJPA* 54:147–51.

Russell, J. C. 1948. *British medieval population.* Albuquerque: University of New Mexico Press.

Sahlins, Marshall. 1968. Notes on the original affluent society, 85–88 in Lee and Devore.

———. 1972. *Stone Age economics.* Chicago: Aldine.

St. Hoyme, Lucille. 1969. On the origins of New World paleopathology. *AJPA* 31: 295–302.

St. Hoyme, L. E., and R. T. Koritzer. 1976. Ecology of dental disease. *AJPA* 45: 673–86.

Saffirio, G., and R. Scaglion. 1982. Hunting efficiency in acculturated and unacculturated Yanomamo villages. *JAR* 38:315–32.

Salzano, F. M. 1972. Genetic aspects of the demography of American Indians and Eskimos, 234–51 in Harrison and Boyce.

Salzano, F. M. et al. 1967. Further studies on the Xavante Indians. *Amer. J. Hum. Gen.* 19: 463–89.

Sanders, W. T., and David Webster. 1978. Unilinealism, multilinealism and the evolution of complex societies, 259–302 in Redman et al.

Sandford, M. K. et al. 1983. Elemental hair analysis: New evidence on the etiology of cribra orbitalia in Sudanese Nubia. *Hum. Biol.* 55:831–44.

Sandison, A. T. 1972. Evidence of infectious disease. *J. Human. Evol.* 1:213–24.

———. 1980. Notes on some skeletal changes in pre-European-contact Australian aborigines. *J. Hum. Evol.* 9:45–47.

———. 1973. Paleopathology of human bones from Murray River region between Mildura and Renmark, Australia. *Mem. Nat. Mus. Victoria.* 34:173–74.

Sandosham, A. A. 1967. Animal parasites of animals which affect man in Malaysia. *Med. J. Malaysia* 22:16–24.

Sarnat, B. G., and I. Schour. 1941. Enamel hypoplasia (chronological enamel aplasia) in relation to systemic disease. *JADA* 28:1989–2000.

Sattenspiel, L., and H. Harpending. 1983. Stable populations and skeletal age. *Amer. Antiq.* 48: 489–98.

Saucier, J-F. 1972. Correlation of long post-partum taboo: A cross cultural study. *CA* 13:238.

Saul, Frank P. 1972. The human skeletal remains of Altar de Sacrificios. *Papers of the Peabody Museum of Arch. and Ethnol.*: 63:2.

——. 1973. Disease in the Maya area: The pre-Columbian evidence, 301–24 in Culbert.

Sawyer, W. A. 1921. Hookworm in Australia. *MJA* 1:148–50.

Scarlett, N. et al. 1982. Bush medicines: The pharmacopoeia of the Yolngu of Arnhemland, 154–92 in Reid.

Schaeffer, Otto. 1970. When the Eskimo comes to town. *Nutrition Today* 6:8–16.

Schapera, Isaac. 1930. *Khoisan peoples of South Africa.* London: Routledge and Sons.

——. 1947. *Migrant labor and tribal life.* London: Oxford.

Schebesta, Paul. 1928. *Among the forest dwarfs of Malaya.* London: Hutchinson.

Schoeninger, Margaret J. 1979. Diet and status at Chalcatzingo: Some empirical and technical aspects of strontium analysis. *AJPA* 51:295–310.

——. 1981. The agricultural revolution and its effects on human diet in the Middle East. *AJPA* 54:275.

——. 1982. Diet and the evolution of modern human form in the Middle East. *AJPA* 55:37–50.

Schoeninger, M. J. et al. 1983. 15n/14n ratios of bone collagen reflect marine and terrestrial composition of prehistoric human diet. *Science* 220:1381–83.

Schofield, Roger. 1984. Population growth in the century after 1750: The rate of mortality decline, 17–40 in Bengtsson et al.

Scholtens, R. G. 1975. Filarial infections, 572–83 in Hubbert et al.

Schrire, Carmel. 1980. An inquiry into the evolutionary status and apparent identity of the San hunter-gatherers. *Hum. Ecol.* 8:9–32.

——, ed. 1984. *Past and present in hunter-gatherer studies.* New York: Academic Press.

Schultz, Adolph. 1967. Diseases and healed fractures of wild apes, 47–55 in Brothwell and Sandison.

Schwanitz, F. 1966. *The origin of cultivated plants.* Cambridge: Harvard University Press.

Schwartz, C. J., and J. A. Casely Smith. 1958. Serum cholesterol levels in atherosclerotic subjects and in Australian aborigines. *MJA* 1:84–86.

Schwartz, C. J. et al. 1957. Serum cholesterol and phospholipid levels of Australian aborigines. *Aust. J. Exp. Biol. Med. Sci.* 35:449–50.

Sciulli, Paul W. 1977. A descriptive and comparative study of the deciduous dentition of prehistoric Ohio Valley Amerindians. *AJPA* 47:71–80.

——. 1978. Developmental abnormalities of the permanent dentition in prehistoric Ohio Valley Amerindians. *AJPA* 48:193–98.

Scrimshaw, N. et al. 1968. *Interactions of nutrition and infection.* Geneva: WHO Monograph 57.

Selby, L. A. 1975a. Blastomycosis, 490–500 in Hubbert et al.

————. 1975b. Coccidioidomyclsis, 517–28 in Hubbert et al.

————. 1975c. Histoplasmosis, 501–16 in Hubbert et al.

Seligmann, C. G., and B. Z. Seligmann. 1911. *The Veddas*. Cambridge: Cambridge University Press.

Sellevold, B. J. et al. 1984. *Iron-Age man in Denmark*. Copenhagen: Detkongelige Nordiske Oldskriftselskag.

Semba, Richard. 1985. Medical care and the survival of the Venezuelan Yanomami, 31–45 in Colchester.

Sen, A. 1981. *Poverty and famines*. Oxford: Oxford University Press.

Sen, B. K., and J. Sen. 1955. Notes on the Birhors. *Man in India* 35:169–75.

Sen Gupta, P. N. 1980. Food consumption, and nutrition of regional tribes of India. *EFN* 9:93–108.

Serjeantson, Susan. 1975. Marriage patterns and fertility in three Papua New Guinea populations. *Hum. Biol.* 47:399–413.

Service, Elman. 1966. *The hunters*. Englewood Cliffs, N.J.: Prentice Hall.

————. 1975. *The origin of the state and civilization*. New York: W. W. Norton.

Sever, Lowell. 1973. *Zinc and human development. Hum. Ecol.* 3:43–57.

Sharp, R. Lauriston. 1940. An Australian aboriginal population. *Hum. Biol.* 12:481–507.

Shipman, P. et al. 1985. *The human skeleton*. Cambridge: Harvard University Press.

Short, R. 1984. Breast feeding. *Sci. Amer.* 250, no. 4:35.

————. 1985. Nature's contraceptive. *J. Biosocial Sci.*, Supp 9:1–3.

Sibajuddin, S. M. 1984. Reproduction and consanguinity among Chenchus of Andhra Pradesh. *Man in India.* 64:181–92.

Sikes, R. K. 1975. Rabies, 871–96 in Hubbert et al.

Silberbauer, George B. 1981a. Hunter-gatherers of the central Kalahari, 455–98 in Harding and Teleki.

————. 1981b. *Hunter and habitat in the central Kalahari*. Cambridge: Cambridge University Press.

Sillen, A., and M. Kavanaugh. 1982. Strontium and paleodietary research: A review. *Yrbk. Phys. Anthrop.* 25:69–90.

Sillen, A., and P. Smith. 1984. Weaning patterns are reflected in strontium-calcium ratios of juvenile skeletons. *J. Arch. Sci.* 11:237–45.

Simon, Julian. 1983. The effects of population on nutrition and economic well-being, 215–39 in Rotberg and Rabb.

Simoons, F. J. 1970. Primary adult lactase deficiency and the milking habit: A problem in biological and cultural interrelations, 2; a cultural-historical hypothesis. *Amer. J. Dig. Dis.* 15:695–710.

Singh, A., and A. de Souza. 1980. *The urban poor*. New Delhi: Manohar.

Sinha, D. P. 1972. The Birhors, 371–403 in Bicchieri.

Smith, D. S. 1977. A homeostatis demographic regime: Patterns in western European family reconstruction studies, 19–52 in R. D. Lee.

Smith, John M. B. 1975. Superficial and cutaneous mycoses, 469–88 in Hubbert et al.

Smith, Patricia et al. 1984a. Diachronic trends in humeral cortical thickness of Near Eastern populations. *JHE* 13:603–11.

Smith, Patricia et al. 1984b. Archaeological and skeletal evidence for dietary change during the late Pleistocene/early Holocene in the Levant, 101–36 in Cohen and Armelagos.

Smith, Phillip E. L. 1972. *The consequences of food production*. Reading, Mass.: Addison-Wesley.

——. 1976. *Food production and its consequences*. Menlo Park, Calif.: Cummings.

Smyth, R. B. 1878. *The aborigines of Victoria*. London: Trubner.

Snow, Charles E. 1948. Indian Knoll skeletons. *University of Kentucky Reports in Anthropology* 4(3):2.

Snow, J. 1936 [1849]. *Snow on cholera*. New York: Commonwealth Fund.

Soffer, Olga. 1985. *The Upper Paleolithic of the central Russian plain*. Orlando, Fla.: Academic Press.

Sorg, M. H., and B. C. Craig. 1981. Patterns of infant mortality in the upper St. Johns River Valley French population, 1791–1838. *AJPA* 54:280.

Sotiroff-Junker J. 1978. Bibliography on behavioral and social and economic aspects of malaria and its control. Geneva: WHO.

Spaeth, R. 1976. Tetanus, 688–701 in Top and Wehrle.

Spencer, Baldwin, and F. J. Gillen. 1904. *The native tribes of central Australia*. London: Macmillan.

——. 1927. *The Arunta*. London: Macmillan.

Speth, J. D. 1983. *Bison kills and bone counts*. Chicago: University of Chicago Press.

——. 1988. Hunter-gatherer diet, resource stress, and the origins of agriculture. Symposium on population growth, disease and the origins of agriculture, Rutgers Univ., New Brunswick.

Spooner, Brian, ed. 1972. *Population growth*. Cambridge: MIT Press.

Stanley, N. F., and R. A. Joske, eds. 1980. *Changing disease patterns and human behavior*. London: Academic Press.

Stanner, J. W., and H. Sheils, eds. 1961. *Australian aboriginal studies*. Melbourne: Oxford University Press.

Steegman, A. T. 1982. Eighteenth century stature: Environmental factors. *AJPA* 57: 232.

——. 1985. Mid-eighteenth century American military stature: Archival and skeletal comparisons. *AJPA* 66:233–34.

Steinbock, R. Ted. 1976. *Paleopathological diagnosis and interpretation*. Springfield, Mass.: C. C. Thomas.

Stephen, L. E. 1975. African trypanosomiasis, 745–64 in Hubbert et al.

Steward, Julian. 1938. Basin-plateau aboriginal sociopolitical groups. Washington, D.C.: Bureau of American Ethnology Bulletin 120.

——. 1955. *Theory of culture change*. Urbana: University of Illinois Press.

Stewart, T. D. 1973. *The people of America*. New York: Charles Scribner's Sons.

——. 1976. A physical anthropologist's view of the peopling of the New World. *SWJA* 16(3):259–73.

——. 1979. *Essentials of forensic anthropology*. Springfield, Mass.: C. C. Thomas.

Stini, William. 1985. Growth rates and sexual dimorphism in evolutionary perspective, 191–226 in Gilbert and Mielke.

Stocks, Anthony. 1983. Cocamilla fishing: Patch modification and environmental buffering in the Amazon, 239–68 in Hames and Vickers.

Stone, Irwin. 1965. Studies of a mammalian enzyme system for producing evolutionary evidence on man. *AJPA* 23:83–86.

Stone, Lawrence. 1977. *The family, sex and marriage in England, 1500–1800*. New York: Harper and Row.

Storey, R. 1985a. An estimate of mortality in a pre-Columbian urban population. *AA* 87:519–35.

———. 1985b. Pre-Columbian child and infant mortality at Teotihuacan and Copan. *AJPA* 66:234.

Story, J. A., and D. Kritchevsky. 1980. Nutrients with special functions: Dietary fiber, 259–79 in Alfin-Slater and Kritchevsky.

Stout, S. D. 1978. Histological structure and its preservation in ancient bone. *Curr. Anthrop.* 19: 600–4.

Stuart-Macadam, P. 1985. Poratic hyperostosis: Representative of a childhood condition. *AJPA* 66:391–98.

Sugarman, B. 1983. Zinc and infection. *RID* 5:137.

Sullivan, Sharon. 1978. Aboriginal diet and food-gathering methods in the Richmond and Tweed river valleys as seen in early settler records, 101–18 in McBryde.

Sussman, R. W. 1972. Child transport, family size and increase in human population during the Neolithic. *CA* 13:258–59.

Suttles, Wayne. 1960. Affinal ties, subsistence and prestige among coast Salish. *Amer. Anthrop.* 62:296–305.

———. 1968. Coping with abundance: Subsistence on the Northwest Coast, 56–68 in Lee and DeVore.

Sweeney, G. 1947. Food supplies of a desert tribe. *Oceania* 17:289–99.

Sweet, W. C. 1924. The intestinal parasites of man in Australia and its dependencies as found by the hookworm campaign. *MJA* 1:405–7.

Symes, Steven. 1984. Harris lines as indicators of stress: An analysis of tibiae from the Crow Creek Massacre. *AJPA* 63:226.

Tanaka, Jiro. 1980. *The San: Hunter-gatherers of the Kalahari*. Tokyo: University of Tokyo Press.

Tanno, T. 1981. Plant utilization of the Mbuti Pygmies with special reference to their material culture and use of wild vegetable foods. *KUASM* 1:1–51.

Taylor, C. E. 1983. Synergy among mass infections, famines and poverty, 285–303 in Rotberg and Rabb.

Taylor, John C. 1977. A pre-contact aboriginal medical system on Cape York Peninsula. *J. Hum. Evol.* 6:419–32.

Terashima, H. 1983. Mota and other hunting activities of the Mbuti archers. *KUASM* 3:71–81.

Thomson, Donald. 1949. *Economic structure and ceremonial exchange in Arnhemland*. Melbourne: Macmillan.

———. 1975. *Bindibu country*. Melbourne: Thomas Nelson.

Tietze, Christopher, and M. C. Murstein. 1975. *Reports on population and family planning*, no. 14. New York: Population Council.

Tilley, L. A. 1983. Food entitlement, famine and conflict, 136–51 in Rotberg and Rabb.

Tindale, Norman B. 1974. *Aboriginal tribes of Australia*. Berkeley: University of California Press.

Tobias, P. V. 1966. The peoples of Africa south of the Sahara, 111–200 in Baker and Weiner.

———. 1978. *The bushmen: San hunters and herders of South Africa*. Capetown: Human and Rousseau.

Tonkinson, Robert. 1978. *The Mardudjara aborigines*. New York: Holt, Rinehart.

Top, F. H. 1976. Rubella, 589–97 in Top and Wehrle.

Top, F. H., and P. F. Wehrle. 1976. Communicable and infectious diseases. St. Louis: C. V. Mosby.

Townsend, P. K. 1971. New Guinea sago gatherers. *EFN* 1:19–24.

Trinkaus, E., and M. R. Zimmerman. 1982. Trauma among Shanidar Neanderthals. *AJPA* 57:61–76.

Trowell, H. C., and D. P. Burkitt, eds. 1981. *Western diseases, their emergence and prevention*. London: Edward Arnold.

Trussell, James. 1980. Statistical flaws in evidence for the Frisch hypothesis that fatness triggers menarche. *Hum. Biol.* 52:711–20.

Truswell, A. S. 1977. Diet and nutrition of hunter-gatherers, 213–26 in CIBA.

Truswell, A. S., and J. D. L. Hansen. 1976. Medical research among the !Kung, 166–95 in Lee and DeVore.

Turnbull, Colin. 1961. *The forest people*. New York: Simon and Schuster.

———. 1965. *Wayward servants*. Garden City, N.Y.: Natural History Press.

———. 1968. The importance of flux in two hunting societies, 132–37 in Lee and DeVore.

———. 1972. The demography of small scale society, 283–312 in Harrison and Boyce.

———. 1983. *The Mbuti Pygmies: Change and adaptation*. New York: Holt, Rinehart.

Turner, V. 1967. The forest of symbols: Aspects of Ndembu ritual. Ithaca, N.Y.: Cornell University Press.

———. 1979. Dental anthropological indicators of agriculture among the Jomon people of central Japan. *AJPA* 51:619–35.

Turner, David H. 1974. *Tradition and transformation: A study of aborigines in the Groote Eylandt area, northern Australia*. Canberra: Australian Institute Behavioral Studies.

Turner, J. A. 1975. Other cestode infections, 708–44 in Hubbert et al.

Turpeinen, Oiva. 1979. Fertility and mortality in Finland since 1750. *Pop. Stud.* 33:101–14.

Tyrrell, D. A. 1977. Aspects of infections in isolated communities, 137–53 in CIBA.

Ubelaker, Douglas. 1978. Human skeletal remains. Chicago: Aldine.

———. 1984. Prehistoric human biology of Ecuador: Possible temporal trends and cultural correlations, 491–514 in Cohen and Armelagos.

Ucko, P. J., and G. W. Dimbleby, eds. 1969. *The domestication and exploitation of plants and animals*. Chicago: Aldine.

Underwood, E. J. 1971. *Trace elements in human and animal nutrition*. New York: Academic Press.

United Nations. 1948. *Demographic Yearbook 1948*. New York: United Nations.

———. 1984. *Demographic Yearbook 1982*. New York: United Nations.

———. 1987. *Demographic Yearbook 1985*. New York: United Nations.

Vallois, H. V. 1937. *Anthropologie* 47:499–532.

Van Arsdale, P. W. 1978. Population dynamics among Asmat hunter-gatherers of New Guinea: Data, methods, comparisons. *Hum. Ecol.* 6:435–67.

Van Etten, C. H., and J. A. Wolf. 1973. Natural sulphur compounds, 210–34 in NAS-NRC.

Van Gerven, D. P., and G. J. Armelagos. 1983. Farewell to paleodemography: A reply. *JHE* 12:352–66.

Van Gerven, D. P. et al. 1981. Mortality and cultural change in Nubia's Batn el Hajar. *AJPA* 54:286.

Van Ness, G. B. 1971. Ecology of anthrax. *Science* 172:1303–7.

Van Veen, A. G., and M. S. Van Veen. 1974. Some present-day aspects of vitamin A problems in developing countries. *EFN* 3:35–54.

Variyam, E. P., and J. G. Banwell. 1982. Hookworm: Nutritional implications. *RID* 4:830–35.

Vayda, A. P., ed. 1969. *Environment and cultural behavior*. Garden City, N.Y.: American Museum.

Vickers, W. T. 1980. An analysis of Amazonian hunting yields as a function of settlement age. *Working papers on South American Indians* 2:7–30.

———. 1988. Game depletion hypothesis of Amazonian adaptation: Data from a native community. *Science* 239: 1521–22.

Vogel, F., and M. Chakravartti. 1971. ABO blood groups and smallpox in rural populations of West Bengal and Bihar (India). In *Natural selection in human populations*, ed. C. J. Bajema, 147–65. New York: John Wiley.

Walker, P. L. 1983. Human biological evolution in the Santa Barbara Channel area: An evaluation of genetic and environmental influences on skeletal morphology. *AJPA* 60:267.

———. 1985. The causes of porotic hyperostosis in the American southwest and in southern California. *AJPA* 66:240.

———. 1986. Porotic hyperostosis in a marine-dependent California Indian population. *AJPA* 69: 345–54.

Walker, P. L., and M. DeNiro. 1986. Stable nitrogen and carbon isotope ratios in bone collagen as indices of prehistoric dietary dependence on marine and terrestrial resources in southern California. *AJPA* 71:51–62.

Wall, Richard et al. 1983. *Family forms in historic Europe*. Cambridge: Cambridge University Press.

Warner, W. L. 1937. *A black civilization*. New York: Harper and Brothers.

Warren, K. S. 1982. Schistosomiasis: Host-pathogen biology. *RID* 4:771–75.

Warren, M. C. 1975. Malaria, 789–98 in Hubbert et al.

Watanabe, H. 1969. Famine as a population check: Comparative ecology of northern peoples. Tokyo: *J. Fac. Sci. Sect.* 5 (anthropology) 3:237–52.

Waterford, J. 1982. A fundamental imbalance: Aboriginal ill health, 8–30 in Reid.

Watts, E., F. E. Johnston, and G. W. Lasker, eds. 1975. *Biosocial interrelations in population adaptation*. The Hague: Mouton.

Wayburne, S. 1968. Malnutrition in Johannesburg. In *Calorie deficiencies and protein deficiencies*, ed. R. A. McCance and Elsie Widdowson, 7–19. Boston: Little, Brown.

Weaver, F. J. 1984. Commentary: Food supply, nutritional status, and nutritional education in Malawi. *EFN* 15:341–47.

Webb, Malcolm. 1984. The state of the art on state origins. *Rev. Anthrop.* 11:270–81.

Webb, Stephen. 1982. Cribra orbitalia: A possible sign of anemia in pre- and post-contact crania from Australia and Papua, New Guinea. *Arch. Oceania* 17:148–56.

———. 1984. Prehistoric stress in Australian aborigines. Thesis, Department of Prehistory, Australian National University.

————. N.d. Intensification, population and social change in southeastern Australia, the skeletal evidence.

Webster, David. 1975. Warfare and the evolution of the state: A reconsideration. *Amer. Antiq.* 40:467–70.

Webster, David, and G. Webster. 1984. Optimal hunting and pleistocene extinctions. *Hum. Ecol.* 12:275–89.

Wehmeyer, A. S., R. B. Lee, and M. Whiting. 1969. The nutrient composition and dietary importance of some vegetable foods eaten by the !Kung Bushmen. *S.A. Tydskrif vir Geneeskunde* 95:1529–30.

Weinberg, E. D. 1974. Iron and susceptibility to infectious disease. *Science* 184: 952–56.

Weiss, K. M. 1973. Demographic models for anthropology. *Mem. Soc. Amer. Arch.* 27 38(2), pt. 2.

————. 1984. On the number of members of the genus Homo who have ever lived and some evolutionary implications. *Hum. Biol.* 56:637–49.

Weiss, K. M. et al. 1984. A syndrome of digestive system diseases with a genetic basis in New World native peoples. *AJPA* 63:233.

Welinder, Stig. 1979. Prehistoric demography. *Acta Arch. Lundensia*, series IN8 Minore, no 8. Bonn: Rudolf Habelt Verlag.

Weller, T. H. 1976. Varicella—Herpes zoster virus, 457–80 in Evans.

Wells, Calvin. 1975. Prehistoric and historical changes in nutritional diseases and associated conditions. *Progress in Food and Nutritional Science* 1:729–79.

Wenlock, R. W. 1979. Social factors, nutrition and child mortality in a rural subsistence economy. *EFN* 8:227–40.

Werner, Dennis. 1983. Why do the Mekranoti trek? 225–38 in Hames and Vickers.

Werner, Dennis et al. 1979. Subsistence productivity and hunting effort in native South America. *Hum. Ecol.* 7:303–16.

Wheeler, Eric. 1980. Nutritional status of savanna peoples, 439–55 in D. Harris.

White H. S. 1980. Iron-hemoglobin, 287–318 in Alfin-Slater and Kritchevsky.

White, Leslie. 1959. The energy theory of cultural development. In M. Fried, *Readings in Anthropology*, 139–46. New York: Crowell.

Whitaker, John. 1983. What causes the disease? In *Multiple sclerosis*. ed. Labe Scheinberg, 7–16. New York: Raven.

White, Christine. 1986. Mayan diet and health status at Lamanai. Paper presented to the nineteenth Chacmool Conference, Calgary.

White, H. S. 1980. Iron and hemoglobin, 287–318 in Alfin-Slater and Kritchevsky.

White, Leslie. 1959. *The evolution of culture.* New York: McGraw Hill.

Whiting, John. 1969. Effects of climate on certain cultural practices, 416–55 in Vayda.

Wilkinson, G. K. et al. 1958. Serum proteins of some central and south Australian aborigines. *MJA* 2:158–60.

Williams, B. J. 1974. A model of band society. *Memoir, Society for American Archaeology* 39:4:2.

Williams, J. A. 1985. Evidence of pre-contact tuberculosis in two Woodland skeletal populations from the northern plains. *AJPA* 66:242–43.

Wilmsen, Edwin. 1978. Seasonal effects of dietary intake on the Kalahari San. *Fed. Proc.* 37: 65–72.

Wilson, B. J., and A. W. Hayes. 1973. Microbial toxins, 372–423 in NAS-NRC.

Wilson, E. O. 1975. *Sociobiology*. Cambridge: Harvard University Press.

Wilson, W. 1953. A dietary survey of aborigines in the Northwest Territory. *MJA* 2: 599–605.

Wing, E. S., and A. B. Brown. 1979. *Paleonutrition*. New York: Academic Press.

Winick, Myron. 1980. *Nutrition in health and disease*. New York: John Wiley.

Winterhalder, Bruce. 1981. Foraging strategies in the boreal forest: An analysis of Cree hunting and gathering, 66–98 in Winterhalder and Smith.

Winterhalder, B., and E. A. Smith, eds. 1981. *Hunter-gatherer foraging strategies*. Chicago: University of Chicago Press.

Wirsing, R. 1985. The health of traditional societies and the effects of acculturation. *CA* 26: 303–22.

Wisseman, C. L. 1976. Rickettsial diseases, 567–84 in Top and Wehrle.

Wittfogel, Karl. 1957. *Oriental despotism*. New Haven and London: Yale University Press.

Wobst, H. M. 1974. Boundary conditions of Paleolithic social systems: A simulation approach. *Amer. Antiquity* 39:147–77.

———. 1975. The demography of finite populations and the origin of the incest taboo. *Amer. Antiquity* 40:75–81.

———. 1976. Locational relationships in Paleolithic society. *J. Hum. Evol.* 5:49–55.

Wolf, George. 1980. Vitamin A, 97–203 in Alfin-Slater and Kritchevsky.

Wolpoff, Milford. 1979. The Krapina dental remains. *AJPA* 50:67–114.

———. 1980. *Paleoanthropology*. New York: Knopf.

Wood, C. S. 1975. New evidence for a late introduction of malaria into the New World. *CA* 16:93–104.

———. 1979. Human sickness and health: A biocultural view. Palo Alto, Calif.: Mayfield.

Wood, James. 1988. Comment. *CA* 29:290.

Wood, James, Patricia Johnson, and Kenneth Campbell. 1985. Demographic and endocrinological aspects of low natural fertility in highland New Guinea. *J. Biosoc. Sci.* 17:57–79.

Wood, James et al. 1985. Lactation and birth spacing in highland New Guinea. *J. Biosoc. Sci.*, Suppl. 9: 159–73.

Woodburn, James. 1968a. An introduction to Hadza ecology, 49–55 in Lee and DeVore.

———. 1968b. Stability and flexibility in Hadza residential groups, 103–10 in Lee and DeVore.

———. 1982. Egalitarian societies. *Man* (N.S.)17:431–51.

Woods, Robert, and John Woodward. 1984. *Urban disease and mortality*. New York: St. Martin's Press.

Work, T. H. 1975. Introduction to arthropod-borne viruses, 922–28 in Hubbert et al.

Wright, H. T., and G. A. Johnson. 1975. Population, exchange, and early state formation in southwestern Iran. *AA* 77:267–89.

Wrigley, E. A. 1966. *An introduction to English historical demography*. New York: Basic.

———. 1969. *Population and history*. New York: McGraw Hill.

Wrigley, E. A., and R. S. Schofield. 1981. *The population history of England, 1541– 1871*. Cambridge: Harvard University Press.

Wurm, H. 1984. The fluctuation of average stature in the course of German history and the influence of protein content in the diet. *JHE* 13:331–34.

y'Edynak, Gloria. 1987. Mesolithic dental reduction as a possible result of sex differences in dental disease and diet. *AJPA* 72:196.

y'Edynak, Gloria, and Sylvia Fleisch. 1983. Microevolution and biological adaptability in the transition from food collecting to food production in the iron gates of Yugoslavia. *JHE* 12:279–96.

Yengoyan, Aram. 1972. Biological and demographic components in aboriginal Australian socio-economic organization. *Oceania* 43:85–95.

Yoffee, N. 1985. Perspectives on the trends toward social complexity in prehistoric Australia and Papua, New Guinea. *Arch. Ocean.* 20:41–49.

Yost, James, and P. M. Kelley. 1983. Shotguns, blowguns and spears: The analysis of technological efficiency, 189–224 in Hames and Vickers.

Young, M. V., and P. L. Pellett. 1985. Wheat proteins in relation to protein requirements and availability of amino acids. *AJCN* 41:1077–90.

Zaino, D. E., and E. C. Zaino. 1975. Cribra orbitalia in the aborigines of Hawaii and Australia. *AJPA* 42:91–94.

Zimmerman, W. J. 1975. Trichinosis, 545–59 in Hubbert et al.

Zivanovic, S. 1982. *Ancient diseases.* Transl. from the Serbian by L. F. Edwards. London: Methuen.

Zubrow, Ezra, ed. 1976. *Demographic anthropology.* Albuquerque: University of New Mexico Press.

Index

ABO blood type, 147n23
Abortion, 198–200n133
Accidents
  archaeological identification and, 109
  as cause of mortality, 92
  in civilized societies, 132
  hunter-gatherers and, 100, 116, 131, 194n123
  in prehistoric farmers, 116
Ache of the Paraguay, 103, 169n4
Acsadi, G., 124, 218n102, 219–20n110, 220n115
Adaptive compromise, 12–15, 146–48n23, 148n25
  newly introduced diseases and, 149n26
  risk in defense against health risks and, 13–14, 149–50n27
Afghanistan, infant mortality in, 198n130
Africa. *See also* Hadza of Tanzania; San of the Kalahari
  caloric intake of hunter-gatherer groups in, 189n78
  meat intake of hunter-gatherer groups in, 185n54
  subsistence farming in, 69
African Pygmies, 93, 193n108
Age at death. *See also* Age estimation
  between A.D. *1400* and *1800*, 123
  adoption of farming and, 122, 218–19n106
  adult, in prehistoric groups, 122, 217–18n102
  in Bronze Age, 123, 219n108
  in later prehistoric American Southwest, 126, 221n132

later prehistoric class distinctions and, 125
  in later prehistoric Israel, 124, 220n123
  for prehistoric aboriginal Australian groups, 209n44
Age estimation
  from adult skeletons, 110–11, 131, 206n29, 210n45, 219n106
  from children's skeletons, 110
  among contemporary hunter-gatherers, 129
Agta of the Philippines, 93, 224n142
AIDS virus (HIV), 9, 38, 162–63n42
Alland, A., 143n3, 149n27
Allison, M. J., 118, 126, 213n70, 214n85, 217n101
American Indians. *See* New World; North America
Ammerman, A. J., 129, 223n141
Anaerobic bacteria, 35
Anemia. *See also* Porotic hyperostosis
  Eskimos and, 95
  in Pleistocene vs. later Australian groups, 114, 209n44
  in prehistoric groups, 107–08, 205n9
  in tropical hunter-gatherers, 94
Angel, J. L., 113, 115, 119, 123, 208n38, 219n108, 221n136
Animal foods
  decay and, 86
  decline in per-capita consumption of, 58, 172n16, 172n17
  domestication of animals and, 119
  fat consumption and, 73
  in nutrition, 58, 173–74n18